A PRACTICAL GUIDE TO COMPREHENSIVE

STROKE CARE

Meeting Population Needs

A PRACTICAL GUIDE TO COMPREHENSIVE
STROKE CARE
Meeting Population Needs

Principal Editor
Lalit Kalra
King's College London, UK

Co-Editors
Charles Wolfe
King's College London, UK

Anthony Rudd
Guy's and St Thomas' Hospital, London, UK

World Scientific

NEW JERSEY · LONDON · SINGAPORE · BEIJING · SHANGHAI · HONG KONG · TAIPEI · CHENNAI

Published by

World Scientific Publishing Co. Pte. Ltd.

5 Toh Tuck Link, Singapore 596224

USA office: 27 Warren Street, Suite 401-402, Hackensack, NJ 07601

UK office: 57 Shelton Street, Covent Garden, London WC2H 9HE

British Library Cataloguing-in-Publication Data
A catalogue record for this book is available from the British Library.

A PRACTICAL GUIDE TO COMPREHENSIVE STROKE CARE
Meeting Population Needs

ISBN-13 978-981-4299-51-0
ISBN-10 981-4299-51-0

Typeset by Stallion Press
Email: enquiries@stallionpress.com

Printed in Singapore.

Foreword

The words "practical" and "comprehensive" do not usually go together in a title; however, under the skillful editorship of Professors Lalit Kalra, Charles Wolfe and Anthony Rudd, this book manages to cover the most important points relating to all phases of stroke succinctly and pragmatically.

It begins with a chapter on the size and changing nature of the problem of stroke, followed by a section on strategies for stroke prevention and chapters that cover the most important aspects of stroke, from presentation to hyperacute management, rehabilitation, long-term management, caregivers needs as well as management, palliative care, stroke services and new horizons in stroke, the latter written by Professor Kalra with clarity and vision. Busy experts seldom have the time to write book chapters, but the editors have recruited a stellar cast to co-author the book.

Anyone involved in stroke care will find something useful in the book, regardless of career stage, discipline or interest. I recommend it highly.

Vladimir Hachinski, CM MD FRCPC DSc Dr hon. causa
Professor of Neurology and
Distinguished University Professor
University of Western Ontario
London, Canada

Contents

List of Contributors

Juliet Addo
King's College London, Division of Health and Social Care Research, London, UK.

Ajay Bhalla
Geriatrics and General Medicine, Guy's and St. Thomas' NHS Foundation Trust, London, UK.

Jonathan Birns
Geriatrics and General Medicine, Guy's and St. Thomas' NHS Foundation Trust, London, UK.

Siobhan Crichton
King's College London, Division of Health and Social Care Research, London, UK.

Anne Forster
Academic Unit of Elderly Care and Rehabilitation, University of Leeds and Bradford Institute for Health Research, Bradford, UK.

Matthew F. Giles
Stroke Prevention Research Unit, NIHR Biomedical Research Centre, Oxford University Department of Clinical Neurology, John Radcliffe Hospital, Oxford, UK.

Ruth Harris
Faculty of Health and Social Care Sciences, Kingston University and St. George's, University of London, UK.

Irene J. Higginson
King's College London
WHO Collaborating Centre for Palliative Care in Older People
Department of Palliative Care, Policy and Rehabilitation, Cicely Saunders Institute, London, UK.

Alex Hoffman
Clinical Standards Department, Royal College of Physicians London.

Lalit Kalra
Academic Neuroscience Centre, King's College London, UK.

Peter Langhorne
University of Glasgow, Academic Section of Geriatric Medicine, Glasgow, UK.

Dulka Manawadu
Department of Stroke Medicine, King's College Hospital NHS Foundation Trust, Denmark Hill, London, UK.

Christopher McKevitt
King's College London, Division of Health and Social Care Research, London, UK.

Keerthi Mohan
King's College London, Division of Health and Social Care Research, London, UK.

Chris Price
Institute for Ageing and Health, Newcastle University Medical School, Newcastle upon Tyne, UK.

Helen Rodgers
Institute for Ageing and Health, Newcastle University Medical School, Newcastle upon Tyne, UK.

Peter M. Rothwell
Stroke Prevention Research Unit, NIHR Biomedical Research Centre, Oxford University Department of Clinical Neurology, John Radcliffe Hospital, Oxford, UK.

Anthony G. Rudd
Clinical Standards Department, Royal College of Physicians London, Stroke Physician Guy's and St. Thomas' Hospital, London, UK.

Kethakie Sumathipala
King's College London, Division of Health and Social Care Research, London, UK.

Ian Wellwood
King's College London, Division of Health and Social Care Research, Guy's Campus, London, UK.

Charles Wolfe
King's College London, Division of Health and Social Care Research, London, UK.

NIHR Biomedical Research Centre, Guy's and St. Thomas' NHS Foundation Trust and King's College London, London, UK.

1   The Size of the Problem

Keerthi Mohan*, Siobhan Crichton*,
Kethakie Sumathipala*, Christopher McKevitt*
and Charles Wolfe*,[†]

Chapter Summary

This chapter explores the changing demographics of stroke incidence and mortality worldwide. It examines the effect which these factors, combined with advances in research, changing national policies and clinical guidance on stroke, have on the provision of high quality cost-effective stroke services.

Both population-based stroke incidence studies and the analysis of routine data identify significant disparities in stroke incidence worldwide, which indicates a widening gap between high income countries with low and declining stroke incidence and mortality rates, and low and middle income countries where rates are high and increasing. Even within the United Kingdom, regional and ethnic differences can be found in stroke incidence and mortality trends.

The management of acute stroke has been influenced by both government policy and subsequent health strategies during the last decade, supplemented by extensive research evidence and clinical guidelines. In particular, studies investigating thrombolytic therapy for appropriately

*King's College London, Division of Health and Social Care Research, London, UK
[†]NIHR Biomedical Research Centre, Guy's and St. Thomas' NHS Foundation Trust and King's College London, London, UK

selected patients after acute infarction, and stroke unit care for all patients after acute stroke have consistently shown better outcomes in both the short term and long term.

The practicalities of implementing nationally-derived standards and guidelines into local stroke services pose a real challenge to healthcare providers and commissioners. However, implementation is essential in order to deliver and maintain stroke services that reach the population they seek to serve, are cost-effective, and of high quality.

Epidemiology of Stroke

The World Health Organization (WHO) estimated that in 2002, 15.3 million people worldwide had a stroke, with more than a third, 5.5 million, resulting in death. Of the 57 million deaths worldwide in 2002, stroke accounted for nearly 10%.[1] Population projections for Europe suggest that the proportion of the population aged 65 and over will increase from 20% to 35% by 2050. During the same time period, the total European population is expected to decrease from 728 million to 705 million.[2] It is predicted that this demographic shift will increase the number of acute stroke episodes from 1.1 to more than 1.5 million per year by 2025.[3]

In a systematic review, Feigin and colleagues identified and analysed 15 population-based stroke incidence studies from around the world and found age-standardised stroke incidence rates for people aged 55 years or more ranged from 4.2 to 11.7 per 1000 person years. The highest incidence rates were recorded in Ukraine, Russia and Japan, with analyses showing that rates in these countries were significantly higher than in other countries studied including Australia, Germany and the United Kingdom.[4]

The European Registers of Stroke (EROS) investigators recorded first-ever strokes in the population-based stroke registers of six European countries with standardised case ascertainment criteria and observation periods. They observed the highest incidences of stroke in Lithuania and the lowest in Italy and Menorca, echoing the high levels of stroke incidence noted in eastern Europe in both previous population-based studies and the WHO Multinational Monitoring of Trends and Determinants in Cardiovascular Disease (MONICA) project in those aged under

75 years.[5-8] A summary of the annual stroke incidence rates for men and women in each EROS study centre is shown in Table 1.

However, data suggest that stroke incidence rates are not increasing in all countries. Data collected in men and women aged 35 to 64 years for the WHO MONICA Project, as well as population-based stroke studies, demonstrate a widening gap between countries with low and declining stroke incidence and mortality rates, and in countries where stroke incidence and mortality is high and increasing.[9-11] In another systematic review, Feigin *et al.* demonstrated that over the last 40 years, age-adjusted stroke incidence rates in high income countries, defined according to the World Bank's country classification, have decreased by 42%. Stroke incidence doubled in middle income countries and increased two-fold in those aged under 75, and four-fold in those aged over 75 years in low-income countries during the same period. They found that from 2000 to 2008, total stroke incidence rates in low to middle income countries exceeded those in high income countries for the first time since these studies were recorded.[11]

Within England and Wales, it is estimated that each year 110,000 people have a first stroke, of whom 30,000 people go on to have further strokes.[12] Mortality data indicate that stroke death rates in people aged under 75 decreased by 30% between 1992 and 2002, and due to both the ageing population and increased survival after stroke, the total cost of stroke care is projected to rise by 30% by 2010 compared to 1991 cost analyses.[13]

In the United Kingdom, regional and temporal differences in stroke incidence, mortality and recurrence rates have been observed. The South London Stroke Register (SLSR) is a population-based stroke register recording first-ever strokes in patients of all age groups for a defined area of South London since 1995. This area comprises 63% white, 28% black, and 9% other ethnic groups, compared with an approximately 90% white population across England and Wales at the time of Census, 2001. In 1999, Stewart *et al.* reported age- and sex-adjusted stroke incidence rates of 1.25 per 1000 population per year. They also noted significantly higher incidence rates in black people compared to white people with a black to white incidence rate ratio, adjusted for age and sex, of 2.21. Their analyses revealed that in people aged 35 to 64, increasing age, male sex, black ethnic group and lower social class were independently associated with an increased incidence of stroke in South London.[15] Longer term analyses

Table 1. Annual stroke incidence rates for the EROS study centres[14]

	Dijon, France	Sesto Fiorentino, Italy	Kaunas, Lithuania	London, UK	Menorca, Spain	Warsaw, Poland
Study period	May 2004 to April 2006	June 2004 to May 2006	June 2004 to May 2005	May 2004 to April 2006	May 2004 to April 2006	January 2005 to December 2005
Estimated source population	152,415	47,236	365,191	326,885	75,135	120,186
Annual stroke incidence rates for men* (95% CI)	122.5 (101.7–146.2)	101.2 (82.5–123.0)	239.3 (209.9–271.6)	121.1 (100.5–144.7)	116.3 (96.1–139.3)	147.2 (124.4–173.0)
Annual stroke incidence rates for women* (95% CI)	75.9 (59.8–95.0)	63.0 (48.5–80.7)	158.7 (135.0–185.7)	78.1 (61.8–97.5)	65.8 (50.9–83.8)	125.9 (104.9–149.9)

*Incidence rates given with 95% Confidence Intervals per 100,000 population adjusted to the European population

conducted between 1995 and 2004 have revealed higher incidence of primary intracerebral haemorrhage (PICH) in the SLSR black Caribbean and African populations, compared to the white population.[16] The excess stroke incidence in the black population reported in the SLSR is similar to the 2.4-fold increase risk reported in both the Atherosclerosis Risk in Communities (ARIC) study and in the Northern Manhattan Stroke Study.[17,18] SLSR analyses reported by Heuschmann *et al.* demonstrated a total stroke incidence decrease of 18% in men from 1.57 to 1.29 per 1000 population and 24% in women from 1.20 to 0.91 per 1000 population per year, over the 10 year study period between 1995–2004.[19]

A decreasing trend in stroke incidence was also reported in comparisons made by the Oxford Vascular Study (OXVASC) in collaboration with the original investigators of the Oxfordshire Community Project (OCSP) in Oxfordshire from 1981 to 1984 and 2002 to 2004. There was little change reported in either the ethnic mix of the 93% white population or in the organisation of primary healthcare during the interim period.[20] Despite a pre-study prediction of a 28% increase in first-ever strokes to account for the higher proportion of people aged over 75 years compared to the original study population, the observed number of strokes recorded decreased in both men and women. Age- and sex-adjusted incidence of first-ever stroke fell by 29% from 2.27 to 1.62 per 1000 population per year between the studies, and significant reductions were reported in the incidence of both disabling and fatal strokes.[20] Further analyses by Lovelock *et al.*, demonstrated a 47% reduction in the incidence of intracerebral haemorrhage (ICH) reported in those aged under 75 years from 1981 to 1984 and 2002 to 2006. However, the total incidence of ICH across all ages remained stable during the study periods, due to increased incidence rates noted amongst those aged over 75 years.[21]

Research from the OCSP found the 30-day case fatality rate after first stroke to be 18%, with patients who survived at least 30 days having an average annual risk of mortality of 9.1%, more than two times the risk of the general population.[22,23] Adjusted mortality rates due to incident stroke (based on survival at one month) decreased by 37% from 0.44/1000 (95% CI: 0.35–0.54) during 1981–1984 to 0.24/1000 (0.20–0.37) during 2002–2004. However, the 30-day case fatality recorded over this period remained the same: 17.2% in 2002–2004 compared to 17.8 in 1981–1984.[20]

In South London, the observed increased risk of stroke incidence in the black population was not shown to translate into an increased case fatality up to eight years after their initial stroke. In general, black patients were 28% more likely to survive than white patients, with current smoking, untreated atrial fibrillation, and a diagnosis of diabetes, whether untreated or treated, associated with reduced survival.[24]

Age-adjusted stroke mortality rates for developed countries have been reported to be between 50 and 100 per 100,000 people per year, yet again substantial differences between high and low income countries have been documented.[25] Projections for 2005 conducted by Strong *et al.* for the WHO Burden of Stroke Programme found stroke mortality rates in people aged 30 to 69 years ranged widely, from 180 per 100,000 people in the Russian Federation, to 15 per 100,000 in Canada and 20 per 100,000 in the United Kingdom.[26] Furthermore, projected trends for stroke mortality between 2002 and 2030 indicate that these inequalities are set to widen due to increasing mortality rates in middle and low-income countries, whilst rates remain stable in high-income countries.[26]

Gross domestic product (GDP) has been found to be the strongest predictor of stroke mortality and burden, exceeding mean blood pressure and the prevalence of obesity and smoking.[27] The highest rates of mortality and burden after stroke have consistently been reported in Eastern Europe, North Asia, Central Africa and the South Pacific, low-income areas previously identified as being at high risk.[9,28] Furthermore, a 4% reduction in stroke mortality was demonstrated for every additional US$1000 in GDP per capita. Problems with poor concordance to secondary prevention measures after stroke in low-income countries have been attributed to lack of equipment and resources for risk factors monitoring, the non-availability of drugs, and a lack of affordable treatment.[29] Guidelines for cost-effective secondary prevention in low-income and middle-income countries proposed by the WHO, highlight the importance of lifestyle modifications and the use of affordable, accessible, and effective pharmacological treatments, such as aspirin, anti-hypertensive medications and statins.[30]

Stroke survivors remain at increased risk of further cerebrovascular events compared to the general population.[31] Recurrent strokes are more likely to be disabling or fatal than first ever strokes, yet studies show considerable variation in estimates of the cumulative risk of stroke recurrence in the early years and long term after first stroke.[32] At one year post-initial stroke, the risk of recurrence was shown to range from 4.7% in The Netherlands[33] to 14% described by different groups based in Sweden.[34,35] Studies have shown the five-year risk of stroke recurrence to range from 12 to 42%.[33,36] By ten years, the risk of stroke recurrence reported is wide-ranging from 16.9% in Sweden[37] and 25% in South London, UK,[38] to 43% in Perth, Australia,[39] 51.3% in Japan[40] and 53.9% in Sweden.[35] These differences in cumulative risk may be explained by varying case ascertainment criteria used between studies, including the definition of stroke recurrence used, differing selection of study samples, i.e. hospital- or population-based, and the length of exclusion period after initial stroke prior to diagnosis of a recurrence.[38]

Whilst different predictors for stroke recurrence have been identified up to ten years after a stroke, little consensus has been reached between studies. At five years after stroke, the major predictors of stroke recurrence were found to be a past history of diabetes and transient ischaemic attack in Rochester[41] and Lehigh Valley[42] respectively, both studied in the USA; older age, diabetes and an initial intracerebral haemorrhage in Perth, Australia[43]; a history of hypertension and atrial fibrillation in South London, UK[38]; and a history of diabetes, atrial fibrillation and a previous transient ischaemic attack in Malmo, Sweden.[44]

Current Acute Service Provision

The last decade has seen important advances in the evidence base for the prevention, treatment and rehabilitation of stroke, resulting in a plethora of local, national and international clinical guidelines ranging from individual clinical practice to stroke service evaluation.[45] Commissioners of healthcare face important decisions about how to extrapolate and implement this evidence most effectively and efficiently both within their population and within the healthcare resources of their local area.

Data from the United Kingdom in the 1990s showed a relatively high cost stroke service with high levels of post-stroke mortality and dependence.[46] Since then, the importance of stroke has been stressed in government policy, and through the publication of Department of Health papers, 'The Health of the Nation' and 'Saving Lives: Our Healthier Nation', targets have been set for the reduction of stroke mortality.[47,48] Furthermore, standard five of the National Service Framework (NSF) for older people published in 2001, states that the NHS should *'take action to prevent strokes, working in partnership with other agencies where appropriate'*, in order to ensure that *'people who are thought to have had a stroke have access to diagnostic services, are treated appropriately by a specialist stroke service, and subsequently, with their carers, participate in a multidisciplinary programme of secondary prevention and rehabilitation'*.[49]

National guidelines on stroke care published by the Intercollegiate Working Party for Stroke and the National Institute of Clinical Excellence (NICE) provide structured guidance on how stroke services and the care they provide can be optimised and maintained.[50,51] However, the practicalities surrounding implementation of these standards within local stroke services provide challenges to healthcare commissioners and providers.[45] The Departments of Health 2006 report, 'Improving Stroke Services: A Guide for Commissioners', in conjunction with the interactive 'Action on Stroke Services: An Evaluation Toolkit for Commissioners (ASSET2)', combines key data and complementary evidence from population-based stroke registers with health economic and statistical modelling to enable commissioners to compare nationally recognised examples of good stroke care to service provision within their area.[52,53] Local stroke services can use this tool to benchmark their current performance against similar Primary Care Trusts (PCTs) and make a broad strategic assessment of need within their locality, in order to highlight areas where increased resources may be required.[52]

The 2006 Helsingborg Declaration on European Stroke Strategies set out that by 2015 all stroke patients in Europe will 'have access to a continuum of care from organised stroke units in the acute phase to appropriate rehabilitation and secondary prevention measures'.[54] Basic requirements for achieving this, as outlined in the Helsingborg declaration, include adapting stroke services to meet local requirements and resources, and the need for evaluation of stroke outcome and assessment of the quality of stroke care provided in all countries.

The Safe Implementation of Thrombolysis in Stroke-Monitoring Study (SITS-MOST) was a prospective, multicentre, multinational observational monitoring study for clinical centres practicing thrombolysis for acute stroke within the member states of the European Union in 2002 and Norway and Iceland.[55] The main aim was to investigate whether thrombolytic therapy with intravenous alteplase (t-PA) within three hours of onset of ischaemic stroke symptoms was as safe in clinical practice across a wide range of acute stroke services as it had been shown to be in randomised controlled trials.[56,57] A key finding of SITS-MOST was that outcomes, including symptomatic intracerebral haemorrhage during three months of follow-up after thrombolysis, were similar between centres regardless of their previous thrombolytic therapy experience level. This suggests that whilst currently fewer than 5% of eligible patients in Europe receive thrombolysis, it should be more widely used.[55,58]

The SITS-MOST investigators identified that older patients, those with a history of high blood pressure, patients with a high score on the National Institute of Health stroke scale, and those with evidence of an infarction on imaging scans, were at an increased risk of a poor outcome after thrombolytic therapy.[59] Identification of patients likely to have a poor outcome after thrombolysis should help even less experienced stroke centres select patients who are most suitable for thrombolytic therapy, therefore reducing the risk of adverse outcomes.

Specific markers to access quality of stroke care at a local level have also been established within some European countries. In Germany, results from the German Registers Study Group (ADSR) in 2000 have shown that 3% of ischaemic stroke patients received thrombolysis within this period.[60] Interestingly, this study found in-hospital mortality to be significantly higher for patients treated with t-PA compared to those not receiving thrombolysis, and noted an inverse relationship between the number of patients treated with t-PA per hospital per year and the subsequent risk of in-hospital death.[61]

The results of both population-based research and national audits since the early 1990s demonstrated large geographic inequalities in access to and patterns of stroke care across Europe.[62] The BIOMED II European Study of Stroke Care found that access to organised stroke care was significantly higher in older rather than younger stroke patients, but was associated with reduced three-month mortality in younger patients only.[63] Discrepancies were also noted between the Eastern and Western European centres investigated, with younger patients in Western Europe more likely to gain access to important components of stroke care such as multidisciplinary therapists and routine investigations, compared with patients in Eastern Europe.[64]

Organised stroke unit care remains the only intervention that is appropriate, and has been shown to improve outcomes in all patients after a stroke. However, the impact of stroke units not only depends on how effective they are, but also on how accessible and available they are to patients, particularly in the acute period after stroke.[65] The National Sentinel Stroke Audit for England, Wales and Northern Ireland reported an increase in the proportion of hospitals with a dedicated stroke unit from 79% in 2004 to 91% in 2006. Results also demonstrated a higher quality of care experienced by patients on a stroke unit compared to other wards, as indicated by higher proportions of patients undergoing earlier therapy assessments and discharge planning.[66] However, despite the overall positive shift, major discrepancies still exist in the provision of stroke services and quality of care provided nationally, with data from Wales indicating very low rates of stroke unit admission compared to the rest of the United Kingdom. The role and importance of monitoring tools such as the National Sentinel Stroke Audit in regulating and improving stroke services will be discussed further in Chapter 12.

'Riks-Stroke', the national quality register for stroke care in Sweden was established in 1994, and since 1998 has covered all 85 hospitals in Sweden admitting acute stroke patients of all ages.[67] The register includes data on patient characteristics, acute stroke management and follow-up at three months post-stroke, allowing comparisons to be made between participating hospitals and to assess the practical implementation of the Swedish national guidelines for stroke care.[68] The proportion of patients treated in a stroke unit was about 40% in 1994, increasing to 83% in 2000, and decreasing to 60% in 2005.[69] Better functional outcome, as measured by the proportion of patients independently mobile and living at home at three months, and independent in their activities of daily living, as well as significantly lower case fatality rates at seven and 27 days, and at three months onset after stroke, were seen in patients admitted to stroke units compared to those admitted to general medical wards.[67] Even two years after the stroke, better outcomes were shown to persist in patients treated in stroke units.[70] More recently, Terent *et al.* demonstrated better long-term survival (up to six years after stroke) in patients treated in a stroke unit regardless of patient age, sex or pathological stroke subtype. The largest mortality risk reduction was noted in patients under 65 years with a primary intracerebral haemorrhage and in those with decreased consciousness on admission to hospital.[71]

Results from 178 German and Austrian hospitals, as part of the European Stroke Facilities Survey, found that minimum care targets, as defined by the European Stroke Initiative, were met in 63% of the surveyed hospitals treating stroke patients, considerably higher than the European average of 48.6%. However, the survey also found that 23% of German and Austrian patients did not have access to a basic level of stroke care, highlighting the importance of accessibility to and availability of good quality stroke services, in order for the best possible care to be administered as quickly as possible to all stroke patients.[72]

In the United States, consensus statements from the Brain Attack Coalition (BAC) in 2000 and 2005, recommended the development of 'primary' stroke centres supported by 'comprehensive' stroke centres in order to provide a full range of services, ranging from acute stroke teams, stroke units, and written protocols for the use of tissue plasminogen activator (t-PA) for thrombolysis, to diagnostic radiological techniques, endovascular therapy and neurovascular and vascular surgery.[73,74] Subsequent quality assessment studies at The Paul Coverdell National Acute Stroke Registry found that 4.5% of ischaemic stroke admissions were treated with t-PA, ranging between 3.0% to 8.5% across sites.[75] An 18-month follow-up study at 32 hospitals in New York after implementation of BAC guidelines in 2002 found significant increases in stroke unit admission rates from 16% to 39%, and in t-PA utilization from 2.4% to 5.2% during this period.[76]

The National Stroke Audit of Acute Services of Australia was undertaken in 2007 and comprised an organisational survey describing the resources available to support the delivery of evidence-based care, and a retrospective case note audit examining the quality of stroke care in Australia.[77] The organisation survey revealed that 21% of hospitals across Australia had a stroke unit. This translated into an increase in access to stroke unit care by patients from 23% to 50% since 2003. However, rates

in 2007 ranged from 34% to 82% between states.[78] The study also found
that 3% of ischaemic stroke patients received thrombolysis. There were
important differences noted between hospitals without a stroke unit where
less than 1% of ischaemic stroke patients underwent thrombolysis and
hospitals with a stroke unit where it occurred in 4% of patients.[77]

Stroke Related Disability

Stroke is increasingly being recognised as a chronic condition which
requires long-term management. Stroke survivors may have multiple
physical, psychological and social problems and one-third are left with
long-term residual disabilities which can persist for many years. The long-
term consequences of stroke can be classified according to the World
Health Organizations' International Classification of Functioning,
Disability and Health (ICF).[79] Proposed in 2001, it provides a unified and
standard language for defining health and health-related outcomes.
Disease and disorder are considered to be an interaction between the four
components (body, activity, participation and contextual factors) and not
solely linked to an individual's functional outcome, and places emphasis
on interaction between its four components. Using the framework of the
ICF, the long-term outcomes and needs of stroke survivors will be
presented in Chapter 9.

Cost of Stroke Care

The sudden onset of stroke combined with the need for acute and long-
term care and loss of income experienced by many stroke patients and
their families result in a significant economic impact.[80] Quantification of
the overall cost attributable to stroke is necessary to aid effective healthcare planning and resource allocation.[81]

The estimated average cost of a stroke varies between countries.[82] A
review of 120 studies of patient-level data estimated that the average cost
of a stroke ranged from US$468 to US$146,149. When studies were
grouped by geographic region, the average costs ranged from US$2,822
in Eastern Europe and US$12,883 in Japan, to US$22,377 in the UK,
US$24,548 in Sweden and US$28,253 in the USA.[83]

Luengo-Fernandez *et al.* estimated the cost of cardiovascular diseases in the United Kingdom. They found that in 2004 cardiovascular disease cost the economy £29.1 billion with cerebrovascular disease accounting for 27% (£8 billion) of the total. Healthcare costs after stroke (including primary care, accident and emergency attendance and drug costs) accounted for £5.2 billion, whilst non-healthcare costs (such as informal care, and loss of working days due to mortality or morbidity) totalled £2.8 billion.[84]

Saka *et al.* used a 'bottom-up' approach to calculate the cost of stroke from a societal perspective in the UK through analysis of patient-level data from the South London Stroke Register. They found that direct care, consisting of diagnosis, inpatient and outpatient care costs, accounted for around 50% of the total cost of a stroke. Informal care and other indirect costs, such as income loss and social benefit payments, each accounted for approximately one quarter of total costs. It was estimated that stroke costs totalled £9 billion per year with productivity losses due to morbidity and mortality accounting for £1.3 billion. A breakdown of the costs is given in Table 2.[85]

Using data from the Oxford Vascular Study (OXVASC), Luengo-Fernandez *et al.* estimated that the cost of acute stroke care ranged from £326 to £19,901 in 346 patients with first or recurrent stroke between

Table 2. Annual cost of stroke care in the United Kingdom[85]

Cost item	Cost in £	Percentage
Diagnosis costs	45.604 m	0.51
Inpatient care costs	865.872 m	9.64
Outpatient costs	109.679 m	1.22
Outpatient drug costs	505.588 m	5.63
Community care costs	2857.113 m	31.82
Annual care costs total	4383.858 m	48.82
Informal care costs total	2420.921 m	26.96
Income lost due to mortality	592.733 m	6.6
Income lost due to morbidity	740.158 m	8.24
Productivity loss total	1332.892 m	14.85
Benefit payments	841.254 m	9.37
Total	8978.926 m	

April 2002 and March 2004. While, in unvariate analysis, they found a history of atrial fibrillation, degree of carotid stenosis and stroke subtype to be the predictors of increased costs in the year after stroke; stroke severity, as measured by the National Institute of Health Stroke Scale (NIHSS) was the most important independent predictor of cost. The mean cost rose with increasing NIHSS score from £3,185 in those with a score <2 to £13,694 in those with a score of 11–20. Average costs then dropped to £3,010 for patients with a score >20 due to increased early case fatality in this group.[86]

Person-level data are also useful to determine the long-term cost effectiveness of new stroke interventions. Saka *et al.* looked at the cost effectiveness of stroke unit care followed by early supported discharge compared to both stroke unit and general medical ward care without early support discharge in the United Kingdom.[87] They used incremental cost-effectiveness ratios (ICERs) to calculate the cost per quality-adjusted life year (QALY) in order to assess the cost-effectiveness of the different discharge strategies. The ICER of stroke unit care followed by early supportive discharge compared with both medical ward and stroke unit care without early supportive discharge was found to be £10,661 and £17,721 respectively. Therefore they found stroke unit care combined with early supportive discharge to be the most cost-effective strategy.[87]

Conclusion

Variations in incidence and mortality rates after stroke represent complex interactions between changing population demographics and risk factors, the availability of improved preventative and curative measures, and differences in methods of case ascertainment worldwide. However, the widening gap between low- and high-income countries remains a significant challenge for long-term stroke strategies and this must be addressed before a true worldwide reduction in stroke incidence and mortality can be demonstrated.

At a local level, the implementation of national policy and clinical guidelines provide challenges for stroke service providers. Accurate identification of the patients most suitable for thrombolytic therapy as soon as possible after the onset of stroke symptoms is essential for the best possible outcome.

Access to good quality organised stroke unit care during the acute period is necessary to improve results and reduce mortality after stroke. Furthermore, the combination of stroke unit care with early supportive discharge has been shown by health economic modelling to not only be an effective management strategy for patients after stroke, but also the most cost-effective approach when compared to both stroke unit and medical ward care without early supportive discharge.

The evidence base for the acute treatment and rehabilitation of stroke patients is vast. The time is now opportune for commissioners of healthcare to extrapolate this evidence into clinical practice in order to optimise and maintain stroke services that are high quality, cost effective, and accessible to their population.

References

1. Johnston SC, Mendis S, Mathers CD. Global variation in stroke burden and mortality: estimates from monitoring, surveillance, and modelling. *Lancet Neurol* 2009 April; 8(4): 345–354.
2. United Nations Population Division. World Population Prospects 2008. Ref Type: Generic.
3. Truelsen T, Piechowski-Jozwiak B, Bonita R, Mathers C, Bogousslavsky J, Boysen G. Stroke incidence and prevalence in Europe: a review of available data. *Eur J Neurol* 2006 June; 13(6): 581–598.
4. Feigin VL, Lawes CM, Bennett DA, Anderson CS. Stroke epidemiology: a review of population-based studies of incidence, prevalence, and case-fatality in the late 20th century. *Lancet Neurol* 2003 January; 2(1): 43–53.
5. Sarti C, Rastenyte D, Cepaitis Z, Tuomilehto J. International trends in mortality from stroke, 1968 to 1994. *Stroke* 2000 July; 31(7): 1588–1601.
6. Incidence of stroke in Europe at the beginning of the 21st century. *Stroke* 2009 May; 40(5): 1557–1563.
7. Feigin VL, Wiebers DO, Nikitin YP, O'Fallon WM, Whisnant JP. Stroke epidemiology in Novosibirsk, Russia: a population-based study. *Mayo Clin Proc* 1995 September; 70(9): 847–852.
8. Mihalka L, Smolanka V, Bulecza B, Mulesa S, Bereczki D. A population study of stroke in West Ukraine: incidence, stroke services, and 30-day case fatality. *Stroke* 2001 October; 32(10): 2227–2231.

9. Sarti C, Rastenyte D, Cepaitis Z, Tuomilehto J. International trends in mortality from stroke, 1968 to 1994. *Stroke* 2000 July; 31(7): 1588–1601.

10. Sarti C, Stegmayr B, Tolonen H, Mahonen M, Tuomilehto J, Asplund K. Are changes in mortality from stroke caused by changes in stroke event rates or case fatality? Results from the WHO MONICA Project. *Stroke* 2003 August; 34(8): 1833–1840.

11. Feigin VL, Lawes CM, Bennett DA, Barker-Collo SL, Parag V. Worldwide stroke incidence and early case fatality reported in 56 population-based studies: a systematic review. *Lancet Neurol* 2009 April; 8(4): 355–369.

12. Department of Health. National Service Framework for Older People in England: Standard Five. 2001.

13. Department of Health. Reducing brain damage: faster access to better stroke care. 2005 Nov 16.

14. Incidence of stroke in europe at the beginning of the 21st century. *Stroke* 2009 May; 40(5): 1557–1563.

15. Stewart JA, Dundas R, Howard RS, Rudd AG, Wolfe CD. Ethnic differences in incidence of stroke: prospective study with stroke register. *BMJ* 1999 April 10; 318(7189): 967–971.

16. Smeeton NC, Heuschmann PU, Rudd AG, McEvoy AW, Kitchen ND, Sarker SJ, Wolfe CD. Incidence of hemorrhagic stroke in black Caribbean, black African, and white populations: the South London stroke register, 1995–2004. *Stroke* 2007 December; 38(12): 3133–3138.

17. Rosamond WD, Folsom AR, Chambless LE, Wang CH, McGovern PG, Howard G, Copper LS, Shahar E. Stroke incidence and survival among middle-aged adults: 9-year follow-up of the Atherosclerosis Risk in Communities (ARIC) cohort. *Stroke* 1999 April; 30(4): 736–743.

18. Sacco RL, Boden-Albala B, Abel G, Lin IF, Elkind M, Hauser WA, Paik MC, Shea S. Race-ethnic disparities in the impact of stroke risk factors: the northern Manhattan stroke study. *Stroke* 2001 August; 32(8): 1725–1731.

19. Heuschmann PU, Grieve AP, Toschke AM, Rudd AG, Wolfe CD. Ethnic group disparities in 10-year trends in stroke incidence and vascular risk factors: the South London Stroke Register (SLSR). *Stroke* 2008 August; 39(8): 2204–2210.

20. Rothwell PM, Coull AJ, Giles MF, Howard SC, Silver LE, Bull LM, Gutnikov SA, Edwards P, Mant D, Sackley CM, Farmer A, Sandercock PA, Dennis MS, Warlow CP, Bamford JM, Anslow P. Change in stroke incidence,

mortality, case-fatality, severity, and risk factors in Oxfordshire, UK from 1981 to 2004 (Oxford Vascular Study). *Lancet* 2004 June 12; 363(9425): 1925–1933.

21. Lovelock CE, Molyneux AJ, Rothwell PM. Change in incidence and aetiology of intracerebral haemorrhage in Oxfordshire, UK, between 1981 and 2006: a population-based study. *Lancet Neurol* 2007 June; 6(6): 487–493.

22. Bamford J, Sandercock P, Dennis M, Burn J, Warlow C. A prospective study of acute cerebrovascular disease in the community: the Oxfordshire Community Stroke Project — 1981–1986. 2. Incidence, case fatality rates and overall outcome at one year of cerebral infarction, primary intracerebral and subarachnoid haemorrhage. *J Neurol Neurosurg Psychiatry* 1990 January; 53(1): 16–22.

23. Dennis MS, Burn JP, Sandercock PA, Bamford JM, Wade DT, Warlow CP. Long-term survival after first-ever stroke: the Oxfordshire Community Stroke Project. *Stroke* 1993 June; 24(6): 796–800.

24. Wolfe CD, Smeeton NC, Coshall C, Tilling K, Rudd AG. Survival differences after stroke in a multiethnic population: follow-up study with the South London stroke register. *BMJ* 2005 August 20; 331(7514): 431.

25. Donnan GA, Fisher M, Macleod M, Davis SM. Stroke. *Lancet* 2008 May 10; 371(9624): 1612–1623.

26. Strong K, Mathers C, Bonita R. Preventing stroke: saving lives around the world. *Lancet Neurol* 2007 February; 6(2): 182–187.

27. Johnston SC, Mendis S, Mathers CD. Global variation in stroke burden and mortality: estimates from monitoring, surveillance, and modelling. *Lancet Neurol* 2009 April; 8(4): 345–354.

28. Yusuf S, Reddy S, Ounpuu S, Anand S. Global burden of cardiovascular diseases: part I: general considerations, the epidemiologic transition, risk factors, and impact of urbanization. *Circulation* 2001 November 27; 104(22): 2746–2753.

29. Brainin M, Teuschl Y, Kalra L. Acute treatment and long-term management of stroke in developing countries. *Lancet Neurol* 2007 June; 6(6): 553–561.

30. WHO. Prevention of recurrent heart attacks and strokes in low- and middle-income populations. Evidence-based recommendations for policy-makers and health professionals. Geneva; 2003.

31. Boysen G, Truelsen T. Prevention of recurrent stroke. *Neurol Sci* 2000 April; 21(2): 67–72.

32. Anderson CS, Carter KN, Brownlee WJ, Hackett ML, Broad JB, Bonita R. Very long-term outcome after stroke in Auckland, New Zealand. *Stroke* 2004; 35(8): 1920–1924.

33. van WI, Kappelle LJ, van GJ, Koudstaal PJ, Franke CL, Vermeulen M, Gorter JW, Algra A. Long-term survival and vascular event risk after transient ischaemic attack or minor ischaemic stroke: a cohort study. *Lancet* 2005 June 18; 365(9477): 2098–2104.

34. Viitanen M, Eriksson S, Asplund K. Risk of recurrent stroke, myocardial-infarction and epilepsy.during long-term follow-up after stroke. *European Neurology* 1988; 28(4): 227–231.

35. Eriksson SE, Olsson JE. Survival and recurrent strokes in patients with different subtypes of stroke: a fourteen-year follow-up study. *Cerebrovasc Dis* 2001; 12(3): 171–180.

36. Sacco RL, Wolf PA, Kannel WB, McNamara PM. Survival and recurrence following stroke. The Framingham study. *Stroke* 1982 May; 13(3): 290–295.

37. Li CR, Hedblad B, Rosvall M, Buchwald F, Khan FA, Engstrom G. Stroke incidence, recurrence, and case-fatality in relation to socioeconomic position — A population-based study of middle-aged Swedish men and women. *Stroke* 2008; 39(8): 2191–2196.

38. Mohan KM, Crichton SL, Grieve AP, Rudd AG, Wolfe CD, Heuschmann PU. Frequency and predictors for the risk of stroke recurrence up to 10 years after stroke: the South London Stroke Register. *J Neurol Neurosurg Psychiatry* 2009 May 21.

39. Hardie K, Hankey GJ, Jamrozik K, Broadhurst RJ, Anderson C. Ten-year risk of first recurrent stroke and disability after first-ever stroke in the Perth Community Stroke Study. *Stroke* 2004 March; 35(3): 731–735.

40. Hata J, Tanizaki Y, Kiyohara Y, Kato I, Kubo M, Tanaka K, Okubo K, Nakamura H, Oishi Y, Ibayashi S, Iida M. Ten-year recurrence after first ever stroke in a Japanese community: the Hisayama study. *J Neurol Neurosurg Psychiatr* 2005; 76(3): 368–372.

41. Petty GW, Brown J, Whisnant JP, Sicks JD, O'Fallon WM, Wiebers DO. Survival and recurrence after first cerebral infarction: a population-based study in Rochester, Minnesota, 1975 through 1989. *Neurology* 1998; 50(1): 208–216.

42. Friday G, Alter M, Lai SM, Sobe E. Transient ischemic attack and risk of stroke recurrence: the Lehigh Valley Recurrent Stroke Study. *J Stroke Cerebrovasc Dis* 1997; 6(6): 410–415.

43. Hankey GJ, Jamrozik K, Broadhurst RJ, Forbes S, Burvill PW, Anderson CS, Stewart-Wynne EG. Long-term risk of first recurrent stroke in the Perth Community Stroke Study. *Stroke* 1998; 29(12): 2491–2500.

44. Elneihoum AM, Goransson M, Falke P, Janzon L. Three-year survival and recurrence after stroke in Malmo, Sweden: an analysis of stroke registry data. *Stroke* 1998 October; 29(10): 2114–2117.

45. Mant J, Wade D, Winner S. Stroke. In Stevens A, Raftery J, Mant J, Simpson S (Eds). *Healthcare Needs Assessment: The Epidemiologically Based Needs Assessment Reviews*. 2nd Edn. Oxford: Radcliffe Publishing Limited; 2004. p. 141–244.

46. Grieve R, Hutton J, Bhalla A, Rastenyte D, Ryglewicz D, Sarti C, Lamassa M, Giroud M, Dundas R, Wolfe CD. A comparison of the costs and survival of hospital-admitted stroke patients across Europe. *Stroke* 2001 July; 32(7): 1684–1691.

47. Department of Health. Our healthier nation a contract for health. 1998. Report No.: 0101385226.

48. Department of Health. Saving lives: our healthier nation. 1999 July 5.

49. Department of Health. National Service Framework for Older People. London: Department of Health; 2001.

50. Royal College of Physicians Intercollegiate Stroke Working Party, 3rd Edn. National Clinical Guidelines for Stroke. London: Royal College of Physicians; 2008.

51. National Institute for Health and Clinical Excellence. *Stroke: Diagnosis and Initial Management of Acute Stroke and Transient Ischaemic Attack (TIA)*. 2008 Jul.

52. Department of Health, Boyle R. Improving stroke services: a guide for commissioners. 2006 Dec 7. Report No.: 278329.

53. Department of Health. Action on stroke services: an evaluation toolkit. 2006 June 4.

54. Kjellstrom T, Norrving B, Shatchkute A. Helsingborg Declaration 2006 on European stroke strategies. *Cerebrovasc Dis* 2007; 23(2–3): 231–241.

55. Wahlgren N, Ahmed N, Davalos A, Ford GA, Grond M, Hacke W, Hennerici MG, Kaste M, Kuelkens S, Larrue V, Lees KR, Roine RO, Soinne L,

Toni D, Vanhooren G. Thrombolysis with alteplase for acute ischaemic stroke in the Safe Implementation of Thrombolysis in Stroke-Monitoring Study (SITS-MOST): an observational study. *Lancet* 2007 January 27; 369(9558): 275–282.

56. Stroke Unit Trialists' Collaboration. Organised inpatient (stroke unit) care for stroke. *Cochrane Database Syst Rev* 2000; (2): CD000197.

57. Stroke Unit Trialists' Collaboration. Organised inpatient (stroke unit) care for stroke. *Cochrane Database Syst Rev* 2002; (1): CD000197.

58. Quinn TJ, Dawson J, Lees KR. Acute stroke: we have the treatments and we have the evidence — we need to use them. *Crit Care* 2007; 11(2): 124.

59. Wahlgren N, Ahmed N, Eriksson N, Aichner F, Bluhmki E, Davalos A, Erila T, Ford GA, Grond M, Hacke W, Hennerici MG, Kaste M, Kohrmann M, Larrue V, Lees KR, Machnig T, Roine RO, Toni D, Vanhooren G. Multivariable analysis of outcome predictors and adjustment of main outcome results to baseline data profile in randomized controlled trials: Safe Implementation of Thrombolysis in Stroke-MOnitoring STudy (SITS-MOST). *Stroke* 2008 December; 39(12): 3316–3322.

60. Heuschmann PU, Berger K, Misselwitz B, Hermanek P, Leffmann C, Adelmann M, Buecker-Nott HJ, Rother J, Neundoerfer B, Kolominsky-Rabas PL. Frequency of thrombolytic therapy in patients with acute ischemic stroke and the risk of in-hospital mortality: the German Stroke Registers Study Group. *Stroke* 2003 May; 34(5): 1106–1113.

61. Heuschmann PU, Berger K. International experience in stroke registries: German Stroke Registers Study Group. *Am J Prev Med* 2006 December; 31(6 Suppl 2): S238–S239.

62. Beech R, Ratcliffe M, Tilling K, Wolfe C. Hospital services for stroke care. A European Perspective. European Study of Stroke Care. *Stroke* 1996 November; 27(11): 1958–1964.

63. Bhalla A, Grieve R, Tilling K, Rudd AG, Wolfe CD. Older stroke patients in Europe: stroke care and determinants of outcome. *Age Ageing* 2004 November; 33(6): 618–624.

64. Bhalla A, Grieve R, Rudd AG, Wolfe CD. Stroke in the young: access to care and outcome; a Western versus eastern European perspective. *J Stroke Cerebrovasc Dis* 2008 November; 17(6): 360–365.

65. Hankey GJ, Warlow CP. Treatment and secondary prevention of stroke: evidence, costs, and effects on individuals and populations. *Lancet* 1999 October 23; 354(9188): 1457–1463.

66. Intercollegiate Stroke Working Party. National Sentinel Stroke Audit. 2006.

67. Asplund K, Hulter AK, Norrving B, Stegmayr B, Terent A, Wester PO. Riks-stroke — a Swedish national quality register for stroke care. *Cerebrovasc Dis* 2003; 15 Suppl 1: 5–7.

68. Terent A, Asplund K, Farahmand B, Henriksson KM, Norrving B, Stegmayr B, Wester PO, Asberg KH, Asberg S. Stroke unit care revisited: who benefits the most? A cohort study of 105,043 patients in Riks-Stroke, the Swedish Stroke Register. *J Neurol Neurosurg Psychiatr* 2009 August; 80(8): 881–887.

69. Appelros P, Samuelsson M, Karlsson-Tivenius S, Lokander M, Terent A. A national stroke quality register: 12 years experience from a participating hospital. *Eur J Neurol* 2007 August; 14(8): 890–894.

70. Glader EL, Stegmayr B, Johansson L, Hulter-Asberg K, Wester PO. Differences in long-term outcome between patients treated in stroke units and in general wards: a 2-year follow-up of stroke patients in sweden. *Stroke* 2001 September; 32(9): 2124–2130.

71. Terent A, Asplund K, Farahmand B, Henriksson K, Norrving B, Stegmayr B, Wester PO, Hulter-Asberg K, Asberg S. Stroke unit care revisited — who benefits the most? A cohort study of 105,043 patients in Riks-Stroke, the Swedish Stroke Register. *J Neurol Neurosurg Psychiatr* 2009 March 29.

72. Ringelstein EB, Meckes-Ferber S, Hacke W, Kaste M, Brainin M, Leys D. European Stroke Facilities Survey: the German and Austrian perspective. *Cerebrovasc Dis* 2009; 27(2): 138–145.

73. Alberts MJ, Hademenos G, Latchaw RE, Jagoda A, Marler JR, Mayberg MR, Starke RD, Todd HW, Viste KM, Girgus M, Shephard T, Emr M, Shwayder P, Walker MD. Recommendations for the establishment of primary stroke centers. Brain Attack Coalition. *JAMA* 2000 June 21; 283(23): 3102–3109.

74. Alberts MJ, Latchaw RE, Selman WR, Shephard T, Hadley MN, Brass LM, Koroshetz W, Marler JR, Booss J, Zorowitz RD, Croft JB, Magnis E, Mulligan D, Jagoda A, O'Connor R, Cawley CM, Connors JJ, Rose-DeRenzy JA, Emr M, Warren M, Walker MD. Recommendations for comprehensive stroke centers: a consensus statement from the Brain Attack Coalition. *Stroke* 2005 July; 36(7): 1597–1616.

75. Reeves MJ, Broderick JP, Frankel M, LaBresh KA, Schwamm L, Moomaw CJ, Weiss P, Katzan I, Arora S, Heinrich JP, Hickenbottom S, Karp H, Malarcher A, Mensah G, Reeves MJ. The Paul Coverdell National Acute

Stroke Registry: initial results from four prototypes. *Am J Prev Med* 2006 December; 31(6 Suppl 2): S202–S209.

76. Gropen TI, Gagliano PJ, Blake CA, Sacco RL, Kwiatkowski T, Richmond NJ, Leifer D, Libman R, Azhar S, Daley MB. Quality improvement in acute stroke: the New York State Stroke Center Designation Project. *Neurology* 2006 July 11; 67(1): 88–93.

77. National Stroke Foundation. National Stroke Audit Clinical Report: Acute Services. 2008.

78. Duffy BK, Phillips PA, Davis SM, Donnan GA, Vedadhaghi ME. Evidence-based care and outcomes of acute stroke managed in hospital specialty units. *Med J Aust* 2003 April 7; 178(7): 318–323.

79. World Health Organization. International Classification of Functioning, Disability and Health (ICF). Geneva: WHO; 2001.

80. National Audit Office. Reducing brain damage: faster access to better stroke care. London: NAO; 2005.

81. Di CA. Human and economic burden of stroke. *Age Ageing* 2009 January; 38(1): 4–5.

82. Evers SM, Struijs JN, Ament AJ, van Genugten ML, Jager JH, van den Bos GA. International comparison of stroke cost studies. *Stroke* 2004 May; 35(5): 1209–1215.

83. Luengo-Fernandez R, Gray AM, Rothwell PM. Costs of stroke using patient-level data: a critical review of the literature. *Stroke* 2009 February; 40(2): e18–e23.

84. Luengo-Fernandez R, Leal J, Gray A, Petersen S, Rayner M. Cost of cardio-vascular diseases in the United Kingdom. *Heart* 2006 October; 92(10): 1384–1389.

85. Saka O, McGuire A, Wolfe C. Cost of stroke in the United Kingdom. *Age Ageing* 2009 January; 38(1): 27–32.

86. Luengo-Fernandez R, Gray AM, Rothwell PM. Population-based study of determinants of initial secondary care costs of acute stroke in the United Kingdom. *Stroke* 2006 October; 37(10): 2579–2587.

87. Saka O, Serra V, Samyshkin Y, McGuire A, Wolfe CC. Cost-effectiveness of stroke unit care followed by early supported discharge. *Stroke* 2009 January; 40(1): 24–29.

2 Strategies for Stroke Prevention

Juliet Addo and Charles Wolfe*

Chapter Summary

Stroke, a leading cause of disability and death worldwide, is largely preventable. Epidemiological studies have identified several modifiable and non-modifiable risk factors associated with stroke. The non-modifiable risk factors for stroke include age, sex, ethnicity/race, and a family history of stroke. Modifiable risk factors include hypertension, diabetes, hyperlipidaemia, atrial fibrillation, cigarette smoking, asymptomatic carotid stenosis, obesity and physical inactivity.

Effective strategies for stroke prevention need to consider prevention at all levels, including the modification of risk factors, appropriate treatment of acute stroke when it does occur, prevention of the complications of stroke, and the prevention of recurrent stroke. These strategies may target the reduction of the risk factors in high-risk individuals and populations and may include the control of hypertension, treatment of hyperlipidaemia, use of antithrombotics, anticoagulation for high-risk patients with atrial fibrillation and the use of endarterectomy in selected patients. The population-based strategy aims to reduce risk factors at the population level through lifestyle and environmental changes and is critical to reducing the overall incidence of cardiovascular disease. The individual-based approach involves detection of individuals at increased

*Division of Health and Social Care Research, Kings College London, London, UK

risk of stroke and taking steps to reduce that risk through lifestyle changes and medications. Effective strategies for stroke prevention require a comprehensive multidisciplinary approach to identify and manage major risk factors and to promote adherence to preventive protocols. Despite the availability of stroke risk assessment tools for identification of individuals at sufficiently increased risk of stroke, and clinical guidelines providing an evidence base to guide modern stroke prevention and treatment, considerable gaps have been reported in the translation of recommendations into practice. Uptake of stroke prevention strategies remains low in most populations and the challenge remains to identify strategies for effective implementation for the benefits of primary and secondary prevention of stroke in different population groups.

Introduction

Stroke is a leading cause of death and disability worldwide.[1,2] It is a preventable and treatable disease which puts a significant burden on society and long-term care resources.[3,4] The impact of stroke is expected to grow rapidly with the increasing proportion of older people in the global population.[1] Clinical trials and observational studies provide evidence for a wide range of interventions for preventing a first or recurrent stroke.[5,6] Guidelines from professional societies and governmental organisations provide an evidence base to guide modern stroke prevention and treatment.[7–9] However, despite these advances and consistent recommendations, considerable gaps exist between the evidence and its translation into actual practice and patient outcomes.[10] Effective prevention remains the best treatment for reducing the burden of stroke.[9] Strategies for stroke prevention need to consider prevention at all levels, including effective modification of risk factors, appropriate treatment of acute stroke when it does occur, prevention of the complications of stroke, and the prevention of recurrent stroke. These strategies may involve a population-based approach to risk factor modification in which the entire distribution of risk factors and risk is shifted toward lower levels through population-wide interventions, or individual-based approach in which individuals' risk are assessed and steps taken to reduce identified risks.[10–12] Stroke prevention requires a long-term effort.[13]

Prevalence of Risk Factors

Epidemiological studies, particularly cohort studies, have identified possible risk factors for stroke and the evidence has been summarised in a useful scientific statement from the American Heart Association.[9] The major risk factors for stroke are similar to those of ischaemic heart disease.[4] Modifiable risk factors (Table 1), with clear supportive epidemiological evidence in addition to evidence of risk reduction with modification as documented by randomised trials, include hypertension, cigarette smoking, diabetes, carotid stenosis, atrial fibrillation, dyslipidaemia (high total cholesterol and low HDL cholesterol), dietary factors (high sodium and low potassium intake), obesity, physical inactivity, postmenopausal hormone therapy, transient ischaemic attacks (TIA) and sickle cell disease.[9,14] Non-modifiable risk factors (Table 2) include age, sex, ethnicity/race, and family history of stroke.[9,14] Although these factors cannot be modified, their presence helps to identify those at increased risk, enabling effective treatment of those risk factors that can be modified.[14] In recent years, epidemiological studies have explored a range of novel risk factors, most of which are thought to operate by accelerating atherosclerosis.[15] These include elevated levels of homocysteine, increased C-reactive protein (and other indices of inflammation), increased fibrinogen and clotting factors.[16-19]

Evidence from the Framingham study, using data collected over 36 years of follow-up in a general population sample, demonstrates that the probability of a stroke depends on the presence and level of risk factors.[13] It is helpful to be able to estimate a person's risk for a first stroke by applying stroke risk assessment tools.[9] The stroke risk profile provides the framework for identification of those individuals at sufficiently increased risk of stroke.[13] Data from the Framingham study demonstrates an increase in the ten-year stroke risk in 70-year-old women and men with borderline hypertension and no associated risk factor abnormalities, from $\leq 9\%$ in women and $\leq 12.3\%$ in men to $>80\%$.[13] The increased risk is observed in the presence of diabetes mellitus, cigarette smoking, antecedent cardiovascular disease, atrial fibrillation, and electrocardiographic abnormalities. Some modifiable risk factors (such as hypertension, diabetes and smoking) are common

Table 1. Modifiable risk factors for stroke

	Population attributable risk (%)	Relative risk	Risk reduction with treatment
Hypertension[22]		Five-fold increase in probability of an ischaemic stroke if BP ≥ 160/95 mmHg compared to BP < 140/90 mmHg.[23] A 20 mmHg lower than usual SBP is associated with more than a two-fold difference in stroke mortality (hazard ratios of 0.36 (CI: 0.32–0.40) at 40–49 years to 0.67 (CI: 0.63–0.71) at 80–89 years.[24]	Dose-response relationship with a 10 mmHg reduction in SBP associated with a 31% reduction in stroke risk.[25]
50–59 years old	48.8		
60–69 years old	53.2		
70–79 years old	48.6		
80–89 years old	33.4		
Diabetes		Relative risk of 2.42 (CI: 1.94–3.02).[26]	The benefit of intensive glucose control over less intensive control on stroke in patients with type 2 diabetes remains unclear.[27] Intensive blood pressure management has however been shown to provide significant benefit on fatal/non-fatal stroke in patients with type 2 diabetes compared to placebo.[28]

(*Continued*)

Table 1. (*Continued*)

	Population attributable risk (%)	Relative risk	Risk reduction with treatment
Smoking		1.5 (95% CI: 1.4–1.6) and increased from 1.37 (CI: 1.24–1.52) in those smoking <10/day to 1.82 (CI: 1.70–1.96) in those smoking >20/day.[29]	The benefit of giving up smoking completely was seen within five years of quitting, with no further consistent decline in risk thereafter, but this was dependent on the amount of tobacco smoked.[30]
Atrial fibrillation[22]			Treatment with warfarin decreased risk of stroke in women by 84% (CI: 55–95%) and 60% (CI: 35–76%) in men.[31]
50–59 years old	1.5	4.0	
60–69 years old	2.8	2.6	
70–79 years old	9.9	3.3	
80–89 years old	23.5	4.5	
Dyslipidaemia		Observational studies have not found a consistent relation between cholesterol levels and incidence of stroke. There have been weak and inconsistent associations reported between ischaemic stroke and the lipid parameters.[32,33]	Randomised trials of statins have consistently demonstrated a reduction of stroke risk with lowering of lipid levels. Treatment with statins decreased total and LDL cholesterol by 22% and 30% respectively with significant reductions in risks of stroke of 29% (95% CI: 14–41%).[34] An absolute risk reduction in stroke rates of 2.2%

(*Continued*)

Table 1. (*Continued*)

	Population attributable risk (%)	Relative risk	Risk reduction with treatment
			(adjusted HR: 0.84; 95% CI: 0.71–0.99) was reported with 80 mg of Atorvastatin daily, associated with a 53% reduction of LDL cholesterol levels.[35]
Asymptomatic carotid stenosis		Crude annual indices of stroke of 0.23% for 0–50% stenosis, 2.48% for 50–75% stenosis and 1.71% for 75–99% stenosis have been reported.[36]	Endarterectomy is reported to be highly beneficial in those with 70% stenosis or greater without near occlusion (16%, $p < 0.001$).[37]
Obesity		Abdominal obesity is associated with an increased risk of stroke (odds ratio: 3.0; CI: 2.1–4.2).[38] Data from prospective studies have reported each 5 kg/m^2 higher BMI to be associated with about 40% higher mortality in the upper BMI groups (25–50 kg/m^2).[39]	Unknown.[9]

(*Continued*)

Table 1. (*Continued*)

	Population attributable risk (%)	Relative risk	Risk reduction with treatment
Physical inactivity		Increasing physical activity is reported to be inversely associated with the risk of stroke with relative risks in the lowest to highest quintile of physical activity level reported as 1.00, 0.98, 0.82, 0.74 and 0.66 (*p*-trend of 0.005).[40] Inverse association is reported between stroke incidence and increasing levels of combined work and leisure activity with a nearly 40% risk reduction in the most active category.[41]	Unknown.[9]

Addo and Wolfe

Table 2. Non-modifiable risk factors

	Relative risk	Ten-year risk of developing stroke[42]:	
		Men	Women
Age (years)	The risk of stroke has been reported to double in each successive decade after 55 years of age.[43,44]		
55		2.9 (2.2–3.6)	2.3 (1.7–2.9)
65		7.0 (5.8–8.2)	4.6 (3.8–5.5)
75		10.4 (8.6–12.1)	10.5 (9.1–11.9)
85		8.5 (5.7–11.3)	13.4 (11.1–15.6)
Sex	Higher incidence rates for stroke have been reported for men; incidence rate ratio adjusted for age of 1.3. (CI: 1.1–1.5)[45]		
Ethnicity	Age- and sex-adjusted stroke incidence rate ratio of 2.18 (95% CI: 1.86–2.56) in the black population compared to the white population.[46]		
Hereditary/ familial factors	There are suggestions of an increased risk of stroke with paternal (RR: 2.4; 95% CI: 0.96–6.03) and maternal (RR: 1.4; 95% CI: 0.60–3.25) histories of stroke, as well as parental history of coronary heart disease (RR: 3.33; 95% CI: 1.27–8.72).[47]		

and affect health in several ways, providing opportunities to modify risk in large numbers of people. Other risk factors such as atrial fibrillation and TIAs are less common and more specific than the common risk factors for stroke.[20] Long-term prospective studies consistently identify people with low levels of risk factors as having lifelong low levels of heart disease and stroke.[21] Models such as the Framingham Stroke Risk Profile have been developed which provide sex specific estimation of the probability of stroke by summing the points represented by individual risk factors for overall risk assessment in clinical practice.[13] The importance of such risk scores in stroke prevention are discussed later in this chapter.

Hypertension

Hypertension is the most prevalent treatable risk factor for the prevention of stroke and its recurrence.[48] The higher the blood pressure (BP), the greater the chances of developing stroke.[49] Hypertension, particularly severe diastolic and malignant hypertension, has long been acknowledged as predisposing to stroke, particularly intracerebral haemorrhage.[50] Available evidence from the combined results of nine major prospective observational studies demonstrate positive, continuous and apparently independent associations between diastolic blood pressure (DBP) and stroke, with no evidence of any 'threshold' below which lower levels of DBP were not associated with lower risk of stroke.[51] Data from the Framingham study demonstrated a five-fold increase in the probability of developing an ischaemic stroke in those with BP ≥ 160/95 mmHg compared to those with BP < 140/90 mmHg.[23] Information obtained from one million adults in 61 prospective observational studies also demonstrated a strong positive association between usual BP and stroke mortality at all ages, without any evidence of a threshold down to at least 115/75 mmHg.[24] A 10 mmHg lower than usual systolic blood pressure (SBP) or 5 mmHg lower than usual DBP from this review was estimated to be associated in the long term with about 40% lower risk of stroke death.[24] There has been evidence from randomised controlled trials for several decades that the control of high BP contributes to the prevention of strokes.[52] A meta-analyses of randomised controlled trials of BP lowering and stroke suggests a dose-response relationship with a 10 mmHg reduction in SBP being associated with a 31% reduction in stroke risk.[53]

The global adult prevalence of hypertension in the year 2000 was estimated to be 26.4%.[54] National surveys conducted in Europe and North America have reported prevalence ranging from 27% to 55%.[55] Prevalence ranging from 11% to 47% has been reported from studies in Africa.[56] The prevalence of hypertension increases with advancing age, with more than half of people aged 60 to 69 years, and approximately 75% of people aged 70 years and older being affected.[57] The odds of hypertension reported has been higher in black men and women as well as South Asian men compared to their white counterparts.[58] The mean SBP determined from reviews of national surveys did not vary significantly by national income category and was 123.2 (95% CI: 122.5–128.2) mmHg in low-income countries and 125.6 (95% CI: 121.6–127.0) mmHg in high-income countries in 2002.[59,60] The majority of people with a stroke in a large Swedish prospective cohort study were those with uncontrolled blood pressure.[61] The crude incidence of stroke during the follow-up period in this study (mean period of six years) was 289/100,000 person-year in controlled hypertensive subjects and 705/100,000 person-year in treated hypertensive subjects with BP ≥ 140/90 mmHg.[61] Treatment and control of hypertension eliminates the excess cardiovascular disease mortality risk observed among the hypertensive population.[62] However, even in developed countries, many patients with hypertension remain undetected or untreated and a large proportion of patients who do receive treatment do not achieve target blood pressure levels.[63,64] Blood pressure is adequately controlled in only 20% of the 50 million hypertensives in the United States and in <10% of hypertensives in most European countries.[50,64] The Euroaspire I, II, and III surveys, designed as cross-sectional studies of patients with coronary heart disease in several centres across Europe over three different time periods, demonstrated no improvement in blood pressure management over time despite large increases in prescriptions of all classes of antihypertensive drugs.[65] Possible explanations for this finding included the use of low-dose prescriptions, inadequate adjustment of doses, and poor patient compliance.[65] In the Cardiovascular Health Study, a cohort study of older adults from four US centres, the control of high BP to levels lower than 140/90 mmHg increased from 37% in

1989–1990 to 49% in 1999.[66] The improvement in control among those treated was achieved in part by a small increase of antihypertensive medications per person over the course of nine years.[66]

Diabetes

Individuals with type 2 diabetes have an increased susceptibility to atherosclerosis and an increased prevalence of atherogenic risk factors, including hypertension, obesity and abnormal lipids.[67] An increase in stroke risk, independent of other cardiovascular disease risk factors, has been reported in those with diabetes.[13,68] A systematic overview of epidemiological studies and surveys observed that 13% of all deaths from stroke worldwide were attributable to higher-than-optimum blood glucose.[69] The relative risk of stroke among Swedish men with diabetes in the Multifactor Primary Prevention Study during a 28-year follow-up period was 2.42 (95%CI: 1.94–3.02).[26] Among Japanese-American men in the Honolulu Heart Program, participants with diabetes had an increased risk of thromboembolic stroke, i.e. 2.45 (95%CI: 1.73–3.47), compared to those without diabetes, over a 22-year follow-up period.[68] The association was largely independent of other cardiovascular disease risk factors. The prevalence of diabetes in 2000 was estimated to be 2.8% worldwide for all age groups and projected to rise to 4.4% in 2030.[70] Reports from the Framingham study suggest a doubling in the incidence of diabetes over the past 30 years.[71] The prevalence of diabetes was 5.6% in men and 4.2% in women in England in 2007, and 7.8% in the US during the period of 2003 to 2006, and higher in Black Americans compared to whites and in those of lower socioeconomic status.[72–74] In 2002, a higher prevalence of diabetes was reported from high-income countries [4.3% (95% CI: 3.0–6.4%)] compared to low-income countries [1.2% (95% CI: 0.6–1.7%)].[59,60] In 2000, 1.1 million persons aged 35 years and above with diabetes in the US were reported to have been diagnosed with a stroke.[75] People with type 2 diabetes generally have additional stroke risk factors, including hypertension, dyslipidaemia, obesity, and atrial fibrillation.[27] A meta-analysis of 27 trials found that antihypertensive regimens based on angiotensin-converting enzyme inhibitors, calcium antagonists, angiotensin receptor blockers and diuretics/beta-blockers, provided significant benefit on fatal/non-fatal stroke in patients with type 2 diabetes compared to placebo.[28] More intensive blood pressure management was significantly more effective than less intensive management.[28] The benefit of intensive glucose control on macrovascular events, including stroke in patients with type 2 diabetes, remains unclear.[27] Over ten years of follow-up in the UK Prospective Diabetes Study (UKPDS), intensive glucose control with insulin and/or sulfonylureas was not associated with a reduced risk of stroke when compared to a less intensive lifestyle intervention.[76] In a supplementary study of overweight patients in the UKPDS, intensive therapy with metformin produced a non-significant reduction in the risk of stroke compared to lifestyle intervention.[77] A meta-analysis of randomised controlled trials of pioglitazone reported a significantly lower risk of stroke among a diverse population of patients with diabetes.[78] The apparent beneficial effects on stroke risk however, remain to be replicated in other large-scale prospective randomised controlled trials with pioglitazone or any other thiazolidinedione.[27]

Smoking

Cigarette smoking has been identified as a potent risk factor for stroke.[79] Smoking possibly contributes to increased stroke risk through both acute effects on the risk of thrombus generation in narrowed arteries and chronic effects related to an increased burden of atherosclerosis.[80] A meta-analysis of 32 studies, including 17 cohort, 14 case-control and 1 hypertension intervention, found an overall relative risk of stroke associated with cigarette smoking of 1.5 (95% CI: 1.4–1.6).[29] The risks of stroke associated with smoking were present in all age groups but reported to be greater in people aged <55 years (RR: 2.94; CI: 2.40–3.59) compared to those aged ≥75 years (RR: 1.11; CI: 0.96–1.28).[29] The cardiovascular risks associated with cigarette smoking increase with the amount smoked and with the duration of smoking.[80,81] In the meta-analysis of 32 studies described earlier, the pooled relative risk estimates indicated a dose response from 1.37 (CI: 1.24–1.52) in those smoking <10/day to 1.82 (CI: 1.70–1.96) in those smoking >20/day.[29] The relative risk of stroke in heavy smokers (greater than 40 cigarettes/day) was twice that of light smokers (fewer than 10 cigarettes/day) in the Framingham study.[81] Cessation of cigarette smoking is reported to reduce stroke risk.[80,81] In the British Regional Heart Study, current smokers were demonstrated to have a four-fold relative risk of stroke compared to never smokers (3.7; CI: 2.0–6.9) during an average follow-up period of 12.75 years after full adjustment of other risk factors.[30] Ex-cigarette smokers showed lower risk than current smokers but showed excess risk compared with never smokers (RR: 1.7; CI: 0.9–3.3).[30] The benefit of giving up smoking completely was seen within five years of quitting, with no further consistent decline in risk thereafter, but this was dependent on the amount of tobacco smoked.[30] Those who smoked <20 cigarettes/day reverted to the risk level of those who had never smoked while heavy smokers retained a more than two-fold risk compared with never smokers (RR: 2.2; CI: 1.1–4.3).[30]

The prevalence of smoking in 2006 was 24% for men and 21% for women in England.[82] In 2005, a higher prevalence of smoking [29.3% (19.6–33.5%)] was reported from upper middle income countries compared to low-income countries [14.7% (9.4–24.3%)].[59,60] Sustained smoking cessation is difficult to achieve mainly because of the powerful addictive qualities of nicotine creating a hurdle even for those with a desire to quit.[9,83] Data from a US national survey of workers' self-reported characteristics showed that moving from no smoking restrictions to a smoke-free workplace decreased the prevalence of smoking by 5.7% (CI: 4.9–6.5) and reduced daily consumption among the remaining smokers by 2.67 cigarettes (CI: 2.28–3.05).[84] A study of the changes in air quality conducted in New York one year after a comprehensive state law requiring almost all indoor workplaces and public places to be smoke-free, demonstrated a substantially lower particulate matter from burning cigarettes (84%) in every venue where smoking or second-hand smoke exposure had been observed at baseline.[85] Meta-analyses in the US Department of Health and Human Services Public Health Service 2008 update of the Treating Tobacco Use and Dependence clinical practice guidelines demonstrate that counselling and medication as interventions to assist smokers to quit smoking work best when used together.[86] A population-based intervention study in Copenhagen that randomised 2408 daily smokers demonstrated a halving of tobacco consumption in the intervention group compared to the background population (odds ratio 2.61; CI: 1.6–4.4).[87] The participants randomised to an intervention involving counselling combined with nicotine replacement therapy had a mean reduction in tobacco consumption of 1.4 g (SD ± 6.3) after one year, compared with 0.03 (SD ± 6.1) in the background population.[87] The 2008 update of the US Public Health Service guideline conducted a meta-analysis of 86 studies that compared various medication combinations to placebo and demonstrated similar effectiveness between the agents.[86] Nicotine replacement therapy is the most common medication used to assist quit attempts.[83] A Cochrane review of interventions to reduce and prevent tobacco use in smokers reported that simple advice from doctors during routine care increased the quit rate (OR: 1.69; CI: 1.45–1.98), with more intensive advice being slightly more effective.[88] Nicotine replacement therapy, available as chewing gum, transdermal patch, nasal spray, inhaler, sublingual tablet and lozenge was found in the review to increase the chances of quitting (1.71; 1.60–1.83), whatever the level of additional support and encouragement.[88,89]

Lipids

Plasma lipids and lipoproteins (total cholesterol, triglycerides, LDL cholesterol, HDL cholesterol, and lipoprotein[s]) are reportedly associated with the risk of ischaemic stroke.[9] In a meta-analysis of prospective studies from the Asia-Pacific region, a 1 mmol/l increase in total cholesterol was associated with a 25% (95% CI: 13–40%) increased risk of fatal or non-fatal ischaemic stroke and a 20% (95% CI: 8–30%) decreased risk of fatal haemorrhagic stroke over 2 million person-years of follow-up, demonstrate an association between total cholesterol and ischaemic but not haemorrhagic strokes.[90] Analysis from a nested case-control study designed from a collaborative project among European cohort studies (EUROSTROKE) demonstrated no significant association between total cholesterol and risk of stroke (odds ratio for increase of 1 mmol/l in cholesterol of 0.98; 95% CI: 0.88–1.09).[91] In men there was a general trend towards a lower risk of stroke, with an increase in HDL cholesterol (odds ratio per 1 mmol/l increase in HDL cholesterol 0.68 (95% CI: 0.40–1.16)) whereas an increase in HDL cholesterol in women was associated with a significant increased risk of non-fatal stroke and of cerebral infarction (odds ratio of 2.46 (95% CI: 1.20–5.04) and 2.52 (95% CI: 1.15–5.50) respectively).[91] During a mean follow-up period of 16.8 years in the British Regional Heart Study, higher levels of HDL cholesterol were associated with a significant decrease in the risk of non-fatal stroke even after adjustment for potential confounders (adjusted relative risk 0.59, 95% CI: 0.39–0.90).[92] Total cholesterol showed no graded association with fatal strokes, but men with levels ≥8.1 mmol/l showed a non-significant increased risk of non-fatal stroke (adjusted RR: 1.46, 95% CI: 0.91–2.32).[92] There was no association seen between triglycerides and the risk of total stroke.[92] Data from the nationally representative Health Survey for England and the Scottish Health Survey report a mean total cholesterol of 5.43 and 5.48 mmol/l in men and women respectively and a mean HDL cholesterol of 1.29 and 1.56 mmol/l respectively. Overall 64.6% of adults had a total cholesterol ≥5 mmol/l.[93] The mean total cholesterol in 2002 was 5.4 (5.2–5.5) mmol/l in high-income countries and 4.3 (4.2–4.8) mmol/l in low-income countries.[59,60] Despite the lack of clear association between serum total cholesterol and risk of stroke in observational epidemiological studies, the results of lipid-lowering trials with statins suggest some benefit for stroke reduction.[34] An overview of 16 published randomised trials of statins, following up subjects for an average of 3.3 years, demonstrated large reductions in total and low-density lipoprotein cholesterol (22% and 30% respectively) and significant reductions in risks of stroke of 29% (95% CI: 14% to 41%) in those assigned to statin drugs.[34] The Stroke Prevention by Aggressive Reduction in Cholesterol Levels (SPARCL) trial randomised patients with a recent TIA or stroke, who had no known coronary heart disease and had a baseline LDL cholesterol between 100–190 mg/dl (2.6–4.9 mmol/l), to atorvastatin 80 mg daily or placebo. The trial demonstrated a 16% reduced relative risk of fatal or non-fatal strokes in the treatment group compared to the placebo group, during a median follow-up of 4.9 years (adjusted hazard ratio 0.84; CI: 0.71–0.99).[35]

Physical Activity

Regular physical activity has well-established benefits for reducing the risk of premature death and cardiovascular disease.[9] The beneficial effects of physical activity for stroke have been documented.[94,95] Over a follow-up period of up to 32 years, the Framingham study investigators reported an increased risk of stroke associated with the lowest levels of physical activity in men.[94] Among men included in this analysis, the crude risk ratios for medium levels of physical activity was 0.36 (95% CI: 0.22–0.59) and 0.33 (95% CI: 0.22–0.50) for high levels of physical activity compared with the lowest level of physical activity.[94] Therefore it can be concluded that there is a beneficial effect of higher levels of physical activity on stroke risk.[94] A strong inverse association between physical activity and the risk of stroke was demonstrated in the British Regional Heart Study after 9.5 years of follow-up that was independent of age, social class, smoking, heavy drinking, SBP, and pre-existing ischaemic heart disease or stroke (RR 1.0 for inactivity, 0.6 for moderate activity, and 0.3 for vigorous activity; test for trend, $p = 0.008$).[96] In 2006, only 40% of men and 28% of women met the physical activity guidelines recommending 30 minutes of physical activity on at least five days a week in England. One-third of English adults were inactive, participating in less than one occasion of 30 minutes activity in a week.[82] The prevalence of physical inactivity among adults in the US in 2003 was 67% (less than 30 minutes of physical activity on at least five days a week).[60] Moderate and moderately vigorous levels of activity in the British Regional Heart Study, such as frequent regular walking plus recreational activity or sporting activity once a week, were associated with a 50% reduction in the risk of stroke.[96] However, vigorous physical activity was associated with a marginally significant increased risk of heart attack compared with moderate and moderately vigorous activity in men with no pre-existing stroke or ischaemic heart disease.[96]

Obesity

Evidence from large-scale prospective studies has documented that increased weight is associated with an increased risk of stroke.[97,98] In the Physician's Health Study, a prospective cohort study of US male physicians, participants with BMI $\geq$ 30 kg/m^2 had an adjusted relative risk of 2.0 (95% CI: 1.48–2.71) for total stroke, 1.95 (95% CI: 1.39–2.72) for ischaemic strokes, and 2.25 (95% CI: 1.01–5.01) for haemorrhagic stroke compared to participants with BMI < 23 kg/m^2 during 12.5 years of follow-up.[97] Each unit increase of BMI was associated with a significant

6% increase in the adjusted relative risks of total, ischaemic and haemorrhagic strokes.[97] The Women's Health Study, a prospective cohort study of female health professionals in the US similarly demonstrated a significant trend for increased risk of total and ischaemic stroke across 7 BMI categories.[99] After a mean follow-up period of ten years, obese women (BMI $\geq$ 30 kg/m^2) had hazard ratios of 1.5 (95% CI: 1.16–1.94) for total stroke, 1.72 (95% CI: 1.30–2.28) for ischaemic stroke and 0.82 (95% CI: 0.43–1.58) for haemorrhagic stroke compared to women with BMI $\leq$ 25 kg/m^2.[99] The World Health Organization (WHO) estimates that there are approximately 350 million obese people (BMI $\geq$ 30 kg/m^2) worldwide.[100] Reports from the National Health and Nutrition Examination Survey (NHANES) suggests that there were 30.4% obese adults (BMI $\geq$ 30 kg/m^2) in the USA in 1999–2002 with 4.9% classified as extremely obese (BMI $\geq$ 40 kg/m^2).[101] In 2006, 24% of men and women in England were classified as obese.[82] The prevalence of overweight and obesity reported in high-income countries in 2002 was 58.5% and 19.3% respectively.[59,60] The WHO estimates that globally there are more than one billion overweight adults (BMI $\geq$ 25 kg/m^2).[100] In 2006, 43% of men and 32% of women were classified as being overweight in England.[82] A review of available literature on patients with obesity-associated medical complications reported weight loss of between 5% and 10% of initial bodyweight to be associated with improvements in cardiovascular risk profiles.[102] Reports from the British Regional Heart Study demonstrates a significantly increased risk of major cardiovascular disease, including stroke (RR: 1.32; 95% CI: 1.07–1.62), over 15 years of follow-up with substantial weight gain (>10%).[103] No significant cardiovascular benefit was seen for weight loss in any group of men, except possibly in considerably overweight (BMI 27.5–29.9 kg/m^2) younger middle-aged men (RR: 0.42; 95% CI: 0.22–0.81).[103] Current lifestyle modifications alone are widely regarded as ineffective.[104] Antiobesity pharmacotherapy is a potentially important adjunctive treatment to lifestyle modification.[104]

Atrial Fibrillation

Atrial fibrillation (AF) is the most common sustained cardiac arrhythmia.[105,106] Data from the Framingham study indicate that AF exerts a significant impact on the risk of stroke that is independent of the often-associated cardiovascular abnormalities.[22] The Framingham study demonstrated a near five-fold excess of stroke over 34 years of follow-up when AF was present.[22] The attributable risk of stroke for AF increased significantly with age, from 1.5% for those aged 50–59 years, to 23.5% for those aged 80–89 years.[22] About 1% of all adults in a large ethnically diverse population were diagnosed with AF.[106] The reported prevalence of AF in England and Wales in 1998 increased from 1/1000 in under 35 year olds to 100/1000 in those aged 85 years and over.[107] The prevalence of AF increases with age, approximately doubling in each decade in individuals older than 50 years.[108] There are an estimated 2.2 million people in the US with AF, with a median age of about 75 years.[109] The prevalence of AF is 2.3% in people older than 40 years and 5.9% in those older than 65 years.[109] In a cross-sectional study of adults enrolled in a large health maintenance organisation in the US, the prevalence of AF increased from 0.1% among persons younger than 55 years to 9.0% in persons aged 80 years or older.[106] Among persons aged 50 years or older, the prevalence of AF was reported to be higher in whites than in blacks (2.2% vs. 1.5%; $p < 0.001$).[106] Randomised controlled trials have demonstrated warfarin therapy to be highly efficacious in reducing risk of ischaemic stroke in patients with AF, with relatively low rates of bleeding.[110,111] Analysis of data from five randomised trials comparing warfarin or aspirin with control in patients with AF demonstrated that warfarin consistently decreases the risk of stroke in patients with AF (a 68% reduction in risk) with virtually no increase in the frequency of major bleeding.[31] The efficacy of aspirin in this study was less consistent, and patients younger than 65 years with AF and without a history of hypertension, previous stroke or transient ischaemic attack, or diabetes were at very low risk of stroke even when untreated (annual rate of stroke is 1% compared to 4.5% for the control group and 1.4% for the warfarin group).[31] The Stroke Prevention in Atrial Fibrillation II study compared the efficacy and safety of aspirin and warfarin in patients with AF.[112] Warfarin proved to be significantly more effective than aspirin in preventing cardioembolic strokes ($p = 0.005$) and strokes of uncertain pathophysiology ($p = 0.01$) but no significant difference was demonstrated for the prevention of non-cardioembolic stroke.[112]

Carotid Stenosis

A carotid stenosis of greater than 50% (diameter reduction) is reported in 5–9% of men and women aged 65 years or older.[113,114] Natural history studies reflect an annual stroke risk between 1% and 3.4% among persons with an asymptomatic carotid artery stenosis between 50% and 99%.[36,115] Results from the North American Symptomatic Carotid Endarterectomy Trial (NASCET) that randomised patients with TIA or a non-disabling stroke to surgery or to medical care, demonstrated a significant advantage of carotid endarterectomy in patients with high-grade stenosis (70–99% narrowing in the luminal diameter) and a moderate reduction of stroke risk in patients with symptomatic moderate carotid stenosis (50–69% narrowing).[116,117] There was a 17% absolute risk reduction of ipsilateral stroke at 18 months in the surgical group ($p < 0.001$) and the risk of any severe stroke or death from any cause was reduced in the surgical group (absolute risk reduction of 7%, $p < 0.01$).[116] In patients with high moderate stenosis (50–69%) in the NASCET trial, the five-year risk of ipsilateral stroke or death for the medical group was 22.2% and was 15.7% for the surgical group (absolute risk reduction of 6.5%).[117] In a pooled analysis of data from NASCET, the European Carotid Surgery Trial (ECST), and Veterans Affairs trial 309 during 35,000 patient-years of follow-up, surgery was reported to increase the five-year risk of ipsilateral ischaemic stroke in patients with less than 30% stenosis (absolute risk reduction −2.2%, $p = 0.05$), have no effect in patients with 30–49% stenosis (3.2%, $p = 0.6$), of marginal benefit in those with 50–69% stenosis (4.6%, $p = 0.04$) and highly beneficial in those with 70% stenosis or greater without near occlusion (16%, $p < 0.001$).[37]

Non-modifiable Risk Factors

Age, sex and socioeconomic status have independent and significant influences on the risk of stroke.[118] The risk of first ever and recurrent strokes have been reported from population-based studies to be strongly associated with increasing age with over 80% of strokes occurring in people over 64 years of age.[119] This is possibly associated with an increase in risk factors, such as hypertension, with age.[57] The cumulative effects of ageing on the cardiovascular system and the progressive nature of stroke risk factors over a prolonged period of time substantially increase stroke risk.[120] The risk of stroke has been reported to double in each successive decade after the age of 55.[43,44]

There is consistent evidence of increased incidence and mortality of stroke in lower socioeconomic groups in different populations.[121,122] Education and poverty index were inversely associated with stroke incidence in whites and blacks in the first National Health and Nutrition Examination Survey (NHANES I) Epidemiologic Follow-up Study with much of the association being mediated by higher levels of risk factors in the lower socioeconomic group.[123] A large cohort study from the US using four equally sized occupational groups to denote socioeconomic status demonstrated a higher mortality rate for stroke in both men and women in the lowest socioeconomic group than the rate in the highest socioeconomic group, with rate ratios of 2.25 (95% CI: 2.14–2.37) and 1.53 (1.44–1.62) respectively.[124]

Epidemiologic reports suggest that ethnic disparities in the impact of stroke are probably associated with the differences in risk factor prevalence, socioeconomic position influencing access to care, as well as environmental, cultural and genetic factors.[125] Ethnic groups including African Caribbean, Black African and South Asian populations are reported to be at increased risk of stroke.[118] In the Atherosclerosis Risk in Communities (ARIC) study, persons of black ethnicity had a 38% greater risk of incident ischaemic stroke compared to those of white ethnicity after accounting for established baseline risk factors.[126] Data from the South London Stroke Register, a prospective community stroke register, demonstrated a 2.18 (95% CI: 1.86–2.56) age- and sex-adjusted incidence rate ratio in the black population compared to the white population.[46] Hypertension and diabetes have been reported to be more common in South Asians, Caribbeans, and West Africans from population-based surveys, obesity rate is high in women of African descent, and serum cholesterol and smoking rates are also higher in these ethnic groups compared to white people.[127]

The percentage of people aged 65 years and above in the UK increased from 13% in 1971 to 16% in 2002 and is projected to rise to 23% in 2031.[128] With an increasing life expectancy in most high-income countries, most adults should expect to grow old and face the risk of developing diseases that are increasingly prevalent with age. An in-depth understanding of these differences will aid and drive more effective stroke prevention programmes in high-risk groups.[129] The number of people from ethnic groups other than white in the UK (25% of black ethnicity), increased by 53% between 1991 and 2001.[128] The ageing and continuing growth of the black population will undoubtedly lead to future increases in the number of blacks with stroke.[130]

Different Strategies for Risk Reduction

Despite improvements in the management of acute stroke and in rehabilitation post-stroke, it is clear that prevention holds the key to decreasing the toll of cerebrovascular disease.[125] The most effective means available for reducing the burden of stroke involve modification and treatment of vascular risk factors.[131] Population-based strategies for the primary prevention of coronary heart disease are also the most cost-effective approaches for prevention of stroke.[132] The potential impact of more effective stroke prevention must be considered in the context of global cardiovascular risk because of the overlap between cerebrovascular and cardiovascular risk.[133] Long-term prospective studies have shown that persons with healthy lifestyles and few risk factors have low risk of heart disease and stroke.[21,134] This suggests that the causes of the vast majority of cases of heart disease and stroke can be attributed to a few deleterious behaviours and lifestyles.[135] A population attributable risk (PAR) for fatal cardiovascular disease (CVD) of 14% among persons with ≥ 2 inadequately controlled risk factors without previous MI or stroke, was demonstrated from a model using data from the Second National Health and Nutrition Examination Survey (NHANES II) Mortality Follow-up Study in the US.[136] Among persons with previous MI or stroke, the PAR was 7% and 8% for one and two inadequately controlled risk factors respectively, demonstrating the need for intensive efforts to be directed toward detection and treatment of CVD risk factors.[136] The probability of a stroke may be quantified by the use of a profile such as the Framingham stroke-risk profile or the SCORE system for risk estimation to identify individuals at sufficiently increased risk of stroke to warrant vigorous risk factor management.[13,137] Strategies for reduction of stroke risk could be targeted at patients and the general population, healthcare providers and healthcare organisations.[138]

Population Approach for Risk Reduction

The population-based strategy to risk factor modification aims to shift the entire distribution of risk factors and risk toward lower levels through population-wide interventions.[12] This strategy aims to reduce risk factors at population level through lifestyle and environmental changes that affect the whole population without requiring medical examination of individuals.[139] Steps to decrease the development of modifiable risk factors associated with stroke would be expected to proportionally reduce their impact on stroke occurrence.[10] As single risk factors, the greatest reduction in stroke would be achieved through a reduction in the population prevalence of hypertension (PAR of 20% at 80 years of age and increasing to 40% at age 50 years).[10] Improvements in facilities and resources in the places where people live and work should enhance the achievements of many goals, including cessation of tobacco use and avoidance of environmental tobacco smoke; reduction in dietary saturated fat, cholesterol, sodium and calories; increased plant-based food intake; increased physical activity; access to preventive healthcare services; and early recognition of symptoms of stroke (discussed in greater detail in Chapter 4).[135] The provision of general education about healthy lifestyles may be beneficial to the entire population.[10] The Stanford Five-City Project conducted in the US provide support for the efficacy of community-wide interventions involving organisation of communities, provision of mass and direct education, and provision of screenings for risk factors, to favourably modify cardiovascular disease risk factors in populations.[140] A Northern Sweden community intervention programme for the prevention of CVD that combined a population strategy with primary care approach demonstrated community-wide behaviour change with sales statistics regarding dairy products for example, showing a significant increase of low fat products.[141] The American Heart Association Guide for 'Improving Cardiovascular Health on the Community Level' outlines an approach for primary prevention and suggests that the engagement of the lay public, the healthcare community, non-governmental voluntary health organisations, and governments is required to affect the types of societal changes necessary to optimise prevention.[135] The guide emphasises the goal to promote lifestyle and behaviour change at the individual and community levels, and policy change at the community level.[135] The population-based or public health approach to risk factor modification is critical to reducing the overall incidence of CVD and has the potential not only to prevent a first stroke in the person at average risk, but also to avoid the need for intensive and expensive pharmacotherapies to control risk factors such as hypertension, hyperlipidaemia and diabetes, once they become established.[135,139]

High-Risk Approach for Prevention

The high-risk approach involves detection of individuals at increased risk of stroke and taking steps to reduce that risk through behaviour modification and medications.[10,133] This includes preventing individuals from having their first stroke and optimising secondary stroke prevention strategies to prevent recurrence and reduce the impact of stroke. Both primary and secondary prevention require a comprehensive multidisciplinary strategy to identify and manage major risk factors and to promote adherence to preventive protocols.[138] Identification of an individual's risk is a necessary first step for their control, but persons at risk for stroke often remain unaware of their risk.[10] Assessment of risk for cardiovascular disease (CVD) by general practitioners is reported to be an effective way to identify unknown cases of patients with CVD.[142] Interventions to reduce CVD risk among high-risk individuals are necessary preventive measures.[142] The European Guidelines on CVD prevention in clinical practice suggests that a quick and easy way of assessing CVD risk is to consider patients who have had a clinical event such as a stroke, or who have markedly increased level of a single risk factor be at increased CVD risk to automatically qualify for intensive risk factor evaluation and management.[139] For all other people, the use of risk charts such as SCORE (a system for risk estimation based on data from 12 European cohort studies which offers direct estimation of total cardiovascular risk) or the Framingham stroke-risk profile,[13,137] can facilitate risk estimation in persons with mildly raised levels of several risk factors that, in combination, can result in unexpectedly high levels of total CVD risk.[139] It is important for the healthcare professional to develop a plan of preventive action together with the patient and create an environment supportive of risk factor change including long-term reinforcement of adherence to lifestyle and drug interventions.[143] Adoption of healthy lifestyles remains the cornerstone of primary prevention, including the avoidance of tobacco, healthy dietary patterns, weight control, and regular, appropriate exercise.[143] Other preventive measures include the control of hypertension with tighter control in patients with diabetes, treatment of hyperlipidaemia, promotion of smoking cessation by the use of non-pharmacological strategies such as counselling or pharmacotherapy with nicotine replacement therapy, use of antithrombotics, anticoagulation for high-risk patients with atrial fibrillation, and use of endarterectomy in selected patients as discussed above.[10,67,142,144] An important role of healthcare providers is to support and reinforce these recommendations for all patients.[143] Information from interviews conducted with key informants from primary healthcare settings in the US report that critical success factors include support for patient self-management and education, interventions integrated easily into the daily work flow and leadership and staff commitment.[145] Data from such practices demonstrated statistically significant improvement in hypertension control rates from 33.1% to 49.7% post-implementation.[146] It is important for primary care professionals to update and maintain their knowledge of national guidelines on the management of the risk factors and implement them in their practice.[7]

Secondary Prevention

The risk of further stroke is highest early after stroke or TIA and may be as high as 10% within the first week, 20% within the first month and increases to 29% at five years.[144,147] Patients with recurrent stroke have on average, poorer outcomes than those with first stroke with 24-month survival, reported to be 48.3% vs. 56.7%, respectively.[148] It is important for appropriate secondary prevention to be implemented as soon as possible and continued in the long term.[144] The non-randomised Early use of eXisting PREventive Strategies for Stroke (EXPRESS) study showed that urgent assessment and treatment after the onset of TIA or minor stroke reduced the 90-day risk of recurrent stroke by about 80%.[149] Effective implementation of secondary stroke preventive measures will not only reduce the rate of recurrent stroke, but also potentially reduce the morbidity and mortality related to coronary heart disease.[10] Effective secondary prevention depends on reliable identification of those at high risk and targeting treatment appropriately as will be discussed in Chapter 3.[150] National consensus guidelines are published to increase provider awareness of evidence-based approaches to disease management with the assumption that increased awareness of guideline content would lead to changes in physician behaviour and ultimately patient behaviour and outcomes.[151] However, despite the availability of published practice guidelines there is evidence to suggest that recommended interventions are frequently not initiated during hospitalisation for acute events.[152] A one-year intervention study to assess performance measure adherence in hospitals, using the 'Get With The Guidelines–Stroke' Program, reported significant improvements from baseline to the fourth quarter in 11 out of 13 measures: use of thrombolytic medications for patients with ischaemic stroke presenting within two hours of onset, 23.5% vs. 40.8% ($p < 0.001$); early use of antithrombotic medications, 88.2% vs. 95.2% ($p < 0.001$); antithrombotic medications prescribed at discharge, 91.0% vs. 97.9% ($p < 0.001$); anticoagulation agents for atrial fibrillation, 81.4% vs. 96.5% ($p < 0.001$); smoking cessation counselling, 38.3% vs. 54.5% ($p < 0.001$); lipid treatment for low-density lipoprotein levels 100 mg/dl or greater, 58.7% vs. 77.0% ($p < 0.001$); diabetes mellitus treatment, 48.5% vs. 83.5% ($p = 0.001$); and weight reduction counselling 32.5% vs. 43.4% ($p < 0.001$).[153] The improvement in the quality of care seen in this project may be related to multiple supportive systems, including a collaborative environment and a customised web-based tool called the Patient Management Tool (PMT) that facilitated concurrent feedback of guideline information at the point of care.[154]

Effectiveness and Uptake of Preventive Strategies

Several guidelines and strategic plans on stroke care, prevention and risk factor management have been developed over the years based on strong evidence of effective interventions and strategies from various epidemiological studies, including randomised controlled trials. These guidelines and strategic plans of action summarise the main evidence on appropriate stroke management and provide stakeholders with a reliable source of the best evidence and aim to inform best practice. However, getting guideline recommendations into practice is a complex process and getting patients' compliance with the recommendations for stroke prevention and management is an even greater challenge. Innovative ways of implementing preventive strategies may be needed to ensure effectiveness of prevention strategies and to promote uptake.[7] An observational study to investigate prior management of risk factors in patients with stroke in a district hospital in the UK reported suboptimal control of vascular risk factors in mainstream practice, despite considerable evidence published in the literature and prioritisation by healthcare planners.[155] Significant increases were observed in the management of risk associated with previous strokes and TIAs (59% to 85%), atrial fibrillation (17% to 61%), and previously asymptomatic carotid artery disease (13% to 85%) over the three-year period of the study.[155]

Interventions to reduce the risk of stroke reported in a review included those to change professional behaviours in preventing and managing stroke, interventions targeted at patients and the public, and interventions targeted at health services.[156] Positive associations were found between skills training and improvements in professional attitude to stroke patients and stroke care. Patient decision-making aids were associated with increased patient choice, which did not necessarily enhance subsequent adherence to treatment. In a study investigating the process of dissemination of locally adapted guidelines on stroke risk factor management to general practitioners, those in the intervention arm reported knowledge and practices more consistent with the guidelines on appropriate aspirin use in stroke prevention and initial investigations for carotid stenosis.[157] Screening and education interventions in a community intervention study were associated with a lower incidence of stroke amongst those in the intervention arm over and above those in the control arm.[158] In a non-randomised trial of a comprehensive risk factor management intervention in people with first-in-lifetime stroke, which involved blood pressure screening and monitoring, counselling- and community-based health education, participants receiving the intervention were less likely to have a recurrence within three years of the initial stroke. There was however, no difference in mortality.[159] A review of randomised controlled trials assessing the effectiveness of multiple risk factor intervention using counselling and/or educational approaches with or without pharmacological interventions found modest reductions in smoking prevalence, systolic blood pressure, and blood cholesterol level in the intervention groups.[5] The authors argued in favour of multiple risk factor interventions for prevention of cardiovascular disease in high-risk groups.[5] In a review of community interventions to manage hypertension among black ethnic groups, health education combined with individualised support for patients to self-manage hypertension were associated with reductions in blood pressure levels and improvements in blood pressure control.[160]

Data from the Health Survey for England have shown steady improvements in population blood pressure control between 1994–2003.[161] Blood pressure monitoring levels of adult patients registered at general practices in England have risen such that by 2007, 88% of the adult population have had their blood pressure measured in the preceding five years.[162] The percentage of men and women prescribed aspirin and anticoagulants in England and Wales increased significantly between 1994 and 1998.[107] Although data on secondary prevention of stroke has shown excellent adherence to stroke prevention strategies in some populations with 84% of patients on aspirin one year after their strokes, lower rates (50–70%) have been achieved in other populations.[163,164] The use of antihypertensives for patients with hypertension and appropriate antiplatelet and anticoagulation therapy for patients with atrial fibrillation are similarly low.[164] In South London, the proportion of patients who still smoke or drink excessively and those who are overweight one year after stroke remained high, with no evidence of improvement in behavioural risk factor control.[165] In a national study of primary care patients in England, only 25.6% of men and 20.8% of women received secondary prevention after a stroke.[166] The Euroaspire surveys conducted in several centres in Europe demonstrates the difficulty in reducing smoking, obesity and cholesterol and controlling blood pressure at the population level in patients with coronary heart disease even in high-income countries.[65] Despite the identification of effective interventions and strategies for preventing stroke and its recurrence, uptake remains considerably low in some populations. Reduced adherence and compliance to any stroke prevention strategies by healthcare providers, patients and organisations could significantly influence the success of such preventive measures. Problems hampering the use of medication for stroke prevention include inadequate prescription of medication, poor adherence to treatment, limited availability of medications and unaffordable cost of treatment.[167] As the number of medications that a patient requires increases, adherence and compliance to therapy are likely to decrease.[168] It has been proposed that a single daily pill (polypill) combining half-doses (to minimise toxicity) of a beta-blocker, thiazide diuretic, and an ACE-inhibitor, together with a statin, folic acid and aspirin administered to people with known cardiovascular disease and everyone aged 55 years and over, would reduce the incidence of stroke by 80%.[169] The use of the 'polypill' which concomitantly reduce multiple risk factors without increasing the pill burden has the potential to improve cardiovascular disease risk management, thereby reducing the incidence of cardiovascular disease.[168] There are however, challenges that need to be addressed for the success of the 'polypill', including the possibility that many patients will remain undertreated, patients' and doctors' acceptability will be less than expected and that potential adverse effects related to some of the cardiovascular 'polypill' components such as aspirin, could lead to the discontinuation of treatment and, therefore, the loss of benefit of all other drugs included in the formulation.[167,168] It is important to determine the best way of implementing prevention strategies for the benefits of primary and secondary prevention to be achieved in different population groups.

Determinants of Successful Implementation

Success in implementation of prevention strategies may be improved if potential barriers are identified and interventions targeted specifically to address these barriers. Barriers to prevention include cultural norms, insufficient attention to health education by healthcare practitioners and school health education, lack of reimbursement for health education services and economic disincentives to healthier lifestyles.[170] Overcoming these barriers would require the involvement of governments, industry, national health authorities, health professionals and society.[2,132]

Clinical guidelines, even when based on the best available evidence from randomised controlled trials, cannot be successfully implemented without the acceptance by the entire health team including physicians, nurses, nutritionists, and other healthcare professionals.[143] The European guidelines on CVD prevention in clinical practice suggest that the implementation of guidelines could possibly be easier if they were made simple and clear and that dissemination of simple, one-sheet versions of risk algorithms and treatment recommendations may facilitate the adherence to the recommendations from the guidelines.[8] Implementation strategies that support physicians in the process of case-finding of potential high-risk patients, such as software programmes to alert practitioners, support in risk communication through training and supporting physicians in deciding jointly with the patient on appropriate action for management may be important.[8,171] Patients need to be well-motivated to take up the challenge of modifying lifestyle and taking prescribed medications regularly and for a lifetime, particularly for an asymptomatic condition. Treatment goals set in collaboration with the patient, taking into account the values and priorities of the patient may facilitate adherence.[8] Barriers to access due to mobility could be overcome by delivering advice and follow-up care to patients in their own homes and making appropriate suggestions for prescription delivery.[172] The workload put on the health system should, however, be affordable for the strategy to be implemented successfully.[8] Involving patients in the decision on appropriate management with the help of educational materials has been found to increase patient satisfaction but not necessarily change risk factor control, emphasising the challenge of patient involvement and behaviour change.[8,173]

Recommendations by health professionals to modify diets or increase physical activity will be hampered by lack of grocery stores or restaurants with heart-healthy choices, and by lack of safe and attractive places to be physically active.[135] Effective implementation of the high-risk preventive strategies requires a functioning and accessible primary health system.[174] The emergency treatment of minor stroke and TIA depends on the swift presentation of patients to specialist services and the capacity of these services to assess, investigate, and treat patients appropriately.[150] However, such services may not be accessible in all cases as there may be people with no health insurance to cover the cost involved, or no legal rights to access the service even when services are free, as occurs in the case of illegal immigrants. Rural institutions may lack the resources for adequate emergency stroke treatment and the extensive community and professional educational services that address stroke awareness and prevention compared with urban areas.[151] Telemedicine is emerging as a tool to support improved rural healthcare, and the acute treatment and primary and secondary prevention of stroke.[175] Only governments can legislate for health warnings on cigarettes, introduce mandatory food standards and labelling or implement national transport policies.[4] Positively helpful government policies with defined prevention strategies, which provide resources and incentives, including remuneration for prevention as well as treatment, may make it easier to implement any prevention strategy.[8] The Quality and Outcomes Framework in the UK includes a number of quality indicators relating to measurement of risk associated with vascular disease.[176] Blood pressure monitoring and control improved substantially after the introduction of these performance indicators and the incorporation of pay for performance into primary care in England in 2004.[162] The linkage of financial incentives to performance targets could possibly have contributed to the overall improvements in monitoring and control of blood pressure in primary care in England in recent years.[162] Civil society and government initiatives in consort with the food and drink manufacturing industry successfully reduced salt content in processed foods in the UK. In Mauritius, cholesterol reduction was achieved largely by a government-led effort switching the main source of cooking oil from palm to soya bean oil.[4] Appropriate government policies, legislation and taxation would provide an enabling environment for health promotion efforts to be effective.

Strategies should be specifically developed, validated and assessed to consider both cultural acceptability, which is likely to affect uptake and compliance, and underlying susceptibility, which may vary the effectiveness of preventive and treatment options in different ethnic groups.[127] Information given should be reviewed to ensure that clear, consistent, culturally sensitive messages are being given to those at high risk.[7]

Conclusions

The burden of cardiovascular disease, particularly strokes and coronary heart disease is certain to increase in the absence of effective prevention strategies, particularly as life expectancy increases in various populations. There has been extensive research into risk factors for stroke and interventions for prevention at all stages of its natural history. Guidelines for prevention of stroke based on the best available evidence are also available to inform practitioners of strategies for effective preventive measures in clinical and public health practice. However, uptake of these strategies remains low in most populations and it is important to identify strategies for effective implementation for the benefits of primary and secondary prevention of stroke to be achieved in different population groups.

References

1. WHO. Burden of disease statistics. http://www.who.int/healthinfo/bod/en/index.html (Accessed June 11, 2009).
2. Beaglehole R, Ebrahim S, Reddy S, Voute J *et al*. Prevention of chronic diseases: a call to action. *Lancet* 2007; 370(9605): 2152–2157.
3. National Institute for Health and Clinical Excellence. Stroke: diagnosis and initial management of acute stroke and transient ischaemic attack. NICE clinical guideline 68 (2008). Available from http://www.nice.org.uk/nicemedia/pdf/CG68FullGuideline.pdf.
4. WHO. Cardiovascular disease: prevention and control. http://www.who.int/dietphysicalactivity/publications/facts/cvd/en.
5. Ebrahim S, Beswick A, Burke M, Davey Smith G. Multiple risk factor interventions for primary prevention of coronary heart disease. *Cochrane Database Syst Rev* 2006; 4: CD001561.
6. Hankey GJ, Warlow CP. Treatment and secondary prevention of stroke: evidence, costs, and effects on individuals and populations. *Lancet* 1999; 354(9188): 1457–1463.
7. Department of Health, National Stroke Strategy 2007. Available at http://www.dh.gov.uk/en/Publicationsandstatistics/Publications/PublicationsPolicyAndGuidance/DH_081062.

8. Fourth Joint Task Force of the European Society of Cardiology Other Societies on Cardiovascular Disease Prevention in Clinical practice, Graham I, Atar D, *et al.* European guidelines on cardiovascular disease prevention in clinical practice: executive summary. *Eur Heart J* 2007; 28(19): 2375–2414.

9. Goldstein LB, Adams R, Alberts MJ, Appel LJ *et al.* Primary prevention of ischemic stroke: a guideline from the American Heart Association/American Stroke Association Stroke Council: cosponsored by the Atherosclerotic Peripheral Vascular Disease Interdisciplinary Working Group; Cardiovascular Nursing Council; Clinical Cardiology Council; Nutrition, Physical Activity, and Metabolism Council; and the Quality of Care and Outcomes Research Interdisciplinary Working Group: the American Academy of Neurology affirms the value of this guideline. *Stroke* 2006; 37(6): 1583–1633.

10. Goldstein LB, How much can be gained by more systematic prevention of stroke? *Int J Stroke* 2008; 3(4): 266–271.

11. Pearson TA, Bazzarre TL, Daniels SR, Fair JM *et al.* American Heart Association guide for improving cardiovascular health at the community level: a statement for public health practitioners, healthcare providers, and health policy makers from the American Heart Association Expert Panel on Population and Prevention Science. *Circulation* 2003; 107(4): 645–651.

12. Rose G. Sick individuals and sick populations. *Int J Epidemiol* 1985; 14(1): 32–38.

13. Wolf PA, D'Agostino RB, Belanger AJ, Kannel WB. Probability of stroke: a risk profile from the Framingham Study. *Stroke* 1991; 22(3): 312–318.

14. Sacco RL, Benjamin EJ, Broderick JP, Dyken M *et al.* American Heart Association Prevention Conference. IV. Prevention and Rehabilitation of Stroke. Risk factors. *Stroke* 1997; 28(7): 1507–1517.

15. Warlow C, Sudlow C, Dennis M, Wardlaw J, Sandercock P. Stroke. *Lancet* 2003; 362(9391): 1211–1224.

16. Ridker PM. Inflammatory biomarkers, statins, and the risk of stroke: cracking a clinical conundrum. *Circulation* 2002; 105(22): 2583–2585.

17. Perry IJ. Homocysteine and risk of stroke. *J Cardiovasc Risk* 1999; 6(4): 235–240.

18. Goldstein LB. Novel risk factors for stroke: homocysteine, inflammation, and infection. *Curr Atheroscler Rep* 2000; 2(2): 110–114.

19. Wolf PA. Prevention of stroke. *Lancet* 1998; 352(Suppl 3): SIII 15–18.
20. Donnan GA, Fisher M, Macleod M, Davis SM. Stroke. *Lancet* 2008; 371(9624): 1612–1623.
21. Stamler J, Stamler R, Neaton JD, Wentworth D *et al.* Low risk-factor profile and long-term cardiovascular and noncardiovascular mortality and life expectancy: findings for 5 large cohorts of young adult and middle-aged men and women. *JAMA* 1999; 282(21): 2012–2018.
22. Wolf PA, Abbott RD, Kannel WB. Atrial fibrillation as an independent risk factor for stroke: the Framingham Study. *Stroke* 1991; 22(8): 983–988.
23. Kannel WB, Dawber TR, Cohen ME, McNamara PM. Vascular disease of the brain — epidemiologic aspects: the FRAMINGHAM study. *Am J Public Health Nations Health* 1965; 55: 1355–1366.
24. Lewington S, Clarke R, Qizilbash N, Peto R *et al.* Age-specific relevance of usual blood pressure to vascular mortality: a meta-analysis of individual data for one million adults in 61 prospective studies. *Lancet* 2002; 360(9349): 1903–1913.
25. Lawes CM, Bennett DA, Feigin VL, Rodgers A. Blood pressure and stroke: an overview of published reviews. *Stroke* 2004; 35(4): 1024.
26. Harmsen P, Lappas G, Rosengren A, Wilhelmsen L. Long-term risk factors for stroke: twenty-eight years of follow-up of 7457 middle-aged men in Goteborg, Sweden. *Stroke* 2006; 37(7): 1663–1667.
27. Sander D, Kearney MT. Reducing the risk of stroke in type 2 diabetes: pathophysiological and therapeutic perspectives. *J Neurol* 2009.
28. Turnbull F, Neal B, Algert C, Chalmers J *et al.* Effects of different blood pressure-lowering regimens on major cardiovascular events in individuals with and without diabetes mellitus: results of prospectively designed overviews of randomized trials. *Arch Intern Med* 2005; 165(12): 1410–1419.
29. Shinton R, Beevers G. Meta-analysis of relation between cigarette smoking and stroke. *BMJ* 1989; 298(6676): 789–794.
30. Wannamethee SG, Shaper AG, Whincup PH, Walker M. Smoking cessation and the risk of stroke in middle-aged men. *JAMA* 1995; 274(2): 155–160.
31. Risk factors for stroke and efficacy of antithrombotic therapy in atrial fibrillation. Analysis of pooled data from five randomized controlled trials. *Arch Intern Med* 1994; 154(13): 1449–1457.

32. Prospective Studies, Lewington CS, Whitlock G, Clarke R *et al.* Blood cholesterol and vascular mortality by age, sex, and blood pressure: a meta-analysis of individual data from 61 prospective studies with 55,000 vascular deaths. *Lancet* 2007; 370(9602): 1829–1839.

33. Shahar E, Chambless LE, Rosamond WD, Boland LL *et al.* Plasma lipid profile and incident ischemic stroke: the Atherosclerosis Risk In Communities (ARIC) study. *Stroke* 2003; 34(3): 623–631.

34. Hebert PR, Gaziano JM, Chan KS, Hennekens CH. Cholesterol lowering with statin drugs, risk of stroke, and total mortality. An overview of randomized trials. *JAMA* 1997; 278(4): 313–321.

35. Amarenco P, Bogousslavsky J, Callahan A, 3rd, Goldstein LB *et al.* High-dose atorvastatin after stroke or transient ischemic attack. *N Engl J Med* 2006; 355(6): 549–559.

36. Autret A, Pourcelot L, Saudeau D, Marchal C *et al.* Stroke risk in patients with carotid stenosis. *Lancet* 1987; 1(8538): 888–890.

37. Rothwell PM, Eliasziw M, Gutnikov SA, Fox AJ *et al.* Analysis of pooled data from the randomised controlled trials of endarterectomy for symptomatic carotid stenosis. *Lancet* 2003; 361(9352): 107–116.

38. Suk SH, Sacco RL, Boden-Albala B, Cheun JF *et al.* Abdominal obesity and risk of ischemic stroke: the Northern Manhattan Stroke Study. *Stroke* 2003; 34(7): 1586–1592.

39. Prospective Studies. Whitlock CG, Lewington S, Sherliker P *et al.* Body-mass index and cause-specific mortality in 900 000 adults: collaborative analyses of 57 prospective studies. *Lancet* 2009; 373(9669): 1083–1096.

40. Hu FB, Stampfer MJ, Colditz GA, Ascherio A *et al.* Physical activity and risk of stroke in women. *JAMA* 2000; 283(22): 2961–2967.

41. Myint PK, Luben RN, Wareham NJ, Welch AA *et al.* Combined work and leisure physical activity and risk of stroke in men and women in the European prospective investigation into Cancer-Norfolk Prospective Population Study. *Neuroepidemiology* 2006; 27(3): 122–129.

42. Seshadri S, Beiser A, Kelly-Hayes M, Kase CS *et al.* The lifetime risk of stroke: estimates from the Framingham Study. *Stroke* 2006; 37(2): 345–350.

43. Brown RD, Whisnant JP, Sicks JD, O'Fallon WM, Wiebers DO. Stroke incidence, prevalence, and survival: secular trends in Rochester, Minnesota, through 1989. *Stroke* 1996; 27(3): 373–380.

44. Wolf PA, D'Agostino RB, O'Neal MA, Sytkowski P *et al.* Secular trends in stroke incidence and mortality. The Framingham Study. *Stroke* 1992; 23(11): 1551–1555.
45. Stewart JA, Dundas R, Howard RS, Rudd AG, Wolfe CD. Ethnic differences in incidence of stroke: prospective study with stroke register. *BMJ* 1999; 318(7189): 967–971.
46. Wolfe CD, Rudd AG, Howard R, Coshall C *et al.* Incidence and case fatality rates of stroke subtypes in a multiethnic population: the South London Stroke Register. *J Neurol Neurosurg Psychiatry* 2002; 72(2): 211–216.
47. Kiely DK, Wolf PA, Cupples LA, Beiser AS, Myers RH. Familial aggregation of stroke. The Framingham Study. *Stroke* 1993; 24(9): 1366–1371.
48. Williams B, Poulter NR, Brown MJ, Davis M *et al.* Guidelines for management of hypertension: report of the fourth working party of the British Hypertension Society, 2004-BHS IV. *J Hum Hypertens* 2004; 18(3): 139–185.
49. Chobanian AV, Bakris GL, Black HR, Cushman WC *et al.* Seventh report of the Joint National Committee on Prevention, Detection, Evaluation, and Treatment of High Blood Pressure. *Hypertension* 2003; 42(6): 1206–1252.
50. Wolf PA, Grotta JC. Cerebrovascular disease. *Circulation* 2000; 102 (20 Suppl 4): IV 75–80.
51. MacMahon S, Peto R, Cutler J, Collins R *et al.* Blood pressure, stroke, and coronary heart disease. Part 1, Prolonged differences in blood pressure: prospective observational studies corrected for the regression dilution bias. *Lancet* 1990; 335(8692): 765–774.
52. Freis ED. The Veterans Administration cooperative study on antihypertensive agents. Implications for stroke prevention. *Stroke* 1974; 5(1): 76–77.
53. Lawes CM, Bennett DA, Feigin VL, Rodgers A. Blood pressure and stroke: an overview of published reviews. *Stroke* 2004; 35(3): 776–785.
54. Kearney PM, Whelton M, Reynolds K, Muntner P *et al.* Global burden of hypertension: analysis of worldwide data. *Lancet* 2005; 365(9455): 217–223.
55. Wolf-Maier K, Cooper RS, Banegas JR, Giampaoli S *et al.* Hypertension prevalence and blood pressure levels in 6 European countries, Canada, and the United States. *JAMA* 2003; 289(18): 2363–2369.
56. Addo J, Smeeth L, Leon DA. Hypertension in sub-saharan Africa: A systematic review. *Hypertension* 2007; 50(6): 1012–1018.

57. Burt VL, Whelton P, Roccella EJ, Brown C *et al.* Prevalence of hypertension in the US adult population. Results from the Third National Health and Nutrition Examination Survey, 1988–1991. *Hypertension* 1995; 25(3): 305–313.

58. Primatesta P, Bost L, Poulter NR. Blood pressure levels and hypertension status among ethnic groups in England. *J Hum Hypertens* 2000; 14(2): 143–148.

59. Johnston SC, Mendis S, Mathers CD. Global variation in stroke burden and mortality: estimates from monitoring, surveillance, and modelling. *Lancet Neurol* 2009; 8(4): 345–354.

60. WHO, WHO Global InfoBase, 2008. http://www.who.int/infobase/comparestart.aspx.

61. Li C, Engstrom G, Hedblad B, Berglund G, Janzon L. Blood pressure control and risk of stroke: a population-based prospective cohort study. *Stroke* 2005; 36(4): 725–730.

62. Gu Q, Burt VL, Paulose-Ram R, Yoon S, Gillum RF. High blood pressure and cardiovascular disease mortality risk among US adults: the third National Health and Nutrition Examination Survey mortality follow-up study. *Ann Epidemiol* 2008; 18(4): 302–309.

63. Hajjar I, Kotchen TA. Trends in prevalence, awareness, treatment, and control of hypertension in the United States, 1988–2000. *JAMA* 2003; 290(2): 199–206.

64. Wolf-Maier K, Cooper RS, Kramer H, Banegas JR *et al.* Hypertension treatment and control in five European countries, Canada, and the United States. *Hypertension* 2004; 43(1): 10–17.

65. Kotseva K, Wood D, De Backer G, De Bacquer D *et al.* Cardiovascular prevention guidelines in daily practice: a comparison of EUROASPIRE I, II, and III surveys in eight European countries. *Lancet* 2009; 373(9667): 929–940.

66. Psaty BM, Manolio TA, Smith NL, Heckbert SR *et al.* Time trends in high blood pressure control and the use of antihypertensive medications in older adults: the Cardiovascular Health Study. *Arch Intern Med* 2002; 162(20): 2325–2332.

67. Goldstein LB, Adams R, Alberts MJ, Appel LJ *et al.* Primary prevention of ischemic stroke: a guideline from the American Heart Association/American Stroke Association Stroke Council: cosponsored by the Atherosclerotic Peripheral Vascular Disease Interdisciplinary Working Group; Cardiovascular Nursing Council; Clinical Cardiology Council; Nutrition, Physical Activity, and Metabolism Council; and the Quality of Care and Outcomes Research Interdisciplinary Working Group: the American Academy of Neurology affirms the value of this guideline. *Stroke* 2006; 37(6): 1583–1633.

68. Burchfiel CM, Curb JD, Rodriguez BL, Abbott RD *et al.* Glucose intolerance and 22-year stroke incidence. The Honolulu Heart Program. *Stroke* 1994; 25(5): 951–957.

69. Danaei G, Lawes CM, Vander Hoorn S, Murray CJ, Ezzati M. Global and regional mortality from ischaemic heart disease and stroke attributable to higher-than-optimum blood glucose concentration: comparative risk assessment. *Lancet* 2006; 368(9548): 1651–1659.

70. Wild S, Roglic G, Green A, Sicree R, King H. Global prevalence of diabetes: estimates for the year 2000 and projections for 2030. *Diabetes Care* 2004; 27(5): 1047–1053.

71. Fox CS, Pencina MJ, Meigs JB, Vasan RS *et al.* Trends in the incidence of type 2 diabetes mellitus from the 1970s to the 1990s: the Framingham Heart Study. *Circulation* 2006; 113(25): 2914–2918.

72. Cheung BM, Ong KL, Cherny SS, Sham PC *et al.* Diabetes prevalence and therapeutic target achievement in the United States, 1999 to 2006. *Am J Med* 2009; 122(5): 443–453.

73. Department of Health, Health Survey for England 2007: Healthy lifestyles: knowledge, attitudes and behaviour. Available at http://www.ic.nhs.uk/statistics-and-data-collections/health-and-lifestyles-related-surveys/

74. Mokdad AH, Ford ES, Bowman BA, Nelson DE *et al.* Diabetes trends in the U.S.: 1990–1998. *Diabetes Care* 2000; 23(9): 1278–1283.

75. Rosamond W, Flegal K, Friday G, Furie K *et al.* Heart disease and stroke statistics — 2007 update: a report from the American Heart Association Statistics Committee and Stroke Statistics Subcommittee. *Circulation* 2007; 115(5): e69–e171.

76. Intensive blood-glucose control with sulphonylureas or insulin compared with conventional treatment and risk of complications in patients with type 2 diabetes (UKPDS 33). UK Prospective Diabetes Study (UKPDS) Group. *Lancet* 1998; 352(9131): 837–853.

77. Effect of intensive blood-glucose control with metformin on complications in overweight patients with type 2 diabetes (UKPDS 34). UK Prospective Diabetes Study (UKPDS) Group. *Lancet* 1998; 352(9131): 854–865.

78. Lincoff AM, Wolski K, Nicholls SJ, Nissen SE. Pioglitazone and risk of cardiovascular events in patients with type 2 diabetes mellitus: a meta-analysis of randomized trials. *JAMA* 2007; 298(10): 1180–1188.

79. Rodriguez BL, D'Agostino R, Abbott RD, Kagan A *et al.* Risk of hospitalized stroke in men enrolled in the Honolulu Heart Program and the

Framingham Study: A comparison of incidence and risk factor effects. *Stroke* 2002; 33(1): 230–236.

80. Burns DM. Epidemiology of smoking-induced cardiovascular disease. *Prog Cardiovasc Dis* 2003; 46(1): 11–29.

81. Wolf PA, D'Agostino RB, Kannel WB, Bonita R, Belanger AJ. Cigarette smoking as a risk factor for stroke. The Framingham Study. *JAMA* 1988; 259(7): 1025–1029.

82. Department of Health, Health Survey for England 2006: CVD and risk factors adults, obesity and risk factors children. Available at http://www.ic.nhs.uk/ statistics-and-data-collections/health-and-lifestyles-related-surveys/.

83. Goodfellow LT, Waugh JB. Tobacco treatment and prevention: what works and why. *Respir Care* 2009; 54(8): 1082–1090.

84. Farrelly MC, Evans WN, Sfekas AE. The impact of workplace smoking bans: results from a national survey. *Tob Control* 1999; 8(3): 272–277.

85. Centers for Disease Control and Prevention. Indoor air quality in hospitality venues before and after implementation of a clean indoor air law — Western New York, 2003. *MMWR Morb Mortal Wkly Rep* 2004; 53(44): 1038–1041.

86. Clinical Practice Guideline Treating Tobacco, UL. Dependence Update Panel, and Staff. A clinical practice guideline for treating tobacco use and dependence: 2008 update. A US Public Health Service report. *Am J Prev Med* 2008; 35(2): 158–176.

87. Pisinger C, Vestbo J, Borch-Johnsen K, Jorgensen T. Smoking reduction intervention in a large population-based study. The Inter 99 study. *Prev Med* 2005; 40(1): 112–118.

88. Lancaster T, Stead L, Silagy C, Sowden A. Effectiveness of interventions to help people stop smoking: findings from the Cochrane Library. *BMJ* 2000; 321(7257): 355–358.

89. Silagy C, Lancaster T, Stead L, Mant D, Fowler G. Nicotine replacement therapy for smoking cessation. *Cochrane Database Syst Rev* 2004(3): CD000146.

90. Zhang X, Patel A, Horibe H, Wu Z *et al.* Cholesterol, coronary heart disease, and stroke in the Asia Pacific region. *Int J Epidemiol* 2003; 32(4): 563–572.

91. Bots ML, Elwood PC, Nikitin Y, Salonen JT *et al.* Total and HDL cholesterol and risk of stroke. EUROSTROKE: a collaborative study among research centres in Europe. *J Epidemiol Community Health* 2002; 56(Suppl 1): i19–i24.

92. Wannamethee SG, Shaper AG, Ebrahim S. HDL-Cholesterol, total choles- terol, and the risk of stroke in middle-aged British men. *Stroke* 2000; 31(8): 1882–1888.

93. Primatesta P, Poulter NR. Lipid levels and the use of lipid-lowering agents in England and Scotland. *Eur J Cardiovasc Prev Rehabil* 2004; 11(6): 484–488.

94. Kiely DK, Wolf PA, Cupples LA, Beiser AS, Kannel WB. Physical activ- ity and stroke risk: the Framingham Study. *Am J Epidemiol* 1994; 140(7): 608–620.

95. Sacco RL, Gan R, Boden-Albala B, Lin IF *et al.* Leisure-time physical activity and ischemic stroke risk: the Northern Manhattan Stroke Study. *Stroke* 1998; 29(2): 380–387.

96. Wannamethee G, Shaper AG. Physical activity and stroke in British middle aged men. *BMJ* 1992; 304(6827): 597–601.

97. Kurth T, Gaziano JM, Berger K, Kase CS *et al.* Body mass index and the risk of stroke in men. *Arch Intern Med* 2002; 162(22): 2557–2562.

98. Rexrode KM, Hennekens CH, Willett WC, Colditz GA *et al.* A prospective study of body mass index, weight change, and risk of stroke in women. *JAMA* 1997; 277(19): 1539–1545.

99. Kurth T, Gaziano JM, Rexrode KM, Kase CS *et al.* Prospective study of body mass index and risk of stroke in apparently healthy women. *Circulation* 2005; 111(15): 1992–1998.

100. WHO. Obesity and overweight fact sheet. 2006. September, http://www. who.int/dietphysicalactivity/publications/facts/obesity/en/

101. Hedley AA, Ogden CL, Johnson CL, Carroll MD *et al.* Prevalence of over- weight and obesity among US children, adolescents, and adults, 1999–2002. *JAMA* 2004; 291(23): 2847–2850.

102. Goldstein DJ. Beneficial health effects of modest weight loss. *Int J Obes Relat Metab Disord* 1992; 16(6): 397–415.

103. Wannamethee SG, Shaper AG, Walker M. Overweight and obesity and weight change in middle aged men: impact on cardiovascular disease and diabetes. *J Epidemiol Community Health* 2005; 59(2): 134–139.

104. Padwal RS, Majumdar SR. Drug treatments for obesity: orlistat, sibutramine, and rimonabant. *Lancet* 2007; 369(9555): 71–77.

105. Valderrama AL, Dunbar SB, Mensah GA. Atrial fibrillation: public health implications. *Am J Prev Med* 2005; 29(5 Suppl 1): 75–80.

106. Go AS, Hylek EM, Phillips KA, Chang Y *et al.* Prevalence of diagnosed atrial fibrillation in adults: national implications for rhythm management and stroke prevention: the AnTicoagulation and Risk Factors in Atrial Fibrillation (ATRIA) Study. *JAMA* 2001; 285(18): 2370–2375.

107. Majeed A, Moser K, Carroll K. Trends in the prevalence and management of atrial fibrillation in general practice in England and Wales, 1994–1998: analysis of data from the general practice research database. *Heart* 2001; 86(3): 284–288.

108. Wolf PA, Mitchell JB, Baker CS, Kannel WB, D'Agostino RB. Impact of atrial fibrillation on mortality, stroke, and medical costs. *Arch Intern Med* 1998; 158(3): 229–234.

109. Feinberg WM, Blackshear JL, Laupacis A, Kronmal R, Hart RG. Prevalence, age distribution, and gender of patients with atrial fibrillation. Analysis and implications. *Arch Intern Med* 1995; 155(5): 469–473.

110. The effect of low-dose warfarin on the risk of stroke in patients with non-rheumatic atrial fibrillation. The Boston Area Anticoagulation Trial for Atrial Fibrillation Investigators. *N Engl J Med* 1990; 323(22): 1505–1511.

111. Adjusted-dose warfarin versus low-intensity, fixed-dose warfarin plus aspirin for high-risk patients with atrial fibrillation: Stroke Prevention in Atrial Fibrillation III randomised clinical trial. *Lancet* 1996; 348(9028): 633–638.

112. Miller VT, Pearce LA, Feinberg WM, Rothrock JF *et al.* Differential effect of aspirin versus warfarin on clinical stroke types in patients with atrial fibrillation. Stroke Prevention in Atrial Fibrillation Investigators. *Neurology* 1996; 46(1): 238–240.

113. O'Leary DH, Polak JF, Kronmal RA, Kittner SJ *et al.* Distribution and correlates of sonographically detected carotid artery disease in the Cardiovascular Health Study. The CHS Collaborative Research Group. *Stroke* 1992; 23(12): 1752–1760.

114. Fine-Edelstein JS, Wolf PA, O'Leary DH, Poehlman H *et al.* Precursors of extracranial carotid atherosclerosis in the Framingham Study. *Neurology* 1994; 44(6): 1046–1050.

115. Nadareishvili ZG, Rothwell PM, Beletsky V, Pagniello A, Norris JW. Long-term risk of stroke and other vascular events in patients with asymptomatic carotid artery stenosis. *Arch Neurol* 2002; 59(7): 1162–1166.

116. Clinical alert: benefit of carotid endarterectomy for patients with high-grade stenosis of the internal carotid artery. National Institute of Neurological

Disorders and Stroke Stroke and Trauma Division. North American Symptomatic Carotid Endarterectomy Trial (NASCET) investigators. *Stroke* 1991; 22(6): 816–817.

117. Barnett HJ, Taylor DW, Eliasziw M, Fox AJ *et al*. Benefit of carotid endarterectomy in patients with symptomatic moderate or severe stenosis. North American Symptomatic Carotid Endarterectomy Trial Collaborators. *N Engl J Med* 1998; 339(20): 1415–1425.

118. NHS England. Health Care for London. *Stroke Prevention Strategy* 2008.

119. Carroll K, Eliahoo J, Majeed A, Murad S. Stroke incidence and risk factors in a population-based prospective cohort study. *Health Stat Q* 2001; 12: 18–26.

120. Goldstein LB, Adams R, Becker K, Furberg CD *et al*. Primary prevention of ischemic stroke: A statement for healthcare professionals from the Stroke Council of the American Heart Association. *Circulation* 2001; 103(1): 163–182.

121. Boden-Albala B, Sacco RL. Socioeconomic status and stroke mortality: refining the relationship. *Stroke* 2002; 33(1): 274–275.

122. Cox AM, McKevitt C, Rudd AG, Wolfe CD. Socioeconomic status and stroke. *Lancet Neurol* 2006; 5(2): 181–188.

123. Gillum RF, Mussolino ME. Education, poverty, and stroke incidence in whites and blacks: the NHANES I Epidemiologic Follow-up Study. *J Clin Epidemiol* 2003; 56(2): 188–195.

124. Steenland K, Hu S, Walker J. All-cause and cause-specific mortality by socioeconomic status among employed persons in 27 US states, 1984–1997. *Am J Public Health* 2004; 94(6): 1037–1042.

125. Wolf PA, Kannel WB. Preventing stroke: does race/ethnicity matter? *Circulation* 2007; 116(19): 2099–2100.

126. Rosamond WD, Folsom AR, Chambless LE, Wang CH *et al*. Stroke incidence and survival among middle-aged adults: 9-year follow-up of the Atherosclerosis Risk in Communities (ARIC) cohort. *Stroke* 1999; 30(4): 736–743.

127. Cappuccio FP, Cook DG, Atkinson RW, Strazzullo P. Prevalence, detection, and management of cardiovascular risk factors in different ethnic groups in south London. *Heart* 1997; 78(6): 555–563.

128. Office for National Statistics. Available at http://www.statistics.gov.uk.

129. Allen CL, Bayraktutan U. Risk factors for ischaemic stroke. *Int J Stroke* 2008; 3(2): 105–116.

130. Sacco RL. Preventing stroke among blacks: the challenges continue. *JAMA* 2003; 289(22): 3005–3007.

131. Romero JR, Morris J, Pikula A. Stroke prevention: modifying risk factors. *Ther Adv Cardiovasc Dis* 2008; 2(4): 287–303.

132. Bonita R, Mendis S, Truelsen T, Bogousslavsky J *et al.* The global stroke initiative. *Lancet Neurol* 2004; 3(7): 391–393.

133. Sacco RL. The 2006 William Feinberg lecture: shifting the paradigm from stroke to global vascular risk estimation. *Stroke* 2007; 38(6): 1980–1987.

134. Stampfer MJ, Hu FB, Manson JE, Rimm EB, Willett WC. Primary prevention of coronary heart disease in women through diet and lifestyle. *N Engl J Med* 2000; 343(1): 16–22.

135. Pearson TA, Bazzarre TL, Daniels SR, Fair JM *et al.* American Heart Association guide for improving cardiovascular health at the community level: a statement for public health practitioners, healthcare providers, and health policy makers from the American Heart Association Expert Panel on Population and Prevention Science. *Circulation* 2003; 107(4): 645–651.

136. Qureshi AI, Suri MF, Kirmani JF, Divani AA. The relative impact of inadequate primary and secondary prevention on cardiovascular mortality in the United States. *Stroke* 2004; 35(10): 2346–2350.

137. Conroy RM, Pyorala K, Fitzgerald AP, Sans S *et al.* Estimation of ten-year risk of fatal cardiovascular disease in Europe: the SCORE project. *Eur Heart J* 2003; 24(11): 987–1003.

138. Miller NH, Hill M, Kottke T, Ockene IS. The multilevel compliance challenge: recommendations for a call to action. A statement for healthcare professionals. *Circulation* 1997; 95(4): 1085–1090.

139. Graham I, Atar D, Borch-Johnsen K, Boysen G *et al.* European guidelines on cardiovascular disease prevention in clinical practice: executive summary. Fourth Joint Task Force of the European Society of Cardiology and other societies on cardiovascular disease prevention in clinical practice (constituted by representatives of nine societies and by invited experts). *Eur J Cardiovasc Prev Rehabil* 2007; 14(Suppl 2): E1–40.

140. Fortmann SP, Flora JA, Winkleby MA, Schooler C *et al.* Community intervention trials: reflections on the Stanford Five-City Project Experience. *Am J Epidemiol* 1995; 142(6): 576–586.

141. Weinehall L, Hellsten G, Boman K, Hallmans G. Prevention of cardiovascular disease in Sweden: the Norsjo community intervention

programme — motives, methods and intervention components. *Scand J Public Health Suppl* 2001; 56: 13–20.

142. Bernard S, Lux L, Lohr K. Healthcare delivery models for prevention of cardiovascular disease. Quest for Quality and Improved Performance Project. *The Health Foundation* 2009.

143. Pearson TA, Blair SN, Daniels SR, Eckel RH *et al.* AHA Guidelines for Primary Prevention of Cardiovascular Disease and Stroke: 2002 Update: Consensus Panel Guide to Comprehensive Risk Reduction for Adult Patients Without Coronary or Other Atherosclerotic Vascular Diseases. American Heart Association Science Advisory and Coordinating Committee. *Circulation* 2002; 106(3): 388–391.

144. The Royal College of Physicians. National Clinical Guidelines for Stroke 2008. Available at http://www.rcplondon.ac.uk/clinical-standards/ceeu/Current-work/stroke/Pages/Guidelines.aspx.

145. Matson Koffman D, Granade SA, Anwuri VV. Strategies for establishing policy, environmental, and systems-level interventions for managing high blood pressure and high cholesterol in health care settings: a qualitative case study. *Prev Chronic Dis* 2008; 5(3): A83.

146. Stroebel RJ, Broers JK, Houle SK, Scott CG, Naessens JM. Improving hypertension control: a team approach in a primary care setting. *Jt Comm J Qual Improv* 2000; 26(11): 623–632.

147. Petty GW, Brown Jr. RD, Whisnant JP, Sicks JD *et al.* Survival and recurrence after first cerebral infarction: a population-based study in Rochester, Minnesota, 1975 through 1989. *Neurology* 1998; 50(1): 208–216.

148. Samsa GP, Bian J, Lipscomb J, Matchar DB. Epidemiology of recurrent cerebral infarction: a medicare claims-based comparison of first and recurrent strokes on 2-year survival and cost. *Stroke* 1999; 30(2): 338–349.

149. Rothwell PM, Giles MF, Chandratheva A, Marquardt L *et al.* Effect of urgent treatment of transient ischaemic attack and minor stroke on early recurrent stroke (EXPRESS study): a prospective population-based sequential comparison. *Lancet* 2007; 370(9596): 1432–1442.

150. Rothwell PM, Buchan A, Johnston SC. Recent advances in management of transient ischaemic attacks and minor ischaemic strokes. *Lancet Neurol* 2006; 5(4): 323–331.

151. Sacco RL, Adams R, Albers G, Alberts MJ *et al.* Guidelines for prevention of stroke in patients with ischemic stroke or transient ischemic attack: a

statement for healthcare professionals from the American Heart Association/American Stroke Association Council on Stroke: co-sponsored by the Council on Cardiovascular Radiology and Intervention: the American Academy of Neurology affirms the value of this guideline. *Stroke* 2006; 37(2): 577–617.

152. Reeves MJ, Arora S, Broderick JP, Frankel M *et al.* Acute stroke care in the US: results from 4 pilot prototypes of the Paul Coverdell National Acute Stroke Registry. *Stroke* 2005; 36(6): 1232–1240.

153. LaBresh KA, Reeves MJ, Frankel MR, Albright D, Schwamm LH. Hospital treatment of patients with ischemic stroke or transient ischemic attack using the "Get With The Guidelines" program. *Arch Intern Med* 2008; 168(4): 411–417.

154. Get With The Guidelines–Stroke. American Stroke Association Web site. http://www.strokeassociation.org/presenter.jhtml?identifier=3002728. Accessed August 17, 2009.

155. Kalra L, Perez I, Melbourn A. Stroke risk management: changes in mainstream practice. *Stroke* 1998; 29(1): 53–57.

156. Redfern J, McKevitt C, Rudd A, Wolfe C. Review of interventions to change patient and professional behaviors in stroke management and prevention. In *Best Practices in the Behavioural Management of Chronic Disease.* Vol. 1, Chapter 3, updated 2006. Trafton J and Gordon WP (Eds.) Institute for Brain Potential, California.

157. Silagy CA, Weller DP, Lapsley H, Middleton P *et al.* The effectiveness of local adaptation of nationally produced clinical practice guidelines. *Fam Pract* 2002; 19(3): 223–230.

158. Fang XH, Kronmal RA, Li SC, Longstreth Jr. WT *et al.* Prevention of stroke in urban China: a community-based intervention trial. *Stroke* 1999; 30(3): 495–501.

159. Jiang B, Wang WZ, Wu SP, Du XL, Bao QJ. Effects of urban community intervention on 3-year survival and recurrence after first-ever stroke. *Stroke* 2004; 35(6): 1242–1247.

160. Connell P, Wolfe C, McKevitt C. Preventing stroke: a narrative review of community interventions for improving hypertension control in black adults. *Health Soc Care Community* 2008; 16(2): 165–187.

161. Primatesta P, Poulter NR. Improvement in hypertension management in England: results from the Health Survey for England 2003. *J Hypertens* 2006; 24(6): 1187–1192.

162. Ashworth M, Medina J, Morgan M. Effect of social deprivation on blood pressure monitoring and control in England: a survey of data from the quality and outcomes framework. *BMJ* 2008; 337: a2030.
163. Hamann GF, Weimar C, Glahn J, Busse O *et al.* Adherence to secondary stroke prevention strategies — results from the German Stroke Data Bank. *Cerebrovasc Dis* 2003; 15(4): 282–288.
164. Rundek T, Sacco RL. Risk factor management to prevent first stroke. *Neurol Clin* 2008; 26(4): 1007–1045, ix.
165. Redfern J, McKevitt C, Dundas R, Rudd AG, Wolfe CD. Behavioral risk factor prevalence and lifestyle change after stroke: a prospective study. *Stroke* 2000; 31(8): 1877–1881.
166. Raine R, Wong W, Ambler G, Hardoon S. *et al.* Sociodemographic variations in the contribution of secondary drug prevention to stroke survival at middle and older ages: cohort study. *BMJ* 2009; 338: b1279.
167. Sanz G, Fuster V. Fixed-dose combination therapy and secondary cardiovascular prevention: rationale, selection of drugs and target population. *Nat Clin Pract Cardiovasc Med* 2009; 6(2): 101–110.
168. Sleight P, Pouleur H, Zannad F. Benefits, challenges, and registerability of the polypill. *Eur Heart J* 2006; 27(14): 1651–1656.
169. Wald NJ, Law MR. A strategy to reduce cardiovascular disease by more than 80%. *BMJ* 2003; 326(7404): 1419.
170. Whelton PK, He J, Appel LJ, Cutler JA *et al.* Primary prevention of hypertension: clinical and public health advisory from The National High Blood Pressure Education Program. *JAMA* 2002; 288(15): 1882–1888.
171. van Steenkiste B, Grol R, van der Weijden T. Systematic review of implementation strategies for risk tables in the prevention of cardiovascular diseases. *Vasc Health Risk Manag* 2008; 4(3): 535–545.
172. Redfern J, Rudd AD, Wolfe CD, McKevitt C. Stop Stroke: development of an innovative intervention to improve risk factor management after stroke. *Patient Educ Couns* 2008; 72(2): 201–209.
173. Ellis G, Rodger J, McAlpine C, Langhorne P. The impact of stroke nurse specialist input on risk factor modification: a randomised controlled trial. *Age Ageing* 2005; 34(4): 389–392.
174. Earnest MP, Norris JM, Eberhardt MS, Sands GH. Report of the AAN Task Force on access to health care: the effect of no personal health insurance on health care for people with neurologic disorders. Task Force on Access to

Health Care of the American Academy of Neurology. *Neurology* 1996; 46(5): 1471–1480.

175. Wang DZ. Editorial comment — telemedicine: the solution to provide rural stroke coverage and the answer to the shortage of stroke neurologists and radiologists. *Stroke* 2003; 34(12): 2957.

176. Majeed A, Lester H, Bindman AB. Improving the quality of care with performance indicators. *BMJ* 2007; 335(7626): 916–918.

3   Transient Ischaemic Attacks

Matthew F. Giles* and Peter M. Rothwell*

Chapter Summary

Recent data on the incidence and prevalence of transient ischaemic attack (TIA) are lacking, but available data suggest that the rate of TIA is higher than previously estimated, and rises with increasing age. The burden of TIA is likely to increase with the ageing of the population. Prospective prognostic studies have shown that the early risk of stroke after TIA is approximately 5% at seven days and 10–15% at 90 days depending on clinical settings and study methodology. This risk can be reliably predicted by risk scores based on clinical features (the ABCD system), TIA aetiology and findings on brain imaging, although the optimal combined prognostic strategy is uncertain because the interaction between individual predictors is not established. Research studies of the urgent assessment and initiation of secondary prevention in specialist centres suggest that the early risk of stroke after TIA can be reduced by up to 80%. In England and Wales, recommendations have been made to acute hospitals by the National Institute for Health and Clinical Excellence (NICE) for high-risk TIA patients to be assessed and treated within 24 hours and others to be assessed within seven days. A variety of inpatient

*Stroke Prevention Research Unit, NIHR Biomedical Research Centre, Oxford University Department of Clinical Neurology, Level 6, West Wing, John Radcliffe Hospital, Oxford OX3 9DU, UK

and outpatient models have been used to meet these recommendations, but the optimal means of service provision is unclear.

Introduction

Previous research is likely to have underestimated the burden of transient ischaemic attack (TIA) in terms of its incidence and prognosis. In this chapter, we review recent work showing that TIA is common, it carries a high early risk of stroke which can be predicted and prevented with acute intervention and it carries a high longer term risk of other vascular disease. Barriers to effective delivery of interventions are also reviewed.

There has been recent controversy about the definition of TIA and whether it should be distinguished from stroke according to time-based or tissue-based criteria. TIA and stroke are defined as an acute loss of focal brain or monocular function of presumed vascular cause. The "traditional" World Health Organization (WHO) definition distinguishes a TIA from a stroke according to time-based criteria, with duration of symptoms of less than 24 hours.[1] More recently, the American Stroke Association has proposed a tissue-based distinction, based on the absence of brain infarction on imaging, preferably by diffusion-weighted MRI (DWI).[2] The WHO definition has the advantages of being clinically-based and can be applied after history taking and examination have been performed, without the need for investigations, and has a well-recognised differential diagnosis. The more recent definition is more consistent with pathophysiological processes. In this chapter, the time-based, WHO definition has been used to reflect its widespread use in the UK and lack of availability of routine MRI in the assessment of TIA patients.

Incidence

There is increasing emphasis on establishing specialist services for TIA patients.[3,4] and measures of incidence are necessary to estimate the capacity required. However, high quality epidemiological studies of TIA incidence are difficult to perform, because, in the absence of a gold standard investigation, early expert assessment is required for reliable diagnosis and TIA patients are managed in a variety of different clinical settings. Previous incidence studies have used stringent definitions of first-ever-in-a-lifetime, definite events which will underestimate the overall 'burden of TIA' which is managed by a dedicated service.[5] Recent data from the Oxford Vascular Study (OXVASC),[6] a population-based study of the incidence and outcome of TIA and stroke, estimated the standardised incidence of any definite or probable TIA to be approximately 1.08 (0.95–1.21) per thousand population, almost double the rate calculated according to the definition of first-ever-in-a-lifetime, definite TIA, as used in previous incidence studies (Table 1).[7]

Furthermore, the rate of all referrals to a dedicated outpatient TIA service, including those for minor stroke or suspected TIA in whom an eventual non-neurovascular diagnosis is made, was 2.98 (2.77–3.2). If these rates are extrapolated to 330,000 people, the population served by an average sized district general hospital in the UK, approximately 1000 referrals to a dedicated TIA clinic would be expected per year, or 20 referrals per week (Table 2).

Equivalent recent data from elsewhere in the world are lacking, but it has been estimated that between 200,000 and 500,000 patients with TIA report to medical attention each year in the United States.[8-10] Reliable data on trends in the incidence of TIA are similarly sparse. Comparisons between OXVASC and the Oxfordshire Community Stroke Project (OCSP)[11] in which both studies used identical definitions and high quality methodology applied in the same population, 20 years apart, suggest that the incidence is not falling.[6] Similar observations have been made in Rochester, USA, between the 1960s and 1980s,[10] in Dijon, France, between 1985 and 1994[12] and in Novosibirsk, Russia between 1987–1988 and 1996–1997.[13]

TIA is more common in the elderly and an increase in overall rates might be expected solely due to the ageing of the population, regardless of any change in age-specific incidence rates.[14] Moreover, recent studies on the prevalence of TIA suggest that many events are not currently reported by patients[15,16] and the impact of public education campaigns may further increase demands for specialist TIA services.[17,18]

Table 1. Crude and standardised (to the 2005 population of England) annual incidence rates per thousand population for definite incident TIA, any probable or definite TIA, all referrals to a dedicated TIA clinic and all stroke in OXVASC (study period 2002–2005)[7]

	Mean age (SD)	Crude figures			Standardised to 2005 population of England
		Males	Females	Total	Total
		Rate (95% CI)	Rate (95% CI)	Rate (95% CI)	Rate (95% CI)
Definite, first-ever-in-a-lifetime TIA	73.8 (13.5)	0.35 (0.26–0.46)	0.47 (0.39–0.56)	0.47 (0.39–0.56)	0.54 (0.44–0.63)
Any probable or definite TIA	73.4 (12.5)	0.79 (0.65–0.96)	1.12 (0.94–1.31)	0.95 (0.84–1.07)	1.08 (0.95–1.21)
Any TIAs, minor strokes and patients referred to clinic with suspected events with eventual non-vascular diagnoses	70.1 (14.6)	2.39 (2.14–2.66)	2.96 (2.67–3.27)	2.67 (2.48–2.87)	2.98 (2.77–3.2)

Table 2. Projected total numbers of events (calculated by applying measured standardised incidence rates to the population of interest and rounded to the nearest ten) for an average district general hospital serving 330,000 people and for the estimated 2005 population of England[7]

	Average district general hospital	Population of England (2005)
Clinic and inpatient events combined		
Incident, definite TIAs	170	26,280
All definite or probable TIAs	360	54,610
All definite or probable strokes	700	107,290
Definite and probable events only		
Clinic TIA and strokes	610	92,570
Inpatient TIA and strokes	450	69,330
Definite, probable and suspected events combined		
Clinic activity overall	980	150,440
Inpatient activity overall	620	94,860

Risk of Stroke and Other Vascular Disease after TIA

The importance of TIA lies in the early risk of stroke and later risk of other vascular events.

Short-term risk

Major stroke is often preceded by TIA,[19] although the symptoms may have neither alarmed the patient, nor have been reported. Early studies indicated that TIA was a relatively benign condition with a low risk of stroke (approximately 1–2% at one week and 2–4% at one month).[20–22] These were underestimates, because they were based on observations from cohort studies or clinical trials where patients were recruited weeks to months after their initial event.[23]

More recently, a number of studies have reported the early risk of stroke following TIA using more reliable methodology and recruiting patients in the acute phase. The first of these studied patients presenting to 16 emergency departments (EDs) within a healthcare maintenance organisation in California, US.[24] Patients were followed up by reviewing medical records and searching computerised databases. From 1997 to 1998, 1707 patients presented with TIA were diagnosed by an ED physician, almost all within 24 hours of the event. About 10.5% (180 patients) returned within 90 days with a stroke, half of which occurred within two days of the index TIA. Of these, 38 strokes were fatal and 115 were disabling.

A number of prospective studies of the early risk of TIA conducted in a range of different clinical settings using a variety of methodologies have since been published. A systematic review and meta-analysis of these studies identified 18 cohorts, all published since 2000, reporting the early stroke risk in 10,126 TIA patients.[25] The pooled risks of stroke were 3.1% (95% CI: 2.0–4.1) at two days and 5.2% (3.9–6.5) at seven days, with risks ranging from 0% to 12.8% at seven days and significant heterogeneity between individual estimates. This heterogeneity was almost fully explained by study setting and method. The lowest risks were seen in studies in specialist stroke services offering emergency access and treatment, intermediate risks were observed in routine clinics and EDs and highest risks in population-based studies without urgent treatment.

A similar meta-analysis of studies of stroke risk over 30–90 days after TIA identified 11 studies including a total of 7238 patients.[26] It calculated pooled risks of 8.0% (5.7–10.2%) and 9.2% (6.8–11.5%) at 30 and 90 days respectively. Various clinical and methodological sources of heterogeneity were tested, but only the method of ascertainment of stroke outcomes was identified as being significant, with higher risks being observed in cohorts in which outcome of strokes were ascertained actively with face-to-face follow-up as opposed to by searching administrative databases.

Medium- and long-term risk

Many studies have addressed the question of medium-term prognosis although some were undermined by non-standardised diagnostic criteria, retrospective case identification, incomplete follow-up and small numbers of cases.[27] However, three prospective population-based studies of the medium-term prognosis of TIA have been published from Söderhamn, Sweden

(97 patients, follow-up over three years),[28] Perugia, Italy (94 patients, follow-up over nine years)[29] and Oxfordshire, UK (184 patients, follow-up over 3.7 years).[30] The mean age of patients in each cohort was 69 years.

In the Söderhamn cohort, the risk of stroke was approximately 5% per year and the overall mortality was 24.7% over a mean of three years. No data were reported on cardiovascular morbidity. In the Perugia cohort, the annual risk of stroke after TIA was 2.4% (0.7–4.7). The actuarial risk of death was 28.6% (19.2–37.8) at five years and 49.5% (38.9–60.0) at ten years with roughly equal numbers of cerebrovascular, cardiovascular and non-vascular deaths. In the Oxfordshire cohort the annual stroke risk was 4.4% (1.5–7.3) although this was 'front-loaded' — being highest in the first year after initial TIA. The risk of death at five years was 31.3% (23.3–39.3) and the annual risk of death was 6.3% (4.7–7.9). Again, there were roughly equal numbers of cerebrovascular, cardiovascular and non-vascular deaths. The risk of either fatal or non-fatal myocardial infarction was 12.1% (5.8–18.4) at five years and the approximate annual risk was 2.4%. There are similarly few high quality prospective hospital-based cohort studies of the longer term prognosis of TIA[31] and because these tend to include younger patients due to referral bias, they report lower risks.[32]

Thus, the risk of stroke and other vascular events is appreciable in the medium term; but a question which has only recently been addressed is the vascular risk in the longer term and whether there is a need for ongoing aggressive secondary prevention. Two studies provide reliable data on prognosis up to 15 years after TIA.

One study determined the long-term vascular risk starting some time after the initial TIA.[33] Two hundred and ninety patients with TIA, diagnosed by a neurologist who had participated either in the OCSP or a contemporaneous hospital referred cohort study, were followed-up over a ten-year period starting in 1988, a median of 3.8 years (IQR: 2.2–5.8) after their most recent TIA. Mean age at baseline was 69 years. At the end of the ten-year follow-up, the risk of stroke was 18.8% (13.6–23.7), the risk of MI or death from coronary heart disease was 27.8% (21.8–33.3) and risk of death from any cause was 50.7%. The risk of any first stroke, myocardial infarction or vascular death was 42.8% (36.4–48.5). The risk of major vascular events was found to be constant throughout the follow-up period.

The Life Long After Cerebral Ischaemia (LILAC) study reported near complete follow-up on 2473 participants from the Dutch TIA Trial.[34] Mean age was 65 years and 759 had a TIA while the remainder suffered a minor stroke (defined as a score of ≤3 on the modified Rankin scale at enrolment). The trial recruited patients, all of whom were assessed by a neurologist, between 1986 and 1989 and randomised to two different doses of aspirin. After a mean follow-up of 10.1 years, 1489 (60%) had died and 1336 (54%) had suffered at least one vascular event. At ten years the cumulative risk of recurrent stroke was 18.4% (16.7–20.1), first major vascular event was 44.1% (42.0–46.1) and death was 46.6% (44.2–51.3). The corresponding figures for those presenting with TIA at inception (as opposed to minor stroke) were 35.8% (32.3–39.3) for first vascular event and 34.1% (30.7–37.4) for death. Importantly, due to the inclusion criteria of the original trial, only 22% of patients were randomised within a week of initial vascular event and the median time to randomisation was 18 days. Therefore much of the very high acute risk described above was missed from these estimates.

In summary, the risk of stroke in the short term after TIA is particularly high, while in medium and long term, this is exceeded by the risk of vascular disease in general.

Risk Stratification

Stroke risk after TIA poses a major dilemma to health services because although the majority of patients will have no acute sequelae, an important minority will go on to suffer a potentially disabling stroke which may be prevented with appropriate treatment. Optimal management in the face of this variation in risk has been uncertain and guidelines have been inconsistent about how rapidly and where patients should be assessed, with some recommending inpatient treatment and others more routine outpatient care.[3,35,36] Uncertainty also surrounds the cost effectiveness of each strategy.[37]

In healthcare systems not offering urgent assessment for all, prognostic scores have been suggested as a means of identifying high (and low) risk patients. Validated models have been available for prediction of long-term stroke risk after TIA or minor stroke for some time.[38,39] More recently, risk prediction tools have been developed to identify those individuals at high risk of stroke in the acute phase after TIA, with the aim of informing public education, triaging referrals to secondary care and targeting early secondary preventive treatments.

Clinical Features and the ABCD System

Several factors were found to be independently associated with high risk of stroke in the studies of early prognosis of TIA.[24,40,41] These were used to derive the ABCD score to predict stroke risk within seven days after TIA.[42]

All clinical features which had previously been found to be predictive of stroke after TIA were tested in a derivation cohort of 209 TIA patients recruited from OCSP.[11] Any variable that was a univariate predictor of the seven-day risk of stroke with a significance of $p \leq 0.1$ was incorporated into the score. The score was then validated in three further independent cohorts recruited from OXVASC and a dedicated neurovascular clinic in Oxfordshire, UK.[42]

The score is based on four clinical features and has a total of six (Table 3).

It was found to be highly predictive, with area under the curve (AUC) for prediction of seven-day risk of stroke of 0.85 (0.78–0.91), 0.91 (0.86–0.95) and 0.80 (0.72–0.89) for each of the validation cohorts.

Although diabetes was found to be predictive of stroke in a pooled analysis of all the cohorts in the initial publication, it was not included in the score.[42] The ABCD system was refined and revalidated in cohorts of patients recruited in California, US and Oxfordshire, UK with the addition of one point for diabetes to make the ABCD2 score (Table 3 and Fig. 1).[43]

The validity of a predictive score depends on its statistical accuracy, especially when used by independent investigators, and its usefulness in providing relevant information to clinicians in an easily calculable way. A number of validation studies have been performed by several independent investigators reporting conflicting results. However, in a systematic review and meta-analysis, 11 studies were identified which reported the performance of one or both scores in 14 cohorts including 5938 subjects with 332 strokes at seven days.[44] Pooled estimates of the AUC for the ABCD and ABCD2 scores were 0.74 (0.68–0.81) and 0.77 (0.63–0.91)

Table 3.   Table listing clinical features and scoring for ABCD system[44,45]

	Element	Category	ABCD score	ABCD2 score
A	Age	Age ≥ 60	1	1
		Age < 60	0	0
B	BP	SBP > 140 or DBP ≥ 90	1	1
		Other	0	0
C	Clinical Features	Unilateral weakness	2	2
		Speech disturbance (no weakness)	1	1
		Other	0	0
D	Duration	≥60 minutes	2	2
		10–59 minutes	1	1
		<10 minutes	0	0
D	Diabetes	Present	NA	1
		Absent		0
	Total		**6**	**7**

BP: Blood pressure measured at time of earliest assessment after TIA; SBP: Systolic blood pressure; DBP: Diastolic blood pressure

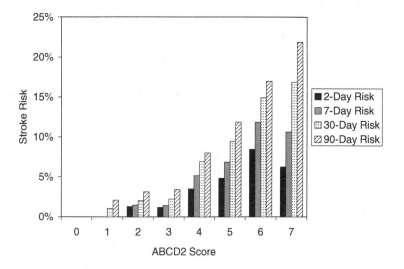

Figure 1.   Observed stroke risk at 2, 7, 30 and 90 days after TIA stratified by ABCD2 score pooled from six validation cohorts. Individual bars refer to risk observed at different intervals from initial TIA.[45]

respectively for seven-day stroke risk after TIA. Predictive power was greater in two cohorts that included patients with both suspected and confirmed TIA compared to cohorts of confirmed TIA patients only, and less good when applied to risk prediction beyond seven days. These findings suggest that the ABCD system works both diagnostically, detecting 'true' TIA patients, and prognostically, identifying those 'true' TIA patients at highest risk. The predictive power of the score was not reduced when validated by independent investigators.

Aetiology

There is evidence that the early risk of stroke after stroke depends on the underlying causal mechanism. A meta-analysis of rates of recurrent stroke according to aetiology among 1709 patients with ischaemic stroke in four population-based studies found highest rates among the large-artery atherosclerotic group, intermediate rates in the cardio-embolic and undetermined groups and lowest rates in the small vessel group.[45]

These findings have since been confirmed in TIA patients. In one study of patients with TIA and ≥50% symptomatic carotid stenosis from OXVASC, a risk of stroke of approximately 20% during the two weeks prior to endarterectomy was reported.[46] In a further two studies including a total of 564 TIA patients who had been admitted to hospital, symptomatic large artery disease, in addition to clinical features, was found to be an independent predictor of early stroke.[47,48]

Imaging

Brain imaging also appears to be of prognostic value. The presence of infarction on computed tomography (CT) brain scanning in patients with TIA has been shown to be associated with an increased risk of stroke recurrence in the medium and long term.[49] Two recent studies of TIA patients who received more acute scanning showed changes on CT to be predictive of early stroke. In one study of 274 TIA patients, the presence of old or new infarction or leukoaraiosis on CT was associated with an almost four-fold increase in stroke risk at 30 days (OR = 3.78, 95% CI: 1.17–12.20, $p = 0.026$), independent of clinical features.[50] In another study of 322 TIA patients scanned with CT within 48 hours of index TIA, the presence of new infarction was associated with similar increase in stroke risk at 90 days (OR = 4.06; 95% CI: 1.16–14.14; p = 0.028).[51]

However, diffusion-weighted magnetic resonance imaging (MRI) is likely to be of greater clinical usefulness than CT.[52,53] In a study of diffusion-weighted imaging (DWI) in patients with TIA, the combination of abnormalities on DWI and symptoms lasting longer than one hour was an independent predictor of further cerebral ischaemic events (OR = 5.02; CI: 1.37–18.3; p = 0.015).[54] A study in which patients were scanned within 24 hours of a TIA reported a higher risk of recurrence in the presence of an acute lesion on DWI as well as an interaction with vessel occlusion, with a 32.6% risk of recurrent stroke at 90 days in those patients with both an ischaemic lesion and an occlusion.[55] In a study of 119 patients with non-disabling stroke who had DWI performed within 24 hours of symptom onset, the presence of multiple acute cerebral infarcts on DWI was an independent predictor of stroke recurrence, vascular events, and death compared to a single acute infarct only.[56] Another study with 360 TIA patients found a higher risk of future stroke in those patients with multiple lesions on DWI, especially if those lesions were of varying ages.[57]

Brain imaging with CT or DWI therefore yields useful prognostic information in addition to informing diagnosis, territory and aetiology of TIA. However, further studies are required to determine whether the presence of an acute ischaemic lesion predicts stroke independently of the clinical characteristics in the risk scores.[58,59]

Territory

Recent evidence suggests that there may not be a major difference in long-term prognosis according to the vascular territory of TIA and the early risk of stroke may be higher after posterior-circulation territory events.[60] In a meta-analysis of cohort studies of stroke risk after TIA, those that recruited during the acute phase found a higher risk of subsequent stroke in patients with posterior circulation events compared to anterior (OR = 1.5; 95% CI: 1.1–2.0, p = 0.014); whereas those mainly recruited after the acute phase found a lower risk (posterior vs. anterior, OR = 0.7; 0.7–0.8, p > 0.001).[60] Observations from OXVASC confirm these findings.[61]

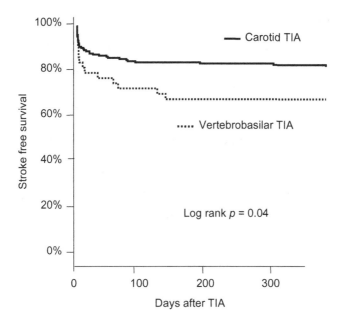

Figure 2. Stroke-free survival curves for consecutive TIA patients with anterior versus posterior circulation events in the OXVASC study.[63]

Among 256 consecutive patients with TIA, 44 (17.1%) with a posterior event and 212 (82.5%) with an anterior event, rates of stroke were 15.9% versus 9.4% (p = 0.22) respectively at seven days, and 31.8% versus 17.0% (p = 0.03) at one year (Fig. 2). Differences in aetiology may explain these observations. In a further series of patients with TIA and minor stroke in OXVASC, the rates of symptomatic large artery stenosis were higher among patients with posterior circulation events as compared to those with carotid territory events.[62]

In summary, a range of clinical, aetiological and imaging factors have been found to predict early stroke risk after TIA. However, the interaction between these predictors and the optimal strategy for combining them is unclear. Larger studies are required to derive such a strategy which is likely to use a staged approach, incorporating initial clinical data and subsequent investigation results, to estimate and then to refine an individual's risk.

Management

The evidence base for secondary prevention after TIA is well-established and several treatments have been shown to prevent stroke in the long-term, including antiplatelet agents, blood-pressure-lowering drugs, statins, anticoagulation and endarterectomy. However, until recently there were few data on the benefits of acute treatment after TIA. Moreover, if the effects of these treatments are independent, results from long-term secondary prevention trials suggest that combined use of these interventions in appropriate patients may reduce the risk of recurrent stroke by approximately 80%.[63] These observations formed the basis of two recent studies of the effect on stroke risk following TIA of combined prevention treatments started urgently in specialist units, the EXPRESS study,[64] and the SOS-TIA study.[65]

The EXPRESS Study

In the EXPRESS study (Early use of EXisting PREventive Strategies for Stroke),[64] the impact of urgent assessment and initiation of secondary prevention treatments for TIA patients in a dedicated, outpatient clinic was studied using a prospective, population-based sequential comparison design, nested within OXVASC.

In the first 30-month phase of the study lasting from 1st April 2002 to 30th September 2004, collaborating GPs were asked to refer all patients with suspected TIA or minor stroke from the study population who did not need hospital admission to a daily dedicated outpatient clinic. The clinic was appointment-based, with inherent delays in receiving referrals and contacting patients, and instead of initiating treatment immediately, recommendations were faxed to the referring physician. In phase 2, lasting from 1st October 2004 to 31st March 2007, an emergency clinic was introduced to which GPs were asked to send all patients immediately after presentation, and treatment was started straight away in the clinic, once the diagnosis had been confirmed.

As the study was nested in OXVASC, all patients with TIA and stroke were ascertained from the study population, regardless of their mode of referral and presentation, including outpatient departments, hospitals or primary care. Throughout both phases, methods of diagnosis, follow-up and adjudication of outcomes were identical, as were treatment recommendations, clinical assessment and mode of imaging. The only difference between the two phases was in the urgency of assessment and initiation of treatment.

Over the five-year study period, 1278 patients with TIA or stroke were recruited from the entire study population. Of these 1278, 620 were referrals to outpatient services (283 with stroke and 337 with TIA), 591 (95.3%) of which were referred directly to the EXPRESS study clinic (310 in phase 1 and 281 in phase 2). Of the 591 referrals to the study clinic, 316 were for TIA and the remaining 275 were for minor stroke. There were no major differences in clinical characteristics between phase 1 and phase 2 that might have been expected to affect the risk of early recurrent stroke after seeking medical attention.

There was no difference between the study periods in the delays from onset of symptoms to the seeking of medical attention, but the median delay from seeking medical attention in primary care to assessment in the clinic decreased from 3 days in phase 1 to less than one day in phase 2 ($p < 0.0001$), with the proportion seen within six hours increasing from 1.7% to 29.0% ($p < 0.0001$). Consequently, there were fewer recurrent strokes after presentation to primary care but before assessment in clinic (11/310 vs. 3/281, $p = 0.048$).

Treatment was initiated more rapidly in phase 2 than in phase 1, with median delay from seeking medical attention to first prescription of recommended treatment falling from 19 days (IQR = 6–48) in phase 1 to one day (IQR = 0–3) in phase 2 ($p < 0.0001$), with corresponding improvement in risk factor control. Reliable 90-day follow-up was available for all presentations with TIA or stroke in the study population. The overall risk of recurrent stroke during the 90 days from first seeking medical attention in all patients referred to the study clinic fell from 10.3% in phase 1 to 2.1% in phase 2 (32/310 vs. 6/281, $p = 0.0001$), and from 10.3% in phase 1 to 0.6% in phase 2 for those referred with TIA (16/156 vs. 1/160, $p = 0.0001$). The overall 90-day risk of non-fatal stroke, MI, or death fell from 11.9% (37/310) in phase 1 to 3.6% (10/281) in phase 2 ($p = 0.0002$). Because the study was nested within a population-based study of all TIA and stroke, irrespective of the mode of presentation (to clinic, hospital or

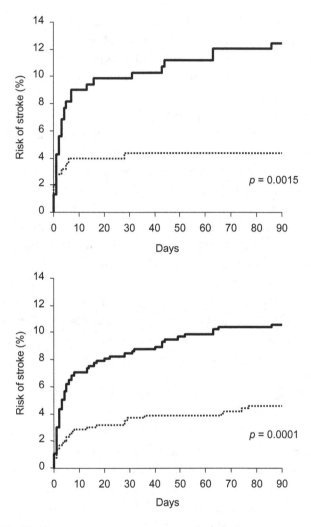

Figure 3. The 90-day risk of recurrent stroke after first seeking medical attention in all patients with TIA (top) and in all patients with TIA or stroke (bottom) in the entire OXVASC study population. The continuous line represents phase 1 of the EXPRESS study and the dotted line represents phase 2.[66]

managed in the community), the impact of the clinic could be assessed in the whole study population. The 90-day risk of recurrent stroke after all TIA presentations in the whole population fell from 12.4% in phase 1 to 4.4% in phase 2 (29/233 vs. 11/252, $p = 0.0015$) and from 9.9% to 4.2%

(63/634 vs. 27/644, p < 0.0001) for all TIA and stroke presentations (Fig. 3). Nearly all of this reduction in rates of recurrent stroke was attributable to changes in the clinic-referred population. There was no difference in rates for either intracranial or extracranial haemorrhage between phases 1 and 2.

Thus, in a rigorous study of all patients presenting with TIA or stroke in the entire study population, the EXPRESS study showed that urgent assessment and initiation of a combination of preventive treatments in a specialist outpatient service can reduce the risk of early recurrent stroke by about 80% after TIA or minor stroke and reduce the total number of all recurrent strokes in the whole population by more than half. This reduction in risk was independent of age and sex, and early treatment did not increase the risk of haemorrhage. Reductions in subsequent hospital bed-days, acute costs, and disability at six months were also observed.[66]

The SOS-TIA Study

The good outcome associated with urgent and intensive treatment was also found in the SOS-TIA study.[65] In 2003, an emergency specialist TIA outpatient clinic was set up in a university teaching hospital in Paris, France, and all 15,000 general practitioners, cardiologists, neurologists, and ophthalmologists in the region were invited to refer to it. The SOS-TIA service offered specialist assessment by a vascular neurologist and investigations within four hours of referral for TIA patients and was available 24 hours a day, seven days a week. The service immediately initiated treatment, including antiplatelet agents, statins and blood pressure lowering treatment, and discharged patients back to the referring doctor unless they fulfilled predefined criteria for admission to the hospital's stroke unit.

Over the three-year study period, the investigators evaluated 1085 patients, including 946 (87%) who were assessed within 24 hours of referral and 574 (53%) who were assessed within 24 hours of symptom onset. Of these, 643 (59%) were definite TIAs, 144 (13%) possible TIAs, 58 (5%) minor ischaemic strokes and 240 (22%) patients had 'other' diagnosis. About 26% (277 patients) were admitted to the stroke unit, and the remaining 74% (808 patients) were discharged home.

Follow-up information at one year was gathered by telephone call and was available in 629 patients with TIA. The observed rate of stroke at 90 days was 1.3% (95% CI: 0.6–2.8) for those without an ischaemic lesion on imaging and 4.8% (95% CI: 2.0–11.1) for those with an ischaemic lesion on brain imaging. The corresponding expected rates of stroke at 90 days according to the ABCD2 score were 6.1% and 7.8% respectively.

The authors concluded that stroke risk observed in the clinic population was substantially lower than expected and attributed the efficacy of SOS-TIA clinic to the short delay to assessment, the immediate start of treatment, and the modification of prevention therapy.

Health Service Perspective and Barriers to Improved Service

Many of the developments in the understanding of stroke risk after TIA, prognostic models and the potential effectiveness of early secondary prevention have occurred in the last five years. Delay in the translation of research findings into routine clinical practice is inevitable but in the case of TIA, there are particular barriers in the patient pathway which may hamper the delivery of effective interventions. These include delays to the correct recognition of symptoms and seeking medical attention by individuals who have a TIA and incorrect diagnosis in the primary or emergency care settings.

Public Knowledge and Education

Individuals' behaviour following stroke has been studied extensively, as has knowledge of stroke among the general public and at risk populations. In contrast, equivalent studies relating to TIA are lacking and the few published studies rarely report TIA patients separately.[67]

One report from OXVASC studied immediate actions after TIA in 241 consecutive patients.[68] Only 107 (44.4%) sought medical attention within hours of the event and a further 107 (44.4%) delayed seeking medical attention for one or more days. Only 24 (10%) attended ED. The main correlate with delay was the day of the week on which the TIA occurred, with longer delays observed when the TIA occurred on a Friday, Saturday or Sunday. Regarding the patients' knowledge of TIA, 231 (95.9%) were able to recall their initial perception of the cause of their symptoms, of whom 98 (42.4%) correctly recognised the cause as TIA or 'mini-stroke' and 82 (35.5%) did not know the cause. The remaining 51 (21.4%) assumed incorrect causes, the most frequent being stress or fatigue, 'eye problems', heart attack and migraine. There was no correlation between correct recognition of symptoms or previous stroke or TIA and seeking medical attention more quickly.

Another report from the Netherlands studied 57 patients with TIA or minor stroke who had attended a specialist clinic, three months after their event by postal questionnaire.[69] Although the majority could identify risk factors which could predispose to stroke, only 15 (26%) correctly identified the brain as the affected organ, and only 21 (37%) could give a correct description of a TIA or stroke.

A recent meta-analysis of patients' actions after TIA identified only nine studies reporting relevant data in 821 patients and eight of these nine studies were predominantly of stroke patients.[67] The country involved, clinical setting and methodology used varied widely. However, incorrect recognition of symptoms was common and delays were shortest among those patients who contacted emergency medical services (EMS) or attended EDs and longest in those who contacted a primary care physician.

Despite the small samples, these observations suggest that knowledge amongst the public about TIA is poor and that education should be focused on both what a TIA is and on what to do in the event. The most effective means of delivering such a message is unclear.

Diagnostic Tools

In the absence of a gold standard investigation, diagnosis of TIA remains clinical and depends on the expertise of the clinician and on accurate recall by the patient. Although clinicians from a variety of clinical settings should expect to encounter TIA patients in the acute phase, reliability in the diagnosis is far from perfect in non-specialist areas,[70] and inter-observer agreement is limited even amongst neurologists and stroke physicians.[71]

Diagnostic tools are designed to improve accuracy, and their performance depends on the differentiation between the condition itself and its mimics and the potential harm caused by an incorrect diagnosis. Such tools have been developed for the diagnosis of stroke in the pre-hospital phase and in ED, but their utility in TIA is uncertain. Such tools may be compromised by the absence of a diagnostic gold standard for TIA, so that any proposed model may simply reflect the clinical features favoured by the investigators for the discrimination of genuine TIA from TIA mimics. Furthermore, their performance may be affected by variation in the patterns of presentation of TIA and its mimics between primary care, outpatient services, and ED.[68]

Patients with genuine TIA have been observed to score higher in the ABCD system than those with TIA mimics, thus some of the ABCD system elements are likely to differentiate genuine TIA from alternative diagnoses.[72,73] However, the use of the ABCD system in diagnosis of (rather than prediction of stroke after) TIA has not been fully studied.

One tool specifically for diagnosis of TIA has been derived and validated in a population of 3216 patients referred to a TIA clinic in Glasgow, UK.[74] Variables likely to be discriminatory in the diagnosis of TIA were identified from previous diagnostic algorithms for stroke and their utility in differentiating neurovascular syndromes (including TIA and minor stroke) from mimics was tested by logistic regression. A model was derived based on age, history of TIA or stroke, headache, diplopia, syncope or pre-syncope, seizure, speech abnormality and limb or facial weakness. Each element was allocated a weighted score according to how strongly its presence or absence was predictive of a neurovascular syndrome or mimic and cut-offs for the total score were weighted to reflect the consequence of an incorrect diagnosis (i.e. missing a genuine TIA). The score was then prospectively validated in a further cohort of patients referred to the same clinic over a subsequent time period and its impact on preventing inappropriate referrals was tested. The tool performed well with positive and negative predictive values of 85% and 54% respectively and 93% and 34% depending on the cut-off used. In order to further assess its validity, its use by independent investigators should be tested as should its performance in cohorts of patients presenting to primary care as opposed to the 'enriched' validation population of referrals to secondary care.

However, the pattern of TIA symptomatology and mimics varies between patient populations presenting to different clinical setting. Another report studied the diagnostic use of certain clinical features in differentiating TIA from its mimics in a cohort of 100 patients with suspected TIA who had been admitted to a stroke unit following assessment by a neurology resident.[75] This was a preselected cohort in which patients with common TIA mimics such as migraine, partial seizure and isolated vertigo due to a peripheral cause had already been excluded. Features which independently distinguished TIA from mimics in this cohort were a prior history of unexplained attacks, gradual onset symptoms and the presence of non-specific symptoms such as light-headedness, pain, memory disturbance and gastrointestinal symptoms.

Service Provision

The standard means of delivering services to patients with suspected TIA in the UK has been by way of weekly hospital-based 'TIA clinics' run either by neurologists or geriatricians. Considerable delays to assessment in such clinics were commonplace due to their frequency, as were delays to investigation and treatment, particularly carotid endarterectomy, leading to an increase in rates of admission for patients with TIA.

In response to the research on the impact of urgent assessment on outcome after TIA and the shortcomings of 'standard' services, the National Institute for Health and Clinical Excellence (NICE) has recommended that patients with suspected TIA who are at high risk of a stroke (ABCD2 score ≥ 4) should receive immediate aspirin and specialist assessment and investigation within 24 hours of symptom onset, including brain and carotid imaging. Other non-high risk patients (ABCD2 score < 4) should be assessed within seven days. Whether the specialist assessment should take place in an inpatient or outpatient setting was not specified.

Such recommendations set considerable challenges to acute hospital and a variety of means have been employed to meet them, depending on the expertise of the referring doctor and the local availability of hospital resources and personnel. Some hospitals provide beds on either a stroke unit or an acute medical unit for the day-case assessment of patients with suspected TIA, often by a stroke physician. Such systems require the flexibility of the specialist physician to be available at short notice and carry the expense of providing a bed-based assessment, but frequently offer a 'one-stop-shop' for clinical assessment and investigations. Other hospitals have adapted the outpatient model and instead of running a single weekly clinic, offer daily 'walk-in' clinic slots in existing clinics throughout the week. This system requires the availability of appointment times and the triage of cases at the time of referral, prior to assessment but avoids the need for hospital admission. Lastly, some centres offer a mobile-phone based service where general practitioners or A&E doctors can contact a stroke physician directly who offers immediate advice about treatment and diagnosis.

Future Perspectives

Research and service provision in TIA have developed considerably in the last five years, but many questions remain unanswered. From a research perspective, these are in the fields of prognostication, treatment and imaging: risk prediction in the acute phase after TIA with clinical and imaging data has been studied, but how these data should be combined and whether these data could be used in longer-term risk prediction is unclear. The prognosis of a large number of patients referred to TIA services in whom a definite vascular diagnosis is not reached or a diagnosis of transient, generalised neurological disturbance is made is the subject of investigation. The optimal drug treatment for secondary prevention is uncertain, and trials of combinations of antiplatelet agents are ongoing. Lastly, the optimal imaging strategy to yield information about differential diagnosis, diagnosis, aetiology and risk will change with emerging technology. From a service perspective, data returned to the Department of Health in England and Wales on the performance of the various models of inpatient and outpatient TIA service delivery will be helpful in determining the best way of meeting the NICE recommendations for urgency of assessment and investigation.

References

1. Hatano S. Experience from a multicentre stroke register: a preliminary report. *Bull World Health Organ* 1976; 54: 541–553.

2. Easton JD, Saver JL, Albers GW *et al.* Definition and evaluation of transient ischemic attack: a scientific statement for healthcare professionals from the American Heart Association/American Stroke Association Stroke Council; Council on Cardiovascular Surgery and Anesthesia; Council on Cardiovascular Radiology and Intervention; Council on Cardiovascular Nursing; and the Interdisciplinary Council on Peripheral Vascular Disease. *Stroke* 2009; 40: 2276–2293.

3. Department of Health. National Stroke Strategy. Crown 2007.

4. Sacco RL, Adams R, Albers G *et al.* Guidelines for prevention of stroke in patients with ischemic stroke or transient ischemic attack: a statement for healthcare professionals from the American Heart Association/American Stroke Association Council on Stroke; co-sponsored by the Council on Cardiovascular Radiology and Intervention; the American Academy of Neurology affirms the value of this guideline. *Stroke* 2006; 37: 577–617.

5. Dennis MS, Bamford JM, Sandercock PA, Warlow CP. Incidence of transient ischemic attacks in Oxfordshire, England. *Stroke* 1989; 20: 333–339.

6. Rothwell PM, Coull AJ, Giles MF *et al.* Change in stroke incidence, mortality, case-fatality, severity, and risk factors in Oxfordshire, UK from 1981 to 2004 (Oxford Vascular Study). *Lancet* 2004; 363: 1925–1933.

7. Giles MF, Rothwell PM. Substantial underestimation of the need fro out-patient services for TIA and minor stroke. *Age Ageing* 2007; 36: 676–680.

8. Johnston SC. Clinical practice. Transient ischemic attack. *N Engl J Med* 2002; 347: 1687–1692.

9. Kleindorfer D, Panagos P, Pancioli A *et al.* Incidence and short-term prognosis of transient ischemic attack in a population-based study. *Stroke* 2005; 36: 720–723.

10. Brown RD Jr, Petty GW, O'Fallon WM *et al.* Incidence of transient ischemic attack in Rochester, Minnesota, 1985–1989. *Stroke* 1998; 29: 2109–2113.

11. Bamford J, Sandercock P, Dennis M *et al.* A prospective study of acute cerebrovascular disease in the community: the Oxfordshire Community Stroke Project 1981–1986. I: methodology, demography and incident cases of first-ever stroke. *J Neurol Neurosurg Psychiatry* 1988; 51: 1373–1380.

12. Lemesle M, Milan C, Faivre J, Moreau T, Giroud M, Dumas R. Incidence trends of ischemic stroke and transient ischemic attacks in a well-defined French population from 1985 through 1994. *Stroke* 1999; 30: 371–377.

13. Feigin VL, Shishkin SV, Tzirkin GM, Vinogradova TE, Tarasov AV, Vinogradov SP, Nikitin YP. A population-based study of transient ischemic attack incidence in Novosibirsk, Russia, 1987–1988 and 1996–1997. *Stroke* 2000; 31: 9–13.

14. Rothwell PM, Coull AJ, Silver LE *et al.* Population-based study of event-rate, incidence, case fatality, and mortality for all acute vascular events in all arterial territories (Oxford Vascular Study). *Lancet* 2005; 366: 1773–1783.

15. Jungehulsing GJ, Muller-Nordhorn J, Nolte CH *et al.* Prevalence of stroke and stroke symptoms: a population-based survey of 28,090 participants. *Neuroepidemiology* 2008; 30: 51–57.

16. Johnston SC, Fayad PB, Gorelick PB *et al.* Prevalence and knowledge of transient ischemic attack among US adults. *Neurology* 2003; 60: 1429–1434.

17. Hodgson C, Lindsay P, Rubini F. Can mass media influence emergency department visits for stroke? *Stroke* 2007; 38: 2115–2122.

18. Reeves MJ, Rafferty AP, Aranha AA, Theisen V. Changes in knowledge of stroke risk factors and warning signs among Michigan adults. *Cerebrovasc Dis* 2008; 25: 385–391.

19. Rothwell PM, Warlow CP. Timing of transient ischaemic attacks preceding ischaemic stroke. *Neurology* 2005; 64: 817–820.

20. Hankey GJ, Slattery JM, Warlow CP. The prognosis of hospital-referred transient ischaemic attacks. *J Neurol Neurosurg Psychiatry* 1991; 54: 793–802.

21. Farrell B, Godwin J, Richards S, Warlow C. The United Kingdom transient ischaemic attack (UK-TIA) aspirin trial: final results. *J Neurol Neurosurg Psychiatry* 1991; 54: 1044–1054.

22. The Dutch TIA trial: protective effects of low dose aspirin and atenolol in patients with transient ischemic attacks or non-disabling stroke. The Dutch TIA Study Group. *Stroke* 1988; 19: 512–517.

23. Rothwell PM. Incidence, risk factors and prognosis of stroke and transient ischaemic attack: the need for high-quality large-scale epidemiological studies. *Cerebrovasc Dis* 2003; 16(Suppl 3): 2–10.

24. Johnston SC, Gress DR, Browner WS, Sidney S. Short-term prognosis after emergency department diagnosis of TIA. *JAMA* 2000; 284: 2901–2906.

25. Giles MF, Rothwell PM. Risk of stroke early after transient ischaemic attack: a systematic review and meta-analysis. *Lancet Neurol* 2007; 6: 1063–1072.

26. Wu CM, McLaughlin K, Lorenzetti DL *et al.* Early risk of stroke after transient ischemic attack: a systematic review and meta-analysis. *Arch Intern Med* 2007; 167: 2417–2422.
27. Kernan WN, Feinstein AR, Brass LM. A methodological appraisal of research on prognosis after transient ischemic attacks. *Stroke* 1991; 22: 1108–1116.
28. Terent A. Survival after stroke and transient ischemic attacks during the 1970's and 1980's. *Stroke* 1990; 21: 848–853.
29. Ricci S, Cantisani AT, Righetti E, Duca E, Spizzichino L. Long-term follow-up of TIA's: the SEPIVAC Study. *Neuroepidemiology* 1998; 17: 54.
30. Dennis M, Bamford J, Sandercock P, Warlow C. Prognosis of transient ischaemic attacks in the Oxfordshire Community Stroke Project. *Stroke* 1990; 21: 1320–1326.
31. Hankey GJ. Long-term outcome after ischaemic stroke/Transient ischaemic attack. *Cerebrovasc Dis* 2003; 16(Suppl 1): 14–19.
32. Hankey GJ, Slattery JM, Warlow CP. The prognosis of hospital-referred transient ischaemic attacks. *J Neurol Neurosurg Psychiatry* 1991; 54: 793–802.
33. Clark TG, Murphy MFG, Rothwell PM. Long term risks of stroke, myocardial infarction, and vascular death in "low risk" patients with a non-recent transient ischaemic attack. *J Neurol Neurosurg Psychiatry* 2003; 74: 577–580.
34. Van Wijk I, Kappelle LJ, van Gijn J, Koudstaal PJ, Franke CL, Vermeulen M, Gorter JW, Algra A, for the LILAC study group. Long-term survival and vascular event risk after transient ischaemic attack or minor stroke: A cohort study. *Lancet* 2005; 365: 2098–2104.
35. Johnston SC, Nguyen-Huynh MN, Schwarz ME *et al.* National Stroke Association guidelines for the management of transient ischemic attacks. *Ann Neurol* 2006; 60: 301–313.
36. Albucher JF, Martel P, Mas JL. Clinical practice guidelines: diagnosis and immediate management of transient ischemic attacks in adults. *Cerebrovasc Dis* 2005; 20: 220–225.
37. Nguyen-Huynh MN, Johnston SC. Is hospitalization after TIA cost-effective on the basis of treatment with tPA? *Neurology* 2005; 65: 1799–1801.
38. Hankey GJ, Slattery JM, Warlow CP. Transient ischaemic attacks: which patients are at high (and low) risk of serious vascular events? *J Neurol Neurosurg Psychiatry* 1992; 55: 640–652.

39. Kernan WN, Viscoli CM, Brass LM *et al.* The stroke prognosis instrument II (SPI-II): a clinical prediction instrument for patients with transient ischemia and nondisabling ischemic stroke. *Stroke* 2000; 31: 456–462.
40. Hill MD, Yiannakoulias N, Jeerakathil T *et al.* The high risk of stroke immediately after transient ischemic attack. A population-based study. *Neurology* 2004; 62: 2015–2020.
41. Gladstone DJ, Kapral MK, Fang J *et al.* Management and outcomes of transient ischaemic attacks in Ontario. *CMAJ* 2004; 1707: 1099–1104.
42. Rothwell PM, Giles MF, Flossman E *et al.* A simple score (ABCD) to identify individuals at high early risk of stroke after transient ischaemic attack. *Lancet* 2005; 366: 29–36.
43. Johnston SC, Rothwell PM, Nguyen-Huynh MN *et al.* Validation and refinement of scores to predict very early stroke risk after transient ischaemic attack. *Lancet* 2007; 369: 283–292.
44. Giles MF, Rothwell PM. Systematic review and meta-analysis of validations of the ABCD and ABCD2 scores in prediction of stroke risk after transient ischaemic attack. *Cereborvasc Dis* 2008; 25(Suppl 2): 59.
45. Lovett JK, Coull AJ, Rothwell PM. Early risk of recurrence by subtype of ischemic stroke in population-based incidence studies. *Neurology* 2004; 62: 569–573.
46. Fairhead JF, Mehta Z, Rothwell PM. Population-based study of delays in carotid imaging and surgery and the risk of recurrent stroke. *Neurology* 2005; 65: 371–375.
47. Ois A, Gomis M, Rodríguez-Campello A, Cuadrado-Godia E, Jiménez-Conde J, Pont-Sunyer C, Cuccurella G, Roquer J. Factors associated with a high risk of recurrence in patients with transient ischemic attack or minor stroke. *Stroke* 2008; 39: 1717–1721.
48. Calvet D, Touzé E, Oppenheim C, Turc G, Meder JF, Mas JL. DWI lesions and TIA etiology improve the prediction of stroke after TIA. *Stroke* 2009; 40: 187–192.
49. van Swieten JC, Kappelle LJ, Algra A, van Latum JC *et al.* for the Dutch TIA Study Group. Hypodensity of cerebral white matter in patients with transient ischaemic attack or minor stroke: influence on the rate of subsequent stroke. *Ann Neurol* 1992; 32: 177–183.
50. Sciolla R, Melis F, SINPAC Group. Rapid identification of high-risk transient ischemic attacks: prospective validation of the ABCD score. *Stroke* 2008; 39: 297–302.

51. Douglas VC, Johnston CM, Elkins J *et al.* Head computed tomography findings predict short-term stroke risk after transient ischemic attack. *Stroke* 2003; 34: 2894–2898.

52. Schulz UG, Briley D, Meagher T *et al.* Diffusion-weighted MRI in 300 patients presenting late with subacute transient ischemic attack or minor stroke. *Stroke* 2004; 35: 2459–2465.

53. Oppenheim C, Lamy C, Touzé E *et al.* Do transient ischemic attacks with diffusion-weighted imaging abnormalities correspond to brain infarctions? *AJNR Am J Neuroradiol* 2006; 27: 1782–1787.

54. Purroy F, Montaner J, Rovira A *et al.* Higher risk of further vascular events among transient ischemic attack patients with diffusion-weighted imaging acute ischemic lesions. *Stroke* 2004; 35: 2313–2319.

55. Coutts SB, Simon JE, Eliasziw M *et al.* Triaging transient ischemic attack and minor stroke patients using acute magnetic resonance imaging. *Ann Neurol* 2005; 57: 848–854.

56. Wen HM, Lam WW, Rainer T *et al.* Multiple acute cerebral infarcts on diffusion-weighted imaging and risk of recurrent stroke. *Neurology* 2004; 63: 1317–1319.

57. Sylaja PN, Coutts SB, Subramaniam S *et al.* Acute ischemic lesions of varying ages predict risk of ischemic events in stroke/TIA patients. *Neurology* 2007; 68: 415–419.

58. Crisostomo RA, Garcia MM, Tong DC. Detection of diffusion-weighted MRI abnormalities in patients with transient ischemic attack: correlation with clinical characteristics. *Stroke* 2003; 34: 932–937.

59. Redgrave JN, Coutts SB, Schulz UG *et al.* Systematic review of associations between the presence of acute ischemic lesions on diffusion-weighted imaging and clinical predictors of early stroke risk after transient ischemic attack. *Stroke* 2007; 38: 1482–1488.

60. Flossmann E, Rothwell PM. Prognosis of vertebrobasilar transient ischaemic attack and minor stroke. *Brain* 2003; 126: 1940–1954.

61. Flossmann E, Touze E, Giles MF, Lovelock CE, Rothwell PM. The early risk of stroke after vertebrobasilar TIA is higher than after carotid TIA. *Cerebrovascular Dis* 2006; 219(Suppl 4): 6.

62. Marquardt L, Kuker W, Chandratheva A, Geraghty O, Rothwell PM. Incidence and prognosis of ≥50% symptomatic vertebral or basilar artery stenosis: prospective population-based study. *Brain* 2009; 132: 982–988.

63. Hackam DG, Spence JD. Combining multiple approaches for the secondary prevention of vascular events after stroke: a quantitative modeling study. *Stroke* 2007; 38: 1881–1885.

64. Rothwell PM, Giles MF, Chandratheva A *et al.* On behalf of the Early use of Existing Preventive Strategies for Stroke (EXPRESS) Study. Major reduction in risk of early recurrent stroke by urgent treatment of TIA and minor stroke: EXPRESS Study. *Lancet* 2007; 370: 1432–1442.

65. Lavallée PC, Meseguer E, Abboud H *et al.* A transient ischaemic attack clinic with round-the-clock access (SOS-TIA): feasibility and effects. *Lancet Neurol* 2007; 6: 953–960.

66. Luengo-Fernandez R, Gray AM, Rothwell PM. Effect of urgent treatment for transient ischaemic attack and minor stroke on disability and hospital costs (EXPRESS study): A prospective population-based sequential comparison. *Lancet Neurol* 2009; 8: 235–243.

67. Sprigg N, Machili C, Otter ME, Wilson A, Robinson T. A systematic review of delays in seeking medical attention after transient ischaemic attack. *J Neurol Neurosurg Psychiatry* 2009; 80: 871–875.

68. Giles MF, Flossman E, Rothwell PM. Patient behavior immediately after transient ischemic attack according to clinical characteristics, perception of the event, and predicted risk of stroke. *Stroke* 2006; 37: 1254–1260.

69. Maasland L, Koudstaal PJ, Habbema JD, Dippel DW. Knowledge and understanding of disease process, risk factors and treatment modalities in patients with a recent TIA or minor ischemic stroke. *Cerebrovasc Dis* 2007; 23: 435–440.

70. Ferro JM, Falcão I, Rodrigues G, Canhão P, Melo TP, Oliveira V, Pinto AN, Crespo M, Salgado AV. Diagnosis of transient ischemic attack by the non-neurologist. A validation study. *Stroke* 1996; 27: 2225–2229.

71. Kraaijeveld CL, van Gijn J, Schouten HJ, Staal A. Interobserver agreement for the diagnosis of transient ischemic attacks. *Stroke* 1984; 15: 723–725.

72. Josephson SA, Sidney S, Pham TN, Bernstein AL, Johnston SC. Higher ABCD2 score predicts patients most likely to have true transient ischemic attack. *Stroke* 2008; 39: 3096–3098.

73. Quinn TJ, Cameron AC, Dawson J, Lees KR, Walters MR. ABCD2 scores and prediction of non-cerebrovascular diagnoses in an outpatient population: a case-control study. *Stroke* 2009; 40: 749–753.

74. Dawson J, Lamb KE, Quinn TJ, Lees KR, Horvers M, Verrijth MJ, Walters MR. A recognition tool for transient ischaemic attack. *QJM* 2009; 102: 43–49.
75. Prabhakaran S, Sliver AJ, Warrior L, McClenathan B, Lee VH. Misdiagnosis of transient ischemic attacks in the emergency room. *Cerebrovasc Dis* 2008; 26: 630–636.

4 Early Identification and Presentation to Hospital

Helen Rodgers* and Chris Price*

Chapter Summary

There are many points along the pathway from the onset of symptoms to stroke unit admission where it is possible to improve timely and appropriate access to specialist assessment and treatment. To optimise emergency care following stroke, it is important to look across all elements of the pathway, including the health-seeking behaviour of patients and witnesses at the onset of symptoms, and the factors which will enable pre-hospital and hospital services to deliver a coordinated rapid response.

Although the public may be aware of the symptoms of stroke and regard stroke as a medical emergency, unfortunately less than half of stroke patients recognise that they are having a stroke at the onset of symptoms and one of the delays in receiving emergency care is failure to seek immediate medical help. Mass media campaigns have been shown to increase public awareness of stroke symptoms but their impact upon health-seeking behaviour at the onset of symptoms remains unclear. Improved understanding of why stroke patients do or do not seek immediate medical help is needed to develop strategies and interventions to change behaviour at the onset of symptoms.

*Institute for Ageing and Health, Newcastle University Medical School, Newcastle upon Tyne NE2 4HH, UK

Pre-hospital and hospital emergency services need to work closely together in order to deliver an effective service. Each need to ensure that they have the skills and systems in place to be able to rapidly identify and prioritise stroke patients. This will involve training programmes, protocols, audit and feedback for ambulance, primary care and hospital teams. Validated screening tools such as the FAST test may improve recognition of stroke by emergency services and enable rapid access to a stroke unit and faster clinical and radiological assessment upon hospital arrival. However, as any screening tool will have false positive and false negative cases, careful clinical assessment upon hospital arrival is needed to identify stroke mimics and atypical presentations of stroke.

The pre-hospital emergency response must be matched by the emergency response upon hospital arrival. Hospitals who receive acute stroke patients should have systems in place to identify patients who require hyperacute interventions such as thrombolysis or urgent surgical intervention, whilst all suspected stroke admissions should have early access to a specialist service.

Introduction

Rapid assessment to a specialist stroke service enables accurate diagnosis; access to acute treatment and multidisciplinary care; neurological, cardiovascular and physiological monitoring; prevention and identification of complications; and early implementation of secondary prevention. Avoiding delay in accessing a specialist service is the most important priority for pre-hospital stroke care. In order to achieve this, patients and witnesses need to be aware that a rapid response to the symptoms of stroke is required and pre-hospital and acute services need to be well organised to provide a coordinated and timely response.

Public Awareness and Response to Acute Stroke

Early recognition and immediate response to the symptoms of stroke by patients and/or witnesses is key to improving access to thrombolysis and acute stroke care. A major cause of delay of admission to hospital following stroke is because the patient and/or witness does not seek immediate help from the emergency services at the onset of symptoms. The delay from symptom onset to presentation is 2–3 times longer for stroke compared to acute coronary syndrome.[1]

There may be a number of reasons why patients and/or witnesses do not contact emergency services immediately, including demography, neurological deficit, cognitive and emotional issues, and lack of awareness about stroke and available treatment.[1,2] Unlike myocardial infarction, age, sex and educational level have not been found to be associated with pre-hospital delay following stroke in most studies. Perception of the severity of symptoms may be a factor in deciding whether or not to contact emergency services as patients with severe stroke or loss of consciousness are more likely to be admitted to hospital quicker.

Knowledge of the symptoms of stroke varies between studies depending upon the population studied and how questions were asked, e.g. open ended or multiple choice, but results from UK studies suggest that the majority of the public were aware of at least one common symptom of stroke such as unilateral weakness of speech disturbance.[3,4] However, being able to recall the symptoms of stroke does not necessarily mean that an individual will be able to recognise them when they occur. Less than 50% of stroke patients recognise they are having a stroke at the onset of symptoms.[5–7] Surprisingly, recognition that symptoms were due to stroke does not reduce the time of presentation to admission.[5,8,9]

There is a disparity between what people say they would do if they had a stroke and what actually happens in practice.[7] Although studies report that the majority of members of the public feel that stroke is an emergency and they would seek immediate medical help if they experienced a stroke, in practice this does not always happen. This may be for a number of reasons, including inability to seek help because of the severity of symptoms or speech disturbance; waiting to see if symptoms resolve; perceiving symptoms as non-serious or urgent; reticence to call for help; and lack of awareness about the availability and benefit of acute treatment. Patients who are alone at the onset of symptoms may not be able to seek help but a number of patients who are able to seek help for themselves initially contact a friend, relative or their general practitioner and this can result in a significant delay to admission. When a family member or witness is present an emergency response is more likely.[7] Further research is needed to improve understanding of why stroke patients do or do not delay in seeking immediate help from emergency service at the onset of symptoms. There is a need to improve not only public knowledge of stroke but also to change behaviour at the onset of symptoms.

Mass Media Campaigns

Effective mass media or educational campaigns should be able to demonstrate improvement in a number of outcomes, including increased awareness of stroke symptoms and the need for an emergency response; increased use of emergency services; reduced time between onset of symptoms and arrival to hospital; and increased use of thrombolysis. Prior to introducing a campaign, stroke services should ensure that they are able to respond to this increased demand and raised expectations.

Mass media campaigns are complex intervention and ideally development and evaluation should follow a structured framework such as the one developed by the Medical Research Council (Fig. 1).[10]

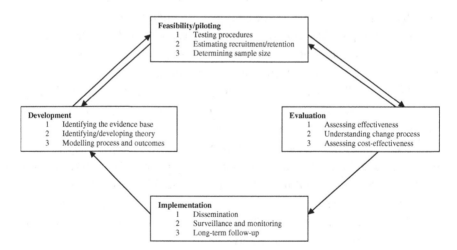

Figure 1. Key elements of the development and evaluation process of complex interventions.

Source: Craig P, Dieppe P, Macintyre S, Michie S, Nazareth I, Petticrew M *et al*. Developing and evaluating complex interventions: the new Medical Research Council guidance. *Br Med J* 2008; 337: a1655.[10]

However, mass media campaigns have rarely been rigorously developed or evaluated. Robust designs include randomised trials, controlled clinical trials, controlled before and after studies and interrupted time series analyses. A recent Cochrane review looking at the effect of mass media interventions upon health service utilisation for a number of conditions identified a total of 20 studies.[11] Grilli *et al.* concluded 'Despite the limited information about key aspects of mass media interventions and the poor quality of the available primary research, there is evidence that these channels of communication may have an important role in influencing the use of healthcare interventions.'

There have been two controlled before and after studies to evaluate campaigns on improving the emergency response to the symptoms of stroke, one from Ontario, Canada and the other from Houston, US.[12–14]

The Canadian campaign had three intervention and one control communities.[12] The intervention communities received either high or low intensity TV advertising or newspaper advertising. The television advertising consisted of a 30-second black and white television advertisement giving the warning signs of a stroke and the print advertisement was based upon the television advert. A telephone poll was undertaken prior to implementation (1999) and three-month post-intervention (2001) in each community using random digit dialling. Approximately 400 respondents in each community were asked 'Can you tell me what warning signs people might experience when they have had a stroke?' A separate sample was used for before and after interviews. The ability to name the warning signs of stroke increased in the two communities who received the television advertising. Intermittent low level television advertising was as effective as continuous high level advertising. The newspaper advertising campaign had no impact and for reasons that were unclear there was a decrease in knowledge in the control population. Importantly, television advertising did not increase knowledge of stroke symptoms in those aged 65 or over, which is the age group who are at greatest risk of stroke and who are most likely to be a witness at the time of stroke. The impact of the campaign upon health-seeking behaviour following stroke was not assessed.

The Texas study used a controlled before-and-after design with matched hospitals in two communities.[13,14] The before phase was undertaken between

February 1998 and October 1998 and the after phase from January 1999 until March 2000. There were five hospitals which admitted stroke patients in each community. The intervention was aimed at influencing both health professionals and the public in order to 'change stroke identification skills, outcome expectations and the community norms of community residents.' The intervention was developed systematically and the local community was involved in identifying issues which may cause delayed admission. The mass media approach included billboard, radio, and television advertising and news stories. Brochures and posters were also produced. Volunteers were trained in stroke recognition and community figures were involved in promoting the importance of calling 911 at the onset of symptoms and the benefits of hyperacute treatment. The advertising campaign also encouraged patients and their families to ask for recombinant tissue-type plasminogen activator (rTPA) treatment. In addition to the advertising campaign, services were reorganised in the intervention community to improve access to thrombolysis. This was accompanied by individual contact, development of guidelines, newsletters and feedback, and an education programme for primary care physicians, acute care physicians and neurologists. Thrombolysis rates for all stroke patients increased from 1.4% to 5.8% in the intervention community compared with 0.5–0.6% in the control community. The benefits were sustained three months after the intervention period. However, it would appear that increased thrombolysis rates were due to a change in professional behaviours and service reorganisation as there was no difference in the time from onset of symptoms to presentation in hospital, although the delay time to hospital presentation decreased significantly in both communities. The study did not measure stroke awareness.

Other studies have evaluated the effect of mass media campaigns but have used less robust deign, e.g. uncontrolled before-and-after studies, making it difficult to be certain if changes in knowledge or behaviour can be directly attributed to the intervention.

Strategies to Improve Professional Awareness

The prompt arrival of stroke patients at an appropriate unit is dependent upon the efficient communication of accurate clinical information between community and hospital professionals from different disciplines. Consequently the American Heart Association recommends that 'education of Emergency Medical Services (EMS) personnel should be provided on a regular basis, perhaps as often as twice per year, to ensure proper recognition, field treatment and delivery of patients to appropriate facilities.'[15] Although services will benefit from developing a comprehensive training strategy, the resources required to provide high quality learning opportunities should not be underestimated. During preparation educators should carefully consider the knowledge and skills appropriate for different roles and include an overview of the whole emergency response to stroke so that learners appreciate the overall context. Traditional classroom-based training may not be an efficient way to maintain current knowledge amongst a very large workforce committed to shift working. This has led to the development of convenient online learning and assessment.[16] Physical examination and communication skills can be learnt in a way more directly transferable to clinical practice during interactive simulation-enhanced courses.[17]

It is also very important that training is not perceived as redundant, i.e. resulting actions are not met by a matching response from the next link in the chain of assessment. For example, a study undertaken in North Carolina reported that a lack of improvement in stroke identification performance after paramedic training was due to their perception that receiving emergency departments had not changed their response accordingly.[18] As suspected stroke is only a small component of emergency services workload, positive feedback to paramedic teams and individuals by post or email directly from the stroke service may overcome misconceptions that their actions have no impact.[19]

In spite of public awareness campaigns, some patients with recent stroke symptoms will continue to present to primary care or directly to emergency departments. Due to delayed presentation and milder deficits, these patients are less likely to benefit from hyperacute care technologies, but it is still appropriate that they have rapid assessment of their secondary prevention needs. Therefore, general practitioners, receptionists and emergency department triage staff should also be able to systematically screen for common symptoms and signs. Such training should not focus solely on knowledge but also explain the implications of assessment and treatments available. A survey of primary care physicians which used clinical case scenarios found that although knowledge of stroke was good, only two-thirds would admit patients with very recent symptoms as an emergency, and even fewer when initial contact was by phone rather than attendance in person.[20] There is no simple explanation for the gap between knowledge and action, but influences include: the views of the patient (who already has not selected an emergency response); a focus on impact of symptoms rather than appreciation of the immediate risk implications; commitment to establishing a diagnosis before referral to a specialty; and distance to the stroke unit. High quality training should consider these additional factors in order to achieve maximum impact.

Early Transfer to Stroke Units

Identification of stroke symptoms

Stroke begins with the sudden onset of stereotypical neurological symptoms whose detection — even without understanding the implications — is the initial vital step in the American Heart Association's 'stroke chain of survival' (Table 1).[21]

As a population of 1 million people can generate up to 400 calls to emergency medical services per day, it is a challenge to accurately and rapidly identify those six patients who, on average, will have suffered a stroke.[22] Many presentations are complicated by speech and cognitive impairments, symptoms which are purely subjective, pre-existing disability and unexpected circumstantial factors at onset. Therefore identification is facilitated by a consistent approach to information collection

Table 1.   Stroke chain of survival

1. Detection	Recognition of stroke signs and symptoms
2. Dispatch	Call 911 and priority EMS dispatch
3. Delivery	Prompt transport and pre-hospital notification to hospital
4. Door	Immediate Emergency Department (ED) triage
5. Data	ED evaluation, prompt laboratory studies, and CT imaging
6. Decision	Diagnosis and decision about appropriate therapy
7. Drug	Administration of appropriate drugs or other interventions

which focused upon the most reliable features of common presentations. When left to unstructured clinical judgement by non-specialists, success in identifying stroke patients is much less likely. For instance, in Copenhagen, it was found that only 30% of patients thought to have suffered a stroke or TIA when seen by critical care physicians in a Mobile Emergency Care Unit were confirmed in hospital.[23] Consequently there are strong recommendations that emergency services should use a validated screening tool based upon typical presentations of stroke, which can then be the gateway to a comprehensive pre-hospital protocol and facilitate audit of urgent response.[24,25]

An ideal screening tool should be specific as well as sensitive, but the variable nature of stroke presentations and similarities to common mimics makes this a difficult balance without demanding a degree of expert knowledge and intensity of assessment, which could make identification of stroke an unattractive priority for emergency medical personnel. Screening tools should also be easy to remember and quick to perform, as many patients have their first contact with a stroke care provider through regional ambulance services for whom suspected stroke typically generates only 2% of overall activity. Rather than speeding up hospital transfer, it has been shown that implementation of stroke screening by paramedics may actually increase the length of time taken from call to hospital arrival by several minutes due to the application of the screening test itself and the resulting protocol-driven actions.[25] The main benefits of pre-hospital identification are faster clinical and radiological assessment in the emergency department after arrival[26] and transport directly to a hyperacute stroke unit should local conditions favour a redirection model.

In the UK, the most commonly used screening tool for stroke symptoms is the Face Arm Speech Test (FAST) (Table 2),[27] which is a refinement of the Cincinnati Prehospital Stroke Scale (CPSS).[28] The 'T' of 'Test' is now often interpreted as 'Time' in order to remind users about the urgency of admission and to prompt ascertaining when symptoms first began or when the patient was last known to be without symptoms. It is important to note that the nature of stroke related impairments combined with features of the population who are at risk, such as social isolation and cognitive impairment, prevents documentation of a reliable onset time for 20–38% of cases.[29,30] Patients who wake up with symptoms should have

Table 2.   Face, arm, speech test (FAST) instructions

Facial Movements

Ask patient to show teeth.

- Is there an unequal smile or grimace?
- Note which side does not move well.

Arm Movements

Lift the patient's arms together to 90° if sitting, 45° if supine.
Ask them to hold the position for 5 seconds before letting go.

- Does one arm drift down or fall rapidly?
- If one arm drifts down or falls, note whether it is the patient's left or right.

Speech

Listen for *new* disturbance of speech.

- Listen for slurred speech.
- Listen for word-finding difficulties with hesitations. This can be confirmed by asking the patient to name objects that may be nearby, such as a cup or chair.
- Check with any person who knows the patient.

---

their onset time backdated to the time they last went to sleep without symptoms, which can require precise questioning and reference to orientation materials such as television and radio broadcasting schedules.

Other screening tools have been developed such as the Los Angeles Prehospital Stroke Screen (LAPSS)[31] and the Melbourne Ambulance Stroke Screen (MASS)[32] (Table 3). They are all very similar to each other but with variations due to the assessment of speech disturbance and grip strength,[33] and inclusion of history elements which might refine diagnosis or help identify a subgroup more likely to be suitable for thrombolysis.[32] All tests tend to favour identification of anterior circulation stroke as posterior circulation symptoms such as dizziness and bilateral in-coordination are common features of vestibular and cardiovascular conditions, which would significantly reduce the specificity of the test. Sensory symptoms are less reliable than motor symptoms due to the difficulty of objective confirmation and the strong association with mimics such as migraine and peripheral nerve lesions. Other screening features found to have no value in the prediction of a final diagnosis of stroke include vomiting, headache, confusion and loss of consciousness.[34]

Table 3. Summary of pre-hospital stroke screening assessments

Test	History	Examination
Cincinnati Prehospital Stroke Scale (CPSS)	None	Facial droop Arm drift Speech abnormal
Los Angeles Prehospital Stroke Screen (LAPSS)	Age > 45 years Seizures history Dependency Blood glucose	Facial asymmetry Arm weakness Hand grip
Face Arm Speech Test (FAST)	None	Facial palsy Arm weakness Speech problems
Melbourne Ambulance Stroke Screen (MASS)	Age > 45 years Seizures history Dependency Blood glucose	Facial droop Arm drift Hand grip Speech problems

In clinical practice, the tests are not as straightforward as they might first appear, as collection of the necessary information — particularly history elements — can be challenging in the unpredictable conditions of emergency scenarios outside of hospital. It is also difficult to make direct comparisons between screening tools as they were constructed and validated in different healthcare settings, supported by variable degrees of training. Even when the same screening test has been used by different ambulance services, very variable balances between sensitivity and specificity have been reported.

When used in its original setting by paramedics as part of a rapid access stroke protocol for 178 unselected patients, the FAST had a positive predictive value for stroke of 78% and an upper estimation of sensitivity of 79%.[27] When examined again in the same setting, according to real-time data the FAST had a sensitivity of 54%, specificity of 91%, positive predictive value of 88% and negative predictive value of 64%.[34] Out of 477 patients in San Diego assessed using the CPSS, 193 had a final discharge diagnosis of stroke, resulting in a sensitivity of 44% and a positive predictive value of 40%.[35] During the development of the CPSS, scoring of any single item by paramedics had shown a sensitivity of 59% and specificity of 89%.[28]

Performance of the LAPSS across all dispatches during the original study period was reported with a sensitivity of 86%, specificity 99%, positive predictive value of 86% and negative predictive value of 99%.[33] These impressive figures have not been repeated and may reflect a study methodology which included the exclusion of comatose and TIA patients, as well as the considerable effort made by the developers to train and certify paramedics in scale application. In Houston, the introduction of the LAPSS as part of a larger stroke awareness initiative was associated with a more modest improvement in the positive predictive value for paramedic stroke prediction from 61% to 79%.[25] An unblinded assessor completing a LAPSS score retrospectively during the validation of the ROSIER score (see below) reported a sensitivity of 59% and specificity of 85%.[34]

When MASS training was given to 18 paramedics, their accuracy for identifying stroke patients improved from a baseline level of 78% to 94%, whereas other paramedics did not show a significant change.[32] In a small study of clinical practice, the MASS had a positive predictive value of 90% compared to 93% for LAPSS and 85% for CPSS, with negative predictive values of 74%, 59% and 79% respectively.[36] These reports reflect how training can influence the decision of when to apply a screening tool as well as how to use it, the impact of variations in healthcare provision, and methodological issues such as certainty about the robustness of the final stroke diagnosis denominator. Rather than assuming that a particular screening test will perform the same as in the original published description, it is very important that its local use is audited after implementation.

A feature of pre-hospital screening tools is the apparent lack of advantage provided by medical training. Paramedics may even demonstrate better performance than primary care and emergency room doctors. During validation of the FAST, paramedics were correct more often (positive predictive value of 78%) than primary care doctors and emergency room doctors (positive predictive value for both of 71%).[27] It has been speculated that paramedics are better at applying protocol led clinical assessment and less distracted by the extraneous information that medical history and examination might reveal. However, it is also likely that medical staff both in the community and emergency room see more atypical presentations and complicated scenarios. For example, during the FAST validation it was observed that paramedics were more likely to admit total anterior circulation strokes than lacunar stroke, whereas doctors were more likely to see presentations later diagnosed as deteriorating dementia and metabolic abnormalities. An observational study from Australia reported that when a medical review in the community triggered a call to the ambulance service because of suspected stroke, those patients were more likely to be older, in residential care and with pre-existing medical conditions.[26]

It should be remembered that pre-hospital screening assessments were developed within well-organised services which may already have raised awareness of stroke symptoms amongst pre-hospital providers because of established operational protocols. It is unclear whether they can maintain their original performance if public awareness campaigns result in more patients with suspected stroke bypassing a medical review before admission. The balance may tip towards greater sensitivity but less specificity, and secondary care teams will have to be prepared to provide an opinion for more patients who do not turn out to have stroke as their primary diagnosis.

Transfer to hospital

There is no doubt that ambulance transportation is associated with quicker arrival at hospital. The largest stroke register in North America, the Paul Coverdell National Acute Stroke Registry, reported that fewer non-ambulance patients (36.2%) arrived within two hours of symptom onset compared with patients transported by ambulance (56.8%).[37] During transport of a patient with possible stroke or TIA to hospital, paramedics should continue to monitor their condition and select the destination according to locally agreed protocols. There is a lack of evidence supporting any specific interventions for stroke during this time, although recommendations exist on the basis of consensus opinion.[38] Table 4 summarises recommendations and practical action points during transportation.

Table 4.   Paramedic response to suspected acute stroke

Documentation
Stroke screening assessment (e.g. FAST)
Onset time (indicate if not known)
Glasgow Coma Score

Actions
If conscious sit up
Remain nil by mouth
Blood glucose reading
Start intravenous saline fluids if hypotensive
Give oxygen if peripheral saturations < 95%
Select destination according to protocol
Pre-notify emergency department

Information
Bring all medications
Enquire about dependency, drug history and medical history
Encourage an informant to accompany the patient or obtain
    telephone number

There is very good evidence that hospital pre-notification speeds up door-doctor and door-imaging times, so this should be included in all stroke response protocols.[26] If appropriate for regional geography and population distribution, studies have reported that registering suspected stroke as a trigger for helicopter dispatch as part of a service improvement programme can improve the speed of arrival at hospital.[39,40] Although projected increases in thrombolysis treatment rates could possibly reduce combined stroke-related health and social care costs,[41] to be affordable this resource would have to be available on the basis that regional circumstances support the general use of air ambulance transport. No direct comparison has been made to a traditional ground response, which generally report favourable call to door times between 30 and 50 minutes on average.

Identification in hospital

Upon arrival at hospital, patients should be urgently assessed by medical staff to confirm the diagnosis, liaising with the stroke team if stroke cannot be quickly excluded. Stroke mimics are, however, very common. In a prospective study of 350 suspected stroke patients referred by emergency services to an established teaching hospital stroke unit, 109 (31%) had a definite (19%) or probable (12%) alternative diagnosis.[42] Many of these were neurological conditions (seizures, tumours, migraine) or the specific combination of previous stroke and sepsis. Mimics were more common if the National Institute of Health (NIH) Stroke Scale was low or if it was not possible to categorise according to the Oxford Community Stroke Project classification (i.e. symptoms did not fit with a typical vascular territory). Lateralising signs in the absence of cognitive impairment were much more reliable. The proportion of definite stroke mimics reported in other settings has ranged from 1.2% to 29% according to the selection of cases, the criteria used for stroke diagnosis and whether the setting was community or specialism focused.[43–45] Overall as many as 1 in 3 referrals for suspected stroke may have an alternative diagnosis despite pre-hospital screening (Table 5). The exclusion of mimics can require a very detailed medical history, repeated examination, laboratory investigations, observation and often additional brain imaging. This is a significant factor to consider when planning local hyperacute services.

Unwitnessed seizures and delirium due to sepsis should be considered in patients with a surprisingly low conscious level for the extent of their focal neurological deficit. Initially it can be very difficult to identify first presentations of acephalgic migraine and somatisation, but the absence of vascular risk factors, previous history of unexplained symptoms and dominance of positive sensory symptoms should increase suspicions that stroke is not the explanation. A diagnosis of stroke will always be more likely if the time can be identified when there was a clear change in the objective focal neurological status of the patient, especially if they have never previously had a neurological diagnosis but do have at least one vascular risk factor.

In order to increase sensitivity to the neurological features of stroke and systematically exclude the most common stroke mimics in emergency departments, the Recognition of Stroke In the Emergency Room (ROSIER) score was developed for use by emergency room staff (Table 6).[34] A score > 0 indicates a high probability of stroke (positive predictive value 90% and negative predictive value 88%) and should trigger specialist team

Table 5. Common stroke mimics and characteristics

Cause	Useful features
Seizures	Previous episodes. Low GCS considering size of focal deficit. Improvement.
Syncope (and cerebral hypoperfusion)	Witnessed. Poor recall. Features improve with volume expansion.
Sepsis (especially after previous stroke)	Fluctuating neurological features. Raised inflammatory markers. Insidious onset.
Sugar (hypoglycaemia and hyperglycaemia)	Disorientated/drowsy with minimal weakness. Medication and past history.
Severe migraine (without headache)	Previous episodes of neurological migraine. Progressive symptoms.
Somatisation	Inconsistent signs. Low vascular risk. History of other unexplained symptoms.
Space occupying lesion	Sub-acute onset. Previous primary tumour. Papilloedema.
Subdural (including unwitnessed falls)	Fluctuating signs. Disorientated/drowsy. Frequent faller. No sepsis.
Single nerve injury (including Bell's palsy)	Sensorimotor deficit in isolated nerve. Dermatomal and lower motor features.
Sclerosis (demyelination)	Previous episodes in different vascular territories. Sub-acute onset.

Table 6. ROSIER score

A total score > 0 indicates high probability of a stroke diagnosis	Yes	No
Has there been loss of consciousness or syncope?	−1	0
Has there been seizure activity?	−1	0
Has there been new acute onset (including on wakening from sleep) of the following:		
Asymmetric facial weakness	+1	0
Asymmetric arm weakness	+1	0
Asymmetric leg weakness	+1	0
Speech disturbance	+1	0
Visual field deficit	+1	0

involvement. It should be remembered that a blood glucose measurement is required for the ROSIER score to be valid and the total is only as trustworthy as the sources used to obtain the necessary information. Supported by training, local ROSIER performance may be adequate to justify initiation of a thrombolysis protocol, direct admission to a stroke unit and brain imaging ahead of specialist review.

In the future, biomarkers may help identify the cause of a stroke (e.g. cardioembolism) but they are currently in developmental stage and may not be of any value in confirming an immediate diagnosis compared to rapid clinical and radiological assessment.[46]

If symptoms completely resolve then patients should not be discharged without considering whether stroke or TIA was the correct initial diagnosis, immediate risk of recurrence, further investigations and secondary prevention. This will often still require review by the local stroke service before discharge or at least urgent referral through an established system according to risk stratification.

In summary, it is important to remember that acute stroke is generally a clinical diagnosis, and in many cases the use of a screening tool by paramedics appears to be equivalent to a pre-hospital non-specialist medical review. FAST remains a very useful quick screening assessment for common presentations — especially those that might be suitable for thrombolysis — with specificity being boosted in hospital by the ROSIER score. No test will be able to cover all possible presentations and patient groups. Thus the effectiveness of these tests will depend upon standardised training, audit and feedback.

Factors Influencing Early Recognition

Stroke presentation

There are clinical and circumstantial influences on the prompt presentation of patients following the onset of stroke symptoms. Severe stroke in a public place is likely to lead to rapid admission, but if unwitnessed, patients with sudden immobility, dysphasia and cognitive impairments may be unable to call for assistance. A witness is also important because patients themselves may be reluctant to call emergency medical services and in many cases only attend after encouragement.[47] It is not unusual for the person making the call to be a third party contacted by a witness for advice, which then prevents essential information being passed onto the dispatcher. It is important that the immediate witness makes contact with the emergency services and stays at the scene to provide paramedics with further information.

Ambulance dispatch

Whilst a lot of emphasis has been placed on paramedic assessment, the first contact with ambulance services is telephone triage by trained dispatchers. Increasingly computerised protocols are used to determine the urgency of dispatch. Until recently stroke did not trigger an immediate 'Category A' ambulance response in the UK unless the caller indicated that the patient might have a low conscious level. Prompts by newer dispatch software packages now guide the operator towards a label of suspected stroke so that patients with less severe presentations can be identified as a priority. Not surprisingly, telephone-based pathways are limited in their ability to identify stroke due to variations in patient presentation and the caller's ability to describe features which distinguish between low conscious level, cardiovascular collapse and confusion. However, they do demonstrate good specificity for straightforward presentations. In the UK, the sensitivity of advanced medical priority dispatch software for detecting stroke was 47% with a specificity of 98%[48] whilst in Los Angeles the dispatcher-assigned Medical Priority Dispatch System codes resulted in a sensitivity of 41% and specificity of 96%.[49] The same dispatch system in San Diego reported a sensitivity of 83% and a positive predictive value of 42%.[35] When dispatcher and paramedic agree on a likely diagnosis of stroke, the patient is more likely to arrive at hospital several minutes faster than if they disagree.[50] This may simply reflect the straightforward nature of those cases when telephone and bedside information is consistent and clearly indicative of stroke, but reaffirms the importance of having a pre-hospital stroke specific protocol.

Analysis of 911 tapes has shown that during the dispatch process, if the caller uses the word 'stroke' there is a greater probability of accurate identification, thus strengthening the case for public awareness campaigns.

Limb and facial weakness or impaired communication are the most reliable symptoms reported about a patient who is conscious.[51] It is important that dispatchers do not classify stroke patients with speech difficulties as 'altered mental status' or leg weakness as 'trouble walking' without attempting to gain more information from the caller.[52]

Pre-hospital protocols

Stroke-specific community protocols are also required to achieve maximum service efficiency. The main features should be: triggering by dispatcher suspicion of stroke, ambulance service response prioritisation, identification of stroke by paramedics, selection of appropriate hospital destination and pre-notification. Even though a pre-hospital medical review might reduce the probability that patients without stroke are directed inappropriately into a hyperacute stroke service, there is no doubt that waiting for this significantly delays hospital admission compared to a direct ambulance service response.[53] Whereas it has been a consistent finding that the involvement of ambulance services in the emergency response to stroke results in a faster medical and radiological assessment of patients when they arrive at the emergency department,[26,37] patients admitted after community medical review are less likely to have rapid brain imaging than those who arrived directly by ambulance.[30] As discussed above, this might reflect greater initial uncertainty about the diagnosis of stroke amongst patients who trigger a medical review before admission, such as subtle symptoms in frail elderly patients. This is unlikely to be a stroke specific observation and reflects differences between the systems set up to deal with the two patient groups and the sense of urgency which emergency department staff associate with different modes of admission.

When a protocol is introduced it should be accompanied by training and monitoring. In Houston it was demonstrated that a combination of education, implementation of a protocol based upon the Los Angeles Prehospital Stroke Scale and competitive benchmarking of performance between six hospitals resulted in an improvement in diagnostic accuracy from 61% to 79%,[25] with thrombolysis delivery across all sites increasing from 10.6% to 12% of total stroke admissions. A regional acute stroke protocol in a mixed urban-rural 20,000 km^2 area of Southeastern Ontario permitted paramedics to by-pass community hospitals without stroke specialists on the basis of their clinical assessment, resulting in 60% of acute stroke patients being redirected to a tertiary centre and a thrombolysis rate of 5.3% of the total regional stroke cases.[54] Both of these initiatives included rapid ambulance dispatch and hospital pre-notification.

Stroke service configuration

As well as providing clinical guidance, protocols should also contain instructions about the selection of hospital destination according to clinical assessment. This requires the analysis of local circumstances, such as geography, organisational distribution of stroke specialists, location of other neuroscience support services and the capacity for sites to assess and treat new patients and stroke mimics at anytime. Published thrombolysis performance figures suggest that overall service design does have an influence upon the early recognition of new cases of acute stroke.[55] Lower rates of treatment are reported by isolated providers who have not collaborated with other organisations compared to those who have reached a regional or sub-regional agreement on the assessment process for acute stroke. Crude comparison suggests that there is no difference in the efficiency of patient assessment for thrombolysis between services which use redirection or telemedicine. The key element appears to be the collaborative aspect, which is likely to be effective through a combination of improved service continuity, whole system staff awareness, training and clear protocols. It is interesting to note that telemedicine systems report less delays in arrival at the emergency department than redirection service designs,[56] but overall are not faster in delivering thrombolysis because of slower door to needle time. The latter may improve with training, protocols and experience, whereas travel times are unlikely to change.

Overall, it appears that multifaceted programmes containing protocols and training to standardise assessment and communication have the greatest effect on the rapid identification of stroke patients both before and after hospital admission (Table 7).[57]

Table 7. Components of a programme to facilitate stroke identification

Public awareness
Primary care education
Ambulance dispatcher training
Pre-hospital stroke protocol
Emergency department stroke protocol
Creation of acute stroke team in hospital
Training sensitive to professional roles
Audit of stroke recognition performance
Feedback to emergency medical services
Stroke service configuration review

Medical review

After arrival at hospital, stroke patients should be admitted as soon as possible to a unit with sufficient resources to offer hyperacute care. Patients without stroke who activated the pre-hospital protocol should also be quickly moved to a suitable environment for their needs. Although direct admission by ambulance to a stroke unit saves time, a rapid specialist review in the emergency department may be a better model for some settings, especially if there is no reliable spare capacity for a protected assessment bed or should patients need to move to a different hospital site because of a stroke mimic diagnosis. The creation of an 'acute stroke team' has been shown to facilitate reliable stroke recognition in the emergency department,[58] whilst hospital based 'Code Stroke' protocols reduce delays before medical review. Protocols can delegate tasks to be performed in parallel according to professional group[59] and avoid delays in thrombolysis delivery through inclusion of instructions such as no routine chest x-ray or coagulation screening unless specifically indicated.[60] A computerised physician order entry system has also been shown to improve the frequency and speed of thrombolysis delivery by alerting staff to the arrival of a potentially treatable patient in the emergency room and subsequently highlighting the relevant clinical, radiological and laboratory information.[61]

In summary, there are many points along the pathway from symptom onset to stroke unit admission where it may be possible to improve the speed and accuracy of diagnosis. There are considerable benefits, including rapid access to specialist assessment, priority imaging and the possibility of urgent treatments. It should not be assumed that implementation of tools and protocols developed elsewhere will generate service improvements without sensitivity to local factors or a significant investment in training, monitoring and feedback.

Location of Early Management

Home or hospital?

Although ten years previously the WHO recommended that all stroke patients should be admitted to hospital,[62] in the 1980s between 25–50% of stroke patients in the UK were not admitted to hospital.[63] There was a view that patients with acute stroke could be cared for at home as 'patients rarely need to be admitted for diagnostic or therapeutic reasons and rehabilitation given in hospital is sometimes inappropriate.'[64] In addition, some patients, particularly those who had a mild stroke or who required palliative care, preferred to remain at home.[65]

Services were established to provide 'hospital at home' for acute stroke patients as it was felt that they could provide care which was equivalent to or better than inpatient services at a lower cost. An alternative model that was developed around this time was early supported discharge, which enabled patients to receive rehabilitation from a specialist community stroke team following a short inpatient stay.[66]

The first controlled trial to evaluate a home care service for acute stroke patients was published in 1985.[67] The service was based in Bristol, UK, and consisted of a district nurse, physiotherapist, occupational therapist, speech and language therapist and social worker. The service was available for both patients who were initially admitted to hospital and those who remained at home and was provided during usual working hours for up to six months post-stroke. Medical care was provided by the patients' general practitioner. The study was not randomised and treatment allocation was according to general practice. Practices in the intervention group were able to refer patients to the new service as they felt appropriate. Unfortunately, the presence of the home care service did not influence admission practices with 66% of patients in the control group and 61% in the intervention group being admitted. Therefore despite recruiting 857 participants from 96 general practices, results were inconclusive as the efficacy of providing a service to enable patients with acute stroke to be cared for at home. The study highlights the challenges of implementing and evaluating changes in service delivery.

Despite American and European guidelines emphasising the importance of stroke unit care, the debate about the pros and cons of admitting stroke patients to hospital persisted. In 1999, a systematic review identified three trials (including the Bristol trial) and concluded that 'there was no evidence to support a radical shift in the care of acute stroke patients from hospital based care.'[68]

In 2000, the results of a landmark trial, which compared the efficacy of stroke unit care with a mobile stroke team and specialist stroke domiciliary care were published.[69] The community stroke team consisted of senior nurses and therapists with stroke expertise. Members of the team provided care to individual patients with support from district nursing and social services. A specialist medical registrar was also part of the team and the patients' GP and a consultant stroke physician shared responsibility for care. The service was available for up to three months. Each patient had an individualised integrated care pathway and weekly multidisciplinary meetings were held.[70] Investigations including CT head scan were undertaken as an outpatient.

Four hundred and fifty-seven patients with moderately severe strokes participated in the study, which was undertaken in Bromley, UK. One hundred and fifty-two were randomised to receive stroke unit care and 153 were randomised to receive domiciliary care. It was not always possible for patients to remain at home and 34% of those who initially received specialist domiciliary care were admitted to hospital within the first two weeks. Reasons included clinical deterioration, need for further investigation, care needs could not be met at home and request from patient or GP. These patients were admitted directly to the stroke unit.

The results of the study clearly demonstrate that following acute stroke, patients who are admitted to a stroke unit have better outcomes than those who remain at home and cared for by a specialist domiciliary team. At one year 24% of patients who were managed at home died or living in an institution compared with 14% of those who received stroke unit care.[70] The difference in mortality was striking. At three months 9.6% of patients who remained at home had died compared to 3.9% who received stroke unit care. The causes of excess mortality were infection, dehydration/renal failure, stroke extension and pulmonary embolism.

Patients who were not admitted to hospital were also more likely to have long-term disability. No differences were seen in levels of anxiety or depression. The costs per patient at one year were £6,840 for those who remained at home and £11,450 for those admitted to a stroke unit.

A further randomised controlled trial undertaken in Turin, Italy evaluated a hospital at home service. This study recruited 120 participants aged 70 and older. Those who were treated at home had lower rates of admission to nursing homes and were less depressed at six months. However, neither the inpatient nor outpatient care was provided by a specialist stroke service.[71]

Rapid admission to hospital following acute stroke is now viewed as an essential component of high quality care. This enables accurate diagnosis, treatment, monitoring and prevention of complications.

Emergency department or acute stroke unit?

Evidence-based practice has been a cornerstone of stroke service development,[72] but research evidence to identify the optimum place for assessment and treatment during the first few hours after stroke is limited. Current NICE guidance recommends that patients with a suspected stroke should be admitted directly to an acute stroke unit, although the authors do acknowledge that rapid admission to a stroke unit has not been shown to reduce mortality, morbidity or length of stay.[24] An acute stroke unit has the following features: policy for direct admission from emergency department/front door; continuous physiological monitoring; rapid access to diagnostic tests and treatment; specialist ward rounds at least five times per week; and acute stroke protocols/guidelines.[73] In 2008, only 16% of hospitals in the UK had an acute stroke unit which fulfilled these criteria and only 17% of patients were admitted to an acute stroke unit within four hours of admission,[74] so considerable reorganisation and investment is required.

Many UK hospitals have reconfigured their acute services so that newly admitted and unstable patients are cared for in a single area. It has been suggested that establishing an alternative pathway for stroke without the same levels of care may be detrimental to stroke patients and may not be an effective use of resources.[75] Another concern is that emphasis on hyperacute units may divert attention away from other aspects of stroke care that have been shown to be effective.[76]

There is however some direct evidence to suggest that the quality of care is better on an acute stroke unit than a general medical ward. In the study undertaken in Bromley, one group of patients were admitted to general medical wards and although they remained under the care of the admitting physician, a specialist team was involved in their care.[69] The team consisted of a doctor, nurse, physiotherapist and occupational therapist with expertise in the care of stroke patients and were involved in planning treatment, goal setting and discharge planning. The three-month mortality of patients who were cared for on a general medical ward with input from a mobile stroke team was 11.9%, which was higher than the mortality of those who were admitted to a stroke unit and similar to those who were treated at home.

Despite involvement of a mobile stroke team, patients who are cared for on general medical wards received inferior care. Patients who were treated on the stroke unit received an earlier and more comprehensive initial assessment and had access to earlier investigations.[77] Those who were treated on general medical wards were less likely to receive some aspects of basic stroke care such as antipyretics, measures to prevent aspiration and early nutrition. Complications such as stroke progression and chest infection were more likely to occur on a general medical ward.

Conclusion

To minimise the time from onset of symptoms to specialist review, patients and witnesses need to be able to respond to the symptoms of stroke as an emergency. Unfortunately, one of the delays in accessing emergency care is failure to seek immediate help from emergency services and further research is needed to understand the reasons for the delay from the perspective of patients and witnesses in order to develop appropriate educational programmes and interventions. Mass media campaigns which aim to increase public awareness and response to the symptoms of stroke have been introduced in many counties but the impact of these campaigns upon behaviour at the time of stroke remains uncertain.

Pre-hospital emergency services also need to be able to identify and prioritise stroke patients, which can be supported by the use of screening tools, training programmes, audit and feedback. Upon arrival at hospital, systems should be in place to identify patients who require hyperacute interventions such as thrombolysis or urgent surgical intervention, whilst all suspected stroke admissions should have early access to a specialist service.

References

1. Moser DK, Kimble LP, Alberts MJ, Alonzo A, Croft JB, Dracup K *et al.* Reducing delay in seeking treatment by patients with acute coronary syndrome and stroke: a scientific statement from the American Heart Association Council on Cardiovascular Nursing and Stroke Council. *Circulation* 2006; 114: 168–182.
2. Mandelzweig L, Goldbourt U, Boyko V, Tanne D. Perceptual, social, and behavioral factors associated with delays in seeking medical care in patients with symptoms of acute stroke. *Stroke* 2006; 37: 1248–1253.
3. Carroll C, Hobart J, Fox C, Teare L, Gibson J. Stroke in Devon: knowledge was good, but action was poor. *J Neurol Neurosurg Psychiatry* 2004; 75: 567–571.
4. Parahoo K, Thompson K, Cooper M, Stringer M, Ennis E, McCollam P. Stroke: awareness of the signs, symptoms and risk factors — a population-based survey. *Cerebrovasc Dis* 2003; 16: 134–140.
5. Salisbury HR, Banks BJ, Footitt DR, Winner SJ, Reynolds DJ. Delay in presentation of patients with acute stroke to hospital in Oxford. *Quar J Med* 1998; 91: 635–640.
6. Shah M, Makinde KA, Thomas P. Cognitive and behavioral aspects affecting early referral of acute stroke patients to hospital. *J Stroke Cerebrovasc Dis* 2007; 16: 71–76.
7. European Stroke Organisation (ESO) Executive Committee and ESO Writing Committee. Guidelines for management of ischaemic stroke and transient ischaemic attack 2008. *Cerebrovasc Dis* 2008; 25: 457–507.

8. Lasserson DS, Chandratheva A, Giles MF, Mant D, Rothwell PM. Influence of general practice opening hours on delay in seeking medical attention after transient ischaemic attack (TIA) and minor stroke: prospective population based study. *Brit Med J* 2008; 337: a1569.

9. Mosley I, Nicol M, Donnan G, Patrick I, Dewey H. Stroke symptoms and the decision to call for an ambulance. *Stroke* 2007; 38: 361–366.

10. Craig P, Dieppe P, Macintyre S, Michie S, Nazareth I, Petticrew M *et al.* Developing and evaluating complex interventions: the new Medical Research Council guidance. *Brit Med J* 2008; 337: a1655.

11. Grilli R, Ramsay C, Minozzi S. Mass media interventions: effects on health services utilisation. *Cochrane Database of Systematic Reviews* 2002; Issue 1 Art No: CD000389 DOI: 101002/14651858 CD000389.

12. Silver FL, Rubini F, Black D, Hodgson CS. Advertising strategies to increase public knowledge of the warning signs of stroke. *Stroke* 2003; 34: 1965–1968.

13. Morgenstern LB, Staub L, Chan W, Wein TH, Bartholomew LK, King M *et al.* Improving delivery of acute stroke therapy: the TLL Temple Foundation Stroke Project. *Stroke* 2002; 33: 160–166.

14. Morgenstern LB, Bartholomew LK, Grotta JC, Staub L, King M, Chan W. Sustained benefit of a community and professional intervention to increase acute stroke therapy. *Arch Intern Med* 2003; 163: 2198–2202.

15. Summers D, Leonard A, Wentworth D, Saver JL, Simpson J, Spilker JA *et al.* Comprehensive overview of nursing and interdisciplinary care of the acute ischemic stroke patient: a scientific statement from the American Heart Association. *Stroke* 2009; 40: 2911–2944.

16. Lellis JC, Brice JH, Evenson KR, Rosamond WD, Kingdon D, Morris DL. Launching online education for 911 telecommunicators and EMS personnel: experiences from the North Carolina Rapid Response to Stroke Project. *Prehospital Emergency Care* 2007; 11: 298–306.

17. Gordon DL, Issenberg SB, Gordon MS, LaCombe D, McGaghie WC, Petrusa ER. Stroke training of prehospital providers: an example of simulation-enhanced blended learning and evaluation. *Medical Teacher* 2005; 27: 114–121.

18. Frendl DM, Strauss DG, Underhill BK, Goldstein LB. Lack of impact of paramedic training and use of the Cincinnati Prehospital Stroke Scale on stroke patient identification and on-scene time. *Stroke* 2009; 40: 754–756.

19. Bray JE, Bladin C. Success with paramedic diagnosis of stroke. *Stroke* 2009; 40: e398.

20. Roebers S, Wagner M, Ritter MA, Dornbach F, Wahle K, Heuschmann PU. Attitudes and current practice of primary care physicians in acute stroke management. *Stroke* 2007; 38: 1298–1303.

21. Adams HP, Jr., del Zoppo G, Alberts MJ, Bhatt DL, Brass L, Furlan A *et al.* Guidelines for the early management of adults with ischemic stroke. *Stroke* 2007; 38: 1655–1711.

22. Rothwell PM, Coull AJ, Silver LE, Fairhead JF, Giles MF, Lovelock CE *et al.* Population-based study of event-rate, incidence, case fatality, and mortality for all acute vascular events in all arterial territories (Oxford Vascular Study). *Lancet* 2005; 366: 1773–1783.

23. Fischer CE, Barnung S, Nielsen SL, Rasmussen LS. Prehospital identification of stroke — room for improvement. *Eur J Neurol* 2008; 15: 792–796.

24. National Collaborating Centre for Chronic Conditions. *Stroke: national clinical guideline for diagnosis and initial management of acute stroke and transient ischaemic attack (TIA).* Royal College of Physicians, London; 2008.

25. Wojner-Alexandrov AW, Alexandrov AV, Rodriguez D, Persse D, Grotta JC. Houston paramedic and emergency stroke treatment and outcomes study (HoPSTO). *Stroke* 2005; 36: 1512–1518.

26. Mosley I, Nicol M, Donnan G, Patrick I, Kerr F, Dewey H. The impact of ambulance practice on acute stroke care. *Stroke* 2007; 38: 2765–2770.

27. Harbison J, Hossain O, Jenkinson D, Davis J, Louw SJ, Ford GA. Diagnostic accuracy of stroke referrals from primary care, emergency room physicians, and ambulance staff using the face arm speech test. *Stroke* 2003; 34: 71–76.

28. Kothari R, Hall K, Brott T, Broderick J. Early stroke recognition: developing an out-of-hospital NIH Stroke Scale. *Acad Emerg Med* 1997; 4: 986–990.

29. Wojner AW, Morgenstern L, Alexandrov AV, Rodriguez D, Persse D, Grotta JC. Paramedic and emergency department care of stroke: baseline data from a citywide performance improvement study. *Am J Crit Care* 2003; 12: 411–417.

30. Rose KM, Rosamond WD, Huston SL, Murphy CV, Tegeler CH. Predictors of time from hospital arrival to initial brain-imaging among suspected stroke patients: the North Carolina Collaborative Stroke Registry. *Stroke* 2008; 39: 3262–3267.

31. Kidwell CS, Saver JL, Schubert GB, Eckstein M, Starkman S. Design and retrospective analysis of the Los Angeles Prehospital Stroke Screen (LAPSS). *Prehosp Emerg Care* 1998; 2: 267–273.
32. Bray JE, Martin J, Cooper G, Barger B, Bernard S, Bladin C. An interventional study to improve paramedic diagnosis of stroke. *Prehosp Emerg Care* 2005; 9: 297–302.
33. Kidwell CS, Starkman S, Eckstein M, Weems K, Saver JL. Identifying stroke in the field. Prospective validation of the Los Angeles prehospital stroke screen (LAPSS). *Stroke* 2000; 31: 71–76.
34. Nor AM, Davis J, Sen B, Shipsey D, Louw SJ, Dyker AG *et al.* The Recognition of Stroke in the Emergency Room (ROSIER) scale: development and validation of a stroke recognition instrument. *Lancet Neurology* 2005; 4: 727–734.
35. Ramanujam P, Guluma KZ, Castillo EM, Chacon M, Jensen MB, Patel E *et al.* Accuracy of stroke recognition by emergency medical dispatchers and paramedics — San Diego experience. *Prehosp Emerg Care* 2008; 12: 307–313.
36. Bray JE, Martin J, Cooper G, Barger B, Bernard S, Bladin C. Paramedic identification of stroke: community validation of the Melbourne Ambulance Stroke Screen. *Cerebrovas Dis* 2005; 20: 28–33.
37. Frankel M, Hinchey J, Schwamm L, Wall H, Rose KM, George MG *et al.* Prehospital and hospital delays after stroke onset — United States, 2005–2006. *Morbidity & Mortality Weekly Report* 2007; 56: 474–478.
38. Clinical Practice Research Unit University of Central Lancashire. *Recognition and emergency management of suspected stroke and TIA. Prepared by the National Pre-hospital Guidelines Group.* Royal College of Physicians, London; 2006.
39. Alberts MJ, Perry A, Dawson DV, Bertels C. Effects of public and professional education on reducing the delay in presentation and referral of stroke patients. *Stroke* 1992; 23: 352–356.
40. Silliman SL, Quinn B, Huggett V, Merino JG. Use of a field-to-stroke center helicopter transport program to extend thrombolytic therapy to rural residents. *Stroke* 2003; 34: 729–733.
41. Silbergleit R, Scott PA, Lowell MJ, Silbergleit R. Cost-effectiveness of helicopter transport of stroke patients for thrombolysis. *Acad Emerg Med* 2003; 10: 966–972.

42. Hand PJ, Kwan J, Lindley RI, Dennis MS, Wardlaw JM. Distinguishing between stroke and mimic at the bedside: the brain attack study. *Stroke* 2006; 37: 769–775.
43. O'Brien PA, Ryder DO, Twomey C. The role of computed tomography brain scan in the diagnosis of acute stroke in the elderly. *Age Ageing* 1987; 16: 319–322.
44. Ellekjaer H, Holmen J, Indredavik B, Terent A. Epidemiology of stroke in Innherred, Norway, 1994 to 1996. Incidence and 30-day case-fatality rate. *Stroke* 1997; 28: 2180–2184.
45. Libman RB, Wirkowski E, Alvir J, Rao TH. Conditions that mimic stroke in the emergency department. Implications for acute stroke trials. *Arch Neurol* 1995; 52: 1119–1122.
46. Montaner J, Perea-Gainza M, Delgado P, Ribo M, Chacon P, Rosell A *et al.* Etiologic diagnosis of ischemic stroke subtypes with plasma biomarkers. *Stroke* 2008; 39: 2280–2287.
47. Kothari R, Jauch E, Broderick J, Brott T, Sauerbeck L, Khoury J *et al.* Acute stroke: delays to presentation and emergency department evaluation. *Annals Emerg Med* 1999; 33: 3–8.
48. Deakin CD, Alasaad M, King P, Thompson F. Is ambulance telephone triage using advanced medical priority dispatch protocols able to identify patients with acute stroke correctly? *Emerg Med J* 2009; 26: 442–445.
49. Buck BH, Starkman S, Eckstein M, Kidwell CS, Haines J, Huang R *et al.* Dispatcher recognition of stroke using the National Academy Medical Priority Dispatch System. *Stroke* 2009; 40: 2027–2030.
50. Ramanujam P, Castillo E, Patel E, Vilke G, Wilson MP, Dunford JV. Prehospital transport time intervals for acute stroke patients. *J Emerg Med* 2009; 37: 40–45.
51. Reginella RL, Crocco T, Tadros A, Shackleford A, Davis SM. Predictors of stroke during 9-1-1 calls: opportunities for improving EMS response. *Prehosp Emerg Care* 2006; 10: 369–373.
52. Rosamond WD, Evenson KR, Schroeder EB, Morris DL, Johnson A-M, Brice JH. Calling emergency medical services for acute stroke: a study of 9-1-1 tapes. *Prehosp Emerg Care* 2005; 9: 19–23.
53. Harbison J, Massey A, Barnett L, Hodge D, Ford GA. Rapid ambulance protocol for acute stroke. *Lancet* 1999; 353: 1935.

54. Riopelle RJ, Howse DC, Bolton C, Elson S, Groll DL, Holtom D *et al.* Regional access to acute ischemic stroke intervention. *Stroke* 2001; 32: 652–655.

55. Price CI, Clement F, Gray J, Donaldson C, Ford GA. Systematic review of stroke thrombolysis service configuration. *Expert Rev Neurother* 2009; 9: 211–233.

56. Audebert HJ, Kukla C, Vatankhah B, Gotzler B, Schenkel J, Hofer S *et al.* Comparison of tissue plasminogen activator administration management between Telestroke Network hospitals and academic stroke centers: the Telemedical Pilot Project for Integrative Stroke Care in Bavaria/Germany. *Stroke* 2006; 37: 1822–1827.

57. Kwan J, Hand P, Sandercock P. Improving the efficiency of delivery of thrombolysis for acute stroke: a systematic review. *Quart J Med* 2004; 97: 273–279.

58. Nazir FS, Petre I, Dewey HM. Introduction of an acute stroke team: an effective approach to hasten assessment and management of stroke in the emergency department. *J Clin Neurosci* 2009; 16: 21–25.

59. Asimos AW, Norton HJ, Price MF, Cheek WM. Therapeutic yield and outcomes of a community teaching hospital code stroke protocol. *Acad Emerg Med* 2004; 11: 361–370.

60. Sattin JA, Olson SE, Liu L, Raman R, Lyden PD. An expedited code stroke protocol is feasible and safe. *Stroke* 2006; 37: 2935–2939.

61. Nam HS, Han SW, Ahn SH, Lee JY, Choi H-Y, Park IC *et al.* Improved time intervals by implementation of computerized physician order entry-based stroke team approach. *Cerebrovasc Dis* 2007; 23: 289–293.

62. World Health Organisation. *Cerebrovascular Diseases: prevention, treatment and rehabilitation.* World Health Organisation, Geneva; 1971.

63. Ebrahim S, Harwood R. *Stroke Epidemiology, Evidence, and Clinical Practice.* 2nd Edn. New York: Oxford University Press; 1999.

64. Wade DT, Hewer RL. Why admit stroke patients to hospital? *Lancet* 1983; 521: 807–809.

65. Bamford J, Sandercock P, Warlow C, Gray M. Why are patients with acute stroke admitted to hospital? *Brit Med J* 1986; 292: 1369.

66. Early Supported Discharge Trialists. Services for reducing duration of hospital care for acute stroke patients. *Cochrane Database of Systematic Reviews*

2005; Issue 2 Art No: CD000443 DOI: 101002/14651858CD000443pub2 CD000443.

67. Wade DT, Langton-Hewer R, Skilbeck CE, Bainton D, Burns-Cox C. Controlled trial of a home-care service for acute stroke patients. *Lancet* 1985; 325: 323–326.

68. Langhorne P, Dennis M, Kalra L, Shepperd S, Wade D, Wolfe C. Services for helping acute stroke patients avoid hospital admission. *Cochrane Database of Systematic Reviews* 1999; Issue 3 Art No: CD000444 DOI: 101002/14651858 CD000444.

69. Kalra L, Evans A, Perez I, Knapp M, Donaldson N, Swift CG. Alternative strategies for stroke care: a prospective randomised controlled trial. *Lancet* 2000; 356: 894–899.

70. Kalra L, Evans A, Perez I, Knapp M, Swift C, Donaldson N. A randomised controlled comparison of alternative strategies in stroke care. *Health Technol Assess* 2005; 9: 1–94.

71. Ricauda NA, Bo M, Molaschi M, Massaia M, Salerno D, Amati D *et al.* Home hospitalization service for acute uncomplicated first ischemic stroke in elderly patients: a randomized trial. *J Am Geriatric Soc* 2004; 52: 278.

72. Langhorne P, Sandercock P, Prasad K. Evidence-based practice for stroke. *Lancet Neurol* 2009; 8: 308–309.

73. Intercollegiate Stroke Working Party. National Sentinel Stroke Audit Phase I (organisational audit) 2008. Royal College of Physicians, London; 2009.

74. Intercollegiate Stroke Working Party. National Sentinel Stroke Audit Phase II (clinical audit) 2008. Royal College of Physicians, London; 2009.

75. Rodgers H, Sudlow M. Commentary: controversies in NICE guidance on acute stroke and transient ischaemic attack. *Brit Med J* 2008; 337: a833.

76. Sudlow C, Warlow C. Getting the priorities right for stroke care. *Brit Med J* 2009; 338: b2083.

77. Evans A, Perez I, Harraf F, Melbourn A, Steadman J, Donaldson N *et al.* Can differences in management processes explain different outcomes between stroke unit and stroke-team care? *Lancet* 2001; 358: 1586–1592.

5   Hyperacute Management of Stroke

Jonathan Birns* and Ajay Bhalla*

Chapter Summary

There have been considerable advances in stroke research leading to translation of drug therapy for stroke into the clinical arena. The key area that has been examined more recently involves the use of thrombolysis for ischaemic stroke that significantly reduces disability. This has revolutionised the manner in which acute stroke is treated as a medical emergency. The use of advanced imaging techniques and adjuncts to thrombolysis may have the potential to improve the ability to select patients who may benefit from reperfusion therapy and allow treatment decisions to be based on individual brain pathophysiology rather than arbitrary time windows. At present, however, there is no drug therapy that has been unequivocally shown to be effective in treating haemorrhagic stroke. Treatment strategies are aimed at limiting haematoma expansion, peri-haematoma inflammation and oedema, reversing coagulopathy and reducing raised intracranial pressure. Larger trials are required to examine the potential benefits of these options. Surgical management is the current option being applied to patients with lobar haemorrhagic stroke but again, trial data is required to identify specifically which patients appear to benefit the most.

*Guy's and St. Thomas' NHS Foundation Trust, London, UK

There is no substitute for organised, coordinated stroke care in stroke units for all patients and the key areas in the management of physiological parameters such as blood pressure, hyperglycaemia, oxygenation, hydration and temperature control are explored. Whether these strategies individually are beneficial in the acute phase of stroke need to be tested in randomised controlled trials. The establishment of stroke networks ensures delivery of hyperacute stroke care from specialist centres to patients within a defined geographical area through a 'hub' and 'spoke' model. Where this may not be possible due to geographical location, adoption of telemedicine technology provides a real opportunity whereby patients gain access to specialist stroke expertise remotely.

Introduction

Until recently, stroke was not considered to be a medical emergency and hospitalisation was considered to be necessary only for nursing, therapy or social care needs.[1] This nihilistic perception has been changed by evidence demonstrating the effectiveness of acute stroke care[2,3] and thrombolysis for selected patients.[4] Management on a specialised acute stroke unit from the time of admission results in 19% more patients being alive and independent at one year compared with being managed on a general medical ward, even with specialist stroke team support.[2,5] Similarly, treatment with thrombolysis within three hours of stroke onset results in 30% more patients being alive and independent at three months.[6]

There has been increasing recognition of the importance of timely medical attention in acute stroke management[7] and the use of fast-track systems with stroke-specific assessment tools has been advocated as a method to evaluate rapidly patients presenting with suspected stroke.[8,9] This leads to patients being prioritised and the early initiation of appropriate clinical assessments and medical investigations. This facilitates early diagnosis and determination of the aetiology of the stroke (ischaemic or haemorrhagic) in addition to planning treatment strategies aimed at reducing the brain damage caused by the stroke and preventing complications.

Acute Care

Clinical assessments

A detailed history is crucial for correct diagnosis and exclusion of mimics in order that appropriate management plans may be employed. Key features pertain to the mode of onset and focal neurologic symptoms, particularly to distinguish stroke from disorders such as migraine, seizure and factitious and psychogenic processes. Attention also needs to be paid to risk factors for stroke in addition to handedness, co-morbidities, medications and social history. Rapid recognition of stroke is critical to hyperacute care pathways and structured assessment tools such as the Face Arm Speech Test (FAST)[10] and Recognition of Stroke in the Emergency Room (ROSIER)[9] have been demonstrated to be effective in the diagnosis of stroke in the pre-hospital and emergency department respectively and have both been implemented in local and national guidelines.[11] These assessment tools have been shown to be accurate in the diagnosis of stroke when used by a variety of healthcare professionals, facilitating the 'fast-tracking' of stroke patients to specialist stroke care.[8,10,12]

Clinical evaluation should assess for conscious level, temperature, heart rate and rhythm, blood pressure, cardiac murmurs, carotid bruits and evidence of aspiration in addition to a detailed neurological examination. The National Institute of Health Stroke Scale (NIHSS) is the most commonly used acute stroke clinical assessment tool and is a 15-item neurologic examination stroke scale that evaluates the effect of acute cerebral infarction on level of consciousness, extraocular movement, visual-field loss, motor strength, ataxia, sensory loss, language, dysarthria and neglect. It provides a quantitative measure of stroke-related neurologic deficit, may serve as a measure of stroke severity, is valid for predicting lesion size, short- and long-term outcome and provides a common language for information exchanges among healthcare providers.[13] Scores may range from a minimum of 0 with no deficit to a maximum of 42. It is designed to be simple, valid, reliable, takes less than 10 minutes to complete and be administered at the bedside consistently by physicians, nurses and therapists trained in its use.

Diagnostic tests

Basic blood tests to assess for derangement of serum haematological or biochemical parameters and an ECG should be undertaken in all suspected stroke patients in addition to brain imaging. The most commonly used modality of brain imaging in the acute assessment of stroke patients is CT scanning due to its ease of use and availability. Computed tomography (CT) in acute stroke is highly sensitive for the detection of intracerebral haemorrhage (ICH) which results in immediate, and easily visible, hyperattenuation. In contrast, acute ischaemic stroke produces hypoattenuation of brain tissue that becomes more apparent over a number of hours. Early ischaemic changes may be difficult to detect and a number of studies have suggested that the sensitivity and reproducibility of early ischaemic change may depend on the quality of the CT scanner used and the experience of the reader.[14,15] Concern about the reliable detection of early ischaemic change on CT and its significance in relation to functional outcome and the risk of symptomatic haemorrhage following thrombolytic therapy led to the development of systematic quantitative measures such as the Alberta Stroke Programme Early CT Score (ASPECTS). ASPECTS is a 10-point scoring system that assesses regional early ischaemic change on CT brain scanning and it has been shown to be simple, valid and reliable (Fig. 1).[16]

MRI is the imaging modality of choice for stroke and can be obtained non-invasively with no exposure to ionising radiation. It has high sensitivity to tissue oedema and ischaemia, particularly in the posterior fossa. Furthermore, MR images may be weighted to augment contrast between tissue types and specialised pulse sequences have been developed to highlight specific tissue properties.[17] For example, information provided by T1 and T2 weighted imaging can be augmented by susceptibility-weighted sequences (sensitive to haemorrhage), diffusion-weighted imaging (tissue destined to infarct without prompt intervention), MR angiography (vascular anatomy) and MR perfusion imaging (cerebral perfusion). However, MRI has a number of limitations including availability, expense, claustrophobia for patients and a contraindication for patients with fragments of metal or with cardiac pacemakers or any other electrically or magnetically implanted device.

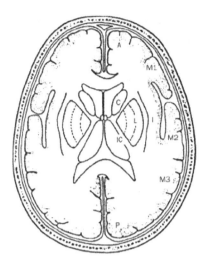 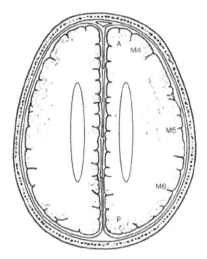

Figure 1. Alberta Stroke Programme Early CT Score (ASPECTS). For ASPECTS score, the territory of the middle cerebral artery is allotted 10 points. 1 point is subtracted for an area of early ischaemic change, such as focal swelling, or parenchymal hypoattenuation, for each of the defined regions. A normal CT scan has an ASPECTS value of 10 points. A score of 0 indicates diffuse ischaemia throughout the territory of the middle cerebral artery. (Used with permission from Elsevier from Barber PA, Demchuk AM, Zhang J, Buchan AM. Validity and reliability of a quantitative computed tomography score in predicting outcome of hyperacute stroke before thrombolytic therapy. ASPECTS Study Group. Alberta Stroke Programme Early CT Score. *Lancet* 2000; 355: 1670–1674.)

General management in acute stroke care

Randomised controlled trials comparing stroke units treating patients in the acute and rehabilitation phase versus conventional care found considerable reductions in early death in patients managed in stroke units.[18,19] The reduction in early death was believed to be due to monitoring and control of abnormal physiological parameters such as hypertension, hyperglycaemia, hypoxia, pyrexia and hydration in the acute phase, which may have aggravated cerebral damage. Significant differences in the management of acute physiology during the first two weeks of admission included the use of intravenous saline in the first 24 hours, antipyretic, antibiotic and oxygen therapy and insulin infusions.[20] Monitoring of acute physiological parameters with treatments aimed at maintaining physiological homeostasis also reduced early neurological progression.[21,22] There is now experimental evidence suggesting that control of these abnormal physiological parameters acts as a form of neuroprotection which may potentially improve the viability of ischaemic neuronal tissue.[23] Interventions aimed at maintaining physiological homeostasis are now recommended by a European review of management of acute stroke care.[24] General management for acute stroke should include strategies not only to maintain physiological homeostasis but also to prevent and treat complications such as urinary incontinence, malnutrition, pressure sores and venous thrombosis.

Oxygenation

More than 60% of stroke patients have been shown to have at least one episode of hypoxia (defined as < 96%) for more than five minutes.[25] Hypoxia following stroke results in anaerobic metabolism and depletion of energy stores, thereby worsening brain injury. Stroke patients are at risk of hypoxia due to abnormalities in respiratory function such as hypoventilation, aspiration pneumonia, atelectasis, sleep apnoea, left ventricular failure, Cheyne-Stroke respiration and pulmonary embolism.[26] Improving oxygen content may therefore prevent neurological deterioration in stroke. Evidence shows that stroke patients have lower oxygen saturations compared to matched controls and that positioning patients upright improves oxygen saturations as well as reducing intracranial pressure (ICP).[27,28] It has been suggested that supplemental oxygen should be administered if oxygen saturations are below 95%.[29]

The use of supplemental oxygen for non-hypoxic patients is however more controversial. In animal models, highly enriched oxygen atmospheres increase mortality.[30] A quasi-randomised controlled study by Ronning and colleagues showed that routine (100%) oxygen supplementation for 24 hours after stroke onset had no benefit in survival.[31] However, in a subgroup of minor to moderate stroke patients, this intervention worsened survival at seven months, possibly as a result of free radical formation during reperfusion. Following these findings, it is not advisable for oxygen therapy to be given routinely to non-hypoxic patients after stroke. Current research is now being directed at examining the effects of supplemental oxygen after acute stroke (2 l/min if baseline saturation > 93% and 3 l/min if ≤ 93%) in a large multi-centre trial.[32]

Hydration

Initial dehydration is frequently hyperosmolar caused by an inadequate intake of water due to drowsiness or dysphagia, a reduction in thirst or the presence of infection. Dehydration, leading to a rise in haematocrit and a reduction in blood pressure (BP) can worsen the ischaemic process during stroke.[33] Stroke patients with high plasma osmolality levels on admission have worse survival at three months.[34] Previously, it was recommended that stroke patients should be 'under-filled' in order to prevent cerebral oedema but studies have shown that early intervention with intravenous saline may contribute to improving functional ability in stroke patients managed in a multidisciplinary environment.[18] It was hypothesised that routine use of saline infusions in the first 24 hours may have improved cerebral blood flow by limiting dips in systemic BP and preventing dehydration. Trials of haemodilution have not shown any clear benefits as yet and require further investigation.[35]

Glucose control

Some 20–50% of acute stroke patients are hyperglycaemic (blood glucose > 8 mmol/l) on presentation[36] and, in the Copenhagen Stroke Study, 20% of patients presenting with stroke were diabetic.[37] Various mechanisms have been suggested to explain the worse prognosis in diabetic and hyperglycaemic patients. These patients have impairment of cerebral blood flow (CBF) and cerebral autoregulation, reduced leukocyte and erythrocyte deformability, increased thrombotic states and endothelial cell activation.[38] Ischaemia leads to a reduction in oxidative glucose metabolism, resulting in production of lactic acid locally, which induces neuronal damage. Hyperglycaemia increases lactic acid production by increasing the available glucose for anaerobic glucose metabolism and also by inhibiting mitochondrial respiration. Most studies agree that high glucose levels after stroke are associated with poor outcome in non-diabetic patients[36,39,40] and this generally holds true with diabetic patients too.[41] Studies have suggested that hyperglycaemia influences stroke outcome independently of stroke severity and diabetic status.[36,42]

The Glucose Insulin in Stroke Trial-UK (GIST-UK) aimed to address the effects of normalising glucose levels (4–7 mmol/l) using glucose/potassium/insulin infusions within 24 hours of stroke in patients with initial glucose levels between 6 and 17 mmol/l.[43] There were no significant differences in mortality or functional disability at three months, although the trial was stopped due to low recruitment (933 patients). Blood glucose levels were only reduced by 0.6 mmol/l in the insulin treated group. Of interest however, the authors stated that there were significantly lower BP recordings (9 mm/Hg) in the insulin treatment arm compared with the control arm. Whether the vasodepressor response of insulin acutely masked the potential benefit of glycaemic control in this trial was unclear. A randomised controlled pilot trial addressing the effects of aggressive glycaemic control with insulin in patients with glucose levels > 8.3 mmol/l post-stroke (Treatment of Hyperglycaemia in Ischaemic Stroke (THIS) study) demonstrated significantly lower glucose levels and non-significant better outcomes in the active treatment arm compared with controls.[44] Further trials are now required to investigate what is the best regimen of delivering insulin therapy practically, what level of glucose should be treated and how aggressive glycaemic control should be with monitoring of hypoglycaemic episodes. European guidelines advocate insulin therapy if glucose levels are > 10 mmol/l[24] whilst American guidelines advocate treatment if glucose levels are > 7.7 mmol/l.[45] The avoidance of glucose containing solutions in the first 24 hours post-stroke has also been advocated.

Blood pressure

Approximately 30% of patients have a history of hypertension prior to ischaemic stroke and 80% have high BP on presentation.[46] Due to spontaneous falls in BP over four to 10 days, approximately 60% are left normotensive.[47] Hypertension may promote early brain oedema and increase in haemorrhagic transformation.[48] Robinson and colleagues demonstrated that an increase in systolic BP by 10 mmHg after stroke was significantly associated with poor outcome.[49] However the International Stroke Trial suggested a U-shaped relationship between BP and mortality.[50] There is paucity of randomised controlled trial evidence of the acute management of high BP after stroke with the potential risk of worsening ischaemia in patients with cerebral infarction.[51] The Acute Candesartan Ciliexitil Evaluation in Stroke Survivors (ACCESS) trial demonstrated that Candesartan given for seven days after acute ischaemic stroke compared with placebo improved outcome but with no significant difference in BP between both groups.[52] The CHHIPS study (Controlling Hypertension and Hypotension Immediately Post Stroke) demonstrated that active BP reduction using lisinopril and labetalol in patients with ischaemic stroke with systolic BP levels > 160 mmHg not only significantly lowered BP acutely but also reduced mortality at three months compared with placebo.[53] American Heart Association (AHA) guidelines suggest that BP post-ischaemic stroke should be lowered if systolic BP is > 220 mmHg and diastolic BP is > 120 mmHg with a goal of reducing BP by 15% during the first 24 hours.[45] The presence of acute heart failure, aortic dissection and hypertensive encephalopathy are other indications for acute BP reduction. Intravenous labetalol, glyceryl trinitrate and sodium nitroprusside are potential agents used. Patients on antihypertensive agents prior to stroke are recommended to continue them if they are physiologically stable. The Continue Or Stop post-Stroke Antihypertensives Collaborative Study (COSSACS) will attempt to address this question.[54] Low BP is uncommon after stroke and may be related to volume loss.[55] Limiting excessive drops in BP by routinely giving patients intravenous saline on admission may be an important element in acute stroke care.[18] Vasopressor drugs such as phenylephrine[56] may be used in treating hypotension; however, randomised controlled trial evidence investigating the use of inotropes is lacking. The treatment of BP after haemorrhagic stroke is discussed below.

Swallowing and feeding

Up to 50% of patients with stroke can present with oropharyngeal dysphagia with 15% left dysphagic at three months.[57] Patients must not be given any fluid or food until they are deemed to be safe to swallow in order to avoid aspiration pneumonia. Bedside swallow assessment involves evaluation of conscious level, bulbar strength, sensation, articulation and the oral and pharyngeal phase of swallowing. Further evaluation can be carried out by videofluoroscopic measurements. As malnutrition is a common finding post-acute stroke (up to 15%),[58] dietary interventions either by nasogastric (NG) or percutaneous gastrostomy (PEG) may be required. The Feed Or Ordinary Diet (FOOD) trial demonstrated that early enteral feeding (with NG) within seven days compared with delayed feeding after seven days was associated with a trend of fewer deaths at six months but with no significant difference in poor outcome.[59] When NG feeding was compared with PEG feeding within seven days of admission, PEG feeding was associated with significant odds for death and poor outcome. PEG feeding is however, the preferred option for patients who require prolonged tube feeding beyond two to four weeks. Routine oral nutritional supplementation in this trial was not found to be associated with improved survival or functional ability.

Temperature control

Pyrexia following ischaemic stroke may be caused by an acute phase response, disturbance of cerebral mechanisms of temperature control or the presence of infection. Evidence suggests that temperatures up to 38°C post-acute stroke are associated with increased mortality and morbidity.[60] Fever is common after ICH and correlates with ICH volume and third ventricular shift, suggesting a role of hypothalamic compression in 'central fever'.[61] A fever > 38.5°C at 72 hours is an independent risk factor for mortality and disability post-ICH.[62] Although there are no clinical data to guide clinicians as to the appropriateness of routine use of antipyretics, recommendations have been made to maintain normothermia (36°C to 37°C) either by using paracetamol when required or treating underlying infection.[24] Induced hypothermia (32°C to 33°C) has been shown to reduce mortality in patients with severe middle cerebral artery stroke[63] but large trials are required to confirm the use of this intervention given the risk of raised ICP on rewarming.

Bladder management

Urinary incontinence affects up to 40–60% of stroke patients.[64] Common causes include detrusor instability, bladder flow obstruction, constipation, urinary sepsis, immobility, confusion and pre-stroke incontinence. Careful assessment is the key feature of managing urinary incontinence and this should include a voiding diary, post-micturition bladder ultrasound to measure residual volume and urine analysis. Structured strategies used to manage urinary incontinence include regular toileting, intermittent catheterisation if residual volumes are greater than 100 ml and treating the underlying cause. Routine catheterisation is to be avoided due to the risk of urinary infection but may be used if pressure areas are under risk of contamination and breakdown. Occasionally urodynamic investigations are required if incontinence persists.

Pressure care

Pressure sores are readily avoidable and if significant can cause pain and limit recovery. Strategies to combat this include initial structured assessment including nutritional, infection and mobility status. Basic nursing care including regular turning, early mobility and the use of pressure relieving mattresses and specialist seating are key approaches.

Prevention of venous thromboembolism

Clinically evident deep vein thrombosis is present in 5% of cases of stroke but up to 50% of cases through fibrinogen-labelled studies.[65] Pulmonary emboli are clinically evident in 2% of cases.[66] Limited data suggest that the risk of re-bleeding in patients with ICH receiving anticoagulants for three months is between 1% and 3% depending on the location of the index haemorrhage and age.[67] Current interventions used to prevent venous thromboembolism include hydration, early mobilisation, anti-platelet use and graduated compression stockings (GCS). Although low dose subcutaneous heparin has been shown to reduce the incidence of both deep vein thrombosis and pulmonary emboli following ischaemic stroke, the benefits are offset by the increase in haemorrhagic infarction rate and is currently not recommended for routine use.[68] Whether the use of low dose heparin is effective in reducing venous thrombosis in patients who are at low risk of haemorrhagic infarction such as lacunar stroke is unclear; however, consensus opinions from both the AHA and European guidelines suggest that low dose heparin may be considered in neurologically stable patients at high risk of venous thrombosis after day 2 from onset.[69,70] Clinical decision-making in these patients remains individualised, taking into account the risk of recurrent ICH and thrombotic risk.

The effectiveness of thigh length GCS compared with avoidance of GCS post-stroke has been evaluated in the large multicentre randomised controlled trial CLOTS-1.[71] This showed no significant difference in deep vein thrombosis incidence between patients with avoidance of or allocated to GCS (10.5% versus 10% respectively). Those patients allocated to thigh length GCS were also more likely to suffer lower limb skin ulcers and blisters. Therefore, currently thigh length GCS are not recommended for routine use post-stroke. CLOTS-2 and CLOTS-3 studies will address the effectiveness of comparing thigh and below knee GCS and intermittent pneumatic compression devices respectively.

Anticonvulsant therapy

Partial or secondary generalised seizures may occur in the acute phase of stroke. The risk of seizures after ICH has been estimated to be 8% at one month.[72] Lobar haemorrhages and midline shift have been reported to be associated with an increased risk of seizure occurrence.[73] No randomised controlled trials have been evaluated investigating this area; however, observational data suggest prophylactic use of phenobarbitone in the acute phase significantly reduces the risk of seizures in patients with lobar supratentorial ICH.[72]

The role of telemedicine

Telemedicine allows a stroke physician to provide remote specialist assessment of patients with real-time clinical evaluation (by two-way audiovisual communication) and interpretation of brain imaging. This interaction can take place within minutes of arrival of a patient to hospital helping to meet the demands of 'time is brain' in acute stroke care. Telemedicine is feasible, acceptable, technically and diagnostically reliable and is associated with improved delivery of thrombolysis.[74] Evidence-based guidelines now recommend that telemedicine can play an important role not only in the delivery of thrombolysis but also in other aspects of stroke care such as pre-hospital emergency assessment, post-stroke rehabilitation and stroke educational programmes.[75,76]

Different models for providing audiovisual interaction between patient and stroke physician have been developed to meet the local needs of a variety of populations[74,77–82] Most systems feature a high-resolution camera in the emergency department (remotely controlled by the stroke specialist) with a microphone, speaker and screen for the patient to view the stroke specialist, linked usually via internet-based connections to the stroke specialist's computer. Brain imaging transmission is usually via a picture and archiving communication system. Privacy and security of the system may be maintained by secure socket layer conditional access, data encryption and intruder alerts.

Whilst some telemedicine systems facilitate 'round-the-clock' stroke care for a single hospital, it is becoming increasingly common for telemedicine-delivered stroke care to exist and be effective within a 'hub and spoke' model in a geographically organised network.[83,84] Stroke specialists acting as telemedicine practitioners require on-site nurses or doctors, as well as willing emergency staff participation to facilitate the clinical evaluation of the patient, and these healthcare professionals need to be trained in working with remote specialists to obtain accurate neurological assessments. Concerns that remote assessment of neurological status acutely is inferior to bedside clinical assessment is unfounded in trial settings[75] and whilst no detailed, economic analyses of the cost-effectiveness of telemedicine for stroke have been performed, budgetary impact and cost-effectiveness of thrombolysis delivery by telestroke networks has been estimated to be dominant to conservative management.

The Effectiveness of Various Interventions for Acute Ischaemic Stroke

Intravenous thrombolysis — the evidence

Thrombolytic agents are plasminogen activators that catalyse the conversion of the precursor plasminogen to plasmin which then acts to break down the dense meshwork of crosslinked fibrin strands in blood clots.

Studies with the thrombolytic agent streptokinase, which had been successful as a thrombolytic drug in myocardial infarction, proved negative with a significant increase in the rate of symptomatic ICH and no improvement in functional outcome.[85–87] It is not clear if the morbidity and mortality observed with streptokinase in these trials was due to the time interval to treatment (up to six hours), the dose of drug, or the agent itself.[88] Nonetheless, based on these studies, streptokinase is not used clinically to treat acute ischaemic stroke.

Recombinant tissue plasminogen activator (rt-PA) was approved for use in acute ischaemic stroke in 1996, largely on the basis of the National Institute of Neurological Disorders and Stroke (NINDS) rt-PA study.[6] In this pivotal study, 624 patients presenting within three hours of symptom onset were randomly assigned treatment with 0.9 mg/kg of intravenous rt-PA or placebo. Whilst neurological improvement did not differ between the two groups after 24 hours, clinical outcome was significantly better in the treated group at three months. More specifically, the trial showed that compared with placebo, rt-PA provided a 14% increase in the chance of being alive and independent and a 13% decrease in the chance of being alive and dependent three months after stroke. Symptomatic ICH occurred in 6.4% of patients treated with rt-PA compared with 0.6% of those given placebo.[6] Across the entire spectrum of outcomes, the number needed to treat to cause significant improvement in one patient was estimated to be 3, and the number needed to treat to cause harm was 30.[89] Benefits of treatment with rt-PA were shown to be cost-effective, sustained at one year and be independent of age, gender or the severity of initial neurologic deficit.[6,90–92]

Based on the positive results of the NINDS trial, investigators attempted to increase the time window in which patients can be treated. Two European Cooperative Acute Stroke Studies (ECASS I and ECASS II)[93,94] investigated a time window of up to six hours while the Alteplase Thrombolysis for Acute Noninterventional Therapy in Ischaemic Stroke trial (ATLANTIS)[95] investigated a time window of between three and five hours after symptom onset. These trials failed to demonstrate efficacy of thrombolytic treatment, as defined by primary outcomes. However, the ECASS I study had a high percentage of protocol violations (17%) and used a higher dose of rt-PA (1.1 mg/kg) that was associated with higher rates of ICH.[88] Also, a post-hoc analysis of the ECASS II trial demonstrated rt-PA to reduce significantly death and dependency compared with placebo (45.7% vs. 54.0%, $p = 0.024$).[94] A pooled analysis of 2775 patients enrolled in the ATLANTIS, ECASS and NINDS trials showed that the earlier the commencement of thrombolytic therapy, the greater the benefit,[96] giving rise to the mantra of 'Time is Brain'.[11] The pooled analysis, however, also suggested a potential benefit of thrombolysis beyond three hours.

In September 2008, the results of the ECASS III trial were reported, showing that compared with placebo, rt-PA administered between three and 4.5 hours after the onset of symptoms significantly improved clinical outcome. This study randomised 821 patients to 0.9 mg/kg of intravenous rt-PA or placebo and demonstrated 52.4% of patients treated with rt-PA to be alive and independent three months after stroke compared with 45.2% of patients receiving placebo.[97] Mortality was not significantly affected and as with all previous stroke thrombolysis trials, rates of ICH were higher in the rt-PA treated patients compared with those receiving placebo. The symptomatic haemorrhage rate, however, was 2.4% in patients treated with rt-PA compared with 0.2% of those given placebo. It should be borne in mind, however, that definitions of ICH differ between thrombolysis trials. The ECASS III definition of symptomatic ICH was any haemorrhage associated with death or neurologic deterioration (as indicated by an increase of at least 4 points on the NIHSS score). The NINDS definition was a haemorrhage not seen on a previous brain scan associated with any decline in neurologic status or any suspicion of haemorrhage.[97]

With the exception of the NINDS trial that included a small number of individuals over the age of 80, trials for acute thrombolysis generally excluded patients older than 80 years. Elderly people have poorer outcomes, but this appears to be due to other co-morbid conditions rather than age alone, and in observational studies, the rate of symptomatic ICH did not differ between patients aged over and under 80 years.[98]

Intravenous thrombolysis in practice

After the approval of rt-PA for the treatment of acute ischaemic stroke in 1996, observational studies in both North America and Europe confirmed that administration of rt-PA was safe and feasible in a variety of clinical settings as long as the NINDS guidelines were strictly followed.[99–101] Indeed, rates of symptomatic ICH were shown to be lower than those demonstrated in the NINDS trial, even in centres with little experience of thrombolysis.[99] In contrast, when protocols and guidelines were violated, rates of symptomatic haemorrhage rose considerably.[101]

In order to ensure timely treatment of acute ischaemic stroke with rt-PA, fast-track systems have been advocated.[12] This involves protocols to be in place that ensure the rapid response of ambulance staff, emergency department clinicians and stroke specialists with early clinical evaluation, venesection, cannula insertion and brain imaging.[12] Recognising the need and development of an evidence-based fast-track stroke protocol applicable locally is central to the successful implementation of an efficient stroke thrombolysis service. Developing this service involves meeting with the relevant stakeholders including emergency, neurology, and neuroradiology departments, all nursing teams delivering acute stroke care, and the hospital directorate. Identifying logistical barriers to the development of a thrombolysis service is important such that strategies to overcome each problem may be formulated between the stakeholders. Reservations amongst stakeholders about the introduction of a thrombolysis service in terms of an increase in emergency costs and utilisation of diagnostic facilities need to be weighed up against the potential for reductions in lengths of stay and improvements in clinical outcome with rt-PA. Stressing the benefits of developing a thrombolysis service is important not only to patient outcome but also in terms of staff satisfaction and morale and hospital profile. Introducing thrombolysis into an existing service may prove challenging but sustaining people's interest may prove more difficult. Maintaining the initial momentum can be achieved by ongoing publicity of the results of the service and feedback to all staff involved in addition to continuing educational programmes and assessment of competencies for all staff concerned.[102]

A number of contraindications to thrombolysis exist (Table 1) and these must be excluded by the stroke specialist prior to commencing rt-PA treatment. ICH is the most feared complication of rt-PA therapy and these contraindications, listed in the NINDS trial, reduce this iatrogenic haemorrhagic risk. Indeed, more recently, scoring systems to predict this risk

Table 1. Contraindications to thrombolysis for stroke

- Symptoms rapidly improving
- History of stroke or head injury in the last three months
- Major surgery or trauma in the last 14 days
- History consistent with subarachnoid haemorrhage
- History of previous intracranial haemorrhage
- History of seizure at stroke onset
- Systolic blood pressure consistently > 185 mmHg
- Diastolic blood pressure consistently > 110 mmHg
- History of gastrointestinal or urinary tract haemorrhage within 21 days
- Recent arterial puncture at a non-compressible site
- Recent lumbar puncture
- Heparin treatment within last two days and an elevated APTT
- Haemoglobin < 10 g/dl
- Platelets < 100×10^9/l
- INR > 1.7
- Glucose < 2.7 mmol/l
- Evidence on brain scanning of haemorrhage or > 1/3 middle cerebral artery territory acute ischaemic change

have been developed.[103] The ECASS I and ECASS II studies showed that the presence of early ischaemic changes occupying more than one-third of the middle cerebral artery territory before thrombolysis was accompanied by an increase in the haemorrhagic transformation risk and poor clinical outcome.[93,94,104] Furthermore, the Multicenter rt-PA Stroke Survey Group demonstrated that the symptomatic ICH rate was multiplied by more than four times in 1205 patients who had early ischaemic changes occupying more than one-third of the middle cerebral artery territory and treated by intravenous rt-PA within three hours.[105] Therefore, patients with extensive early ischaemic changes are excluded from intravenous thrombolysis. In the absence of contraindications, rt-PA is infused, via a peripheral cannula, over one hour at a dose of 0.9 mg/kg, with 10% of the total dose being given as a bolus over two minutes. In the immediate period after the commencement of thrombolysis, BP is measured regularly and intravenous hypotensive treatment instituted if the BP exceeds 180/105 mmHg, in order to reduce the risk of haemorrhagic transformation. Patients should be managed on an acute stroke unit, in line with national guidelines, with adherence to the aforementioned multidisciplinary policies.[11,29] Antithrombotic drugs are withheld for 24 hours until repeat brain imaging to exclude ICH and assess for residual structural damage (Figs. 2 and 3).

Intra-arterial thrombolysis

Acute ischaemic stroke from large vessel intracranial artery occlusion within the internal carotid artery, middle cerebral artery or basilar artery carries a high mortality if left untreated and has a reduced therapeutic response to intravenous thrombolysis.[88] Indeed, over 80% of patients with an NIHSS of 10 or more have persisting arterial occlusion lesions on

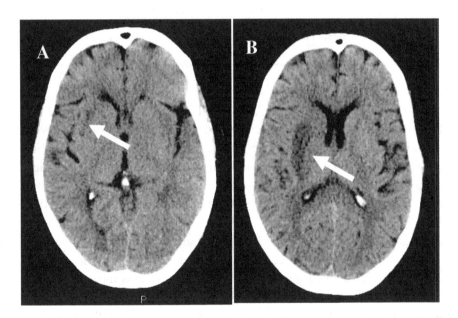

Figure 2. (A) Admission CT brain scan demonstrating minimal early subcortical ischaemic change within the right middle cerebral artery territory (arrow) in a 64-year-old man with acute left-sided sensorimotor deficit and inattention (NIHSS 14). (B) Post-thrombolysis scan showing a residual right lentiform nucleus infarct (arrow) but salvage of the rest of the right middle cerebral artery territory. The patient made good recovery with the only residual deficit being minor right facial paralysis (NIHSS 1).

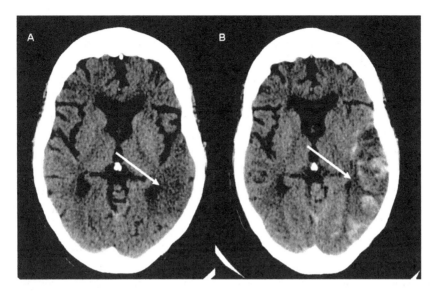

Figure 3. (A) Admission CT brain scan demonstrating early ischaemic change within the posterior third of the left middle cerebral artery territory (arrow) in a 74-year-old woman with an acute onset of aphasia, gaze paresis and right-sided hemianopia, hemineglect, hemiplegia and hemianaesthesia (NIHSS 25). (B) Post-thrombolysis scan showing haemorrhagic transformation of early ischaemic tissue (arrow).

subsequent angiography, even after initial treatment with intravenous rt-PA.[106] Theoretically, administering thrombolytic agents directly to the area of clot may increase efficacy and reduce the risk of bleeding because a high concentration of thrombolytic agents may be delivered into the thrombus.[107]

A small randomised, multicentre trial compared intravenous urokinase with intra-arterial urokinase within the first six hours of acute ischaemic stroke but the study was terminated prematurely because four out of the 14 patients in the intravenous group and three out of 13 in the intra-arterial group died.[108] A further study randomised 16 patients with angiographic evidence of posterior circulation vascular occlusion who presented within 24 hours of symptom onset to either intra-arterial prourokinase or conservative management. Some imbalance between groups existed, with greater severity of deficit at baseline observed in the treatment arm. Good outcomes were observed in four of eight patients who received intra-arterial urokinase compared with one of eight patients in the control group and this led to suggestions that intra-arterial therapy may be used in this setting.[45,109]

The Prolyse in Acute Cerebral Thromboembolism Trials (PROACT I and II) investigated the efficacy and safety of intra-arterial thrombolysis for acute middle cerebral artery territory stroke with prourokinase.[110,111] Despite showing no significant difference in 90-day functional outcome or mortality and an increased symptomatic ICH rate (15.4% versus 7.1%), PROACT I demonstrated improved recanalisation rates (57% versus 0%) in 40 patients with acute ischaemic stroke of less than six hours duration caused by angiographically proven middle cerebral artery occlusion who received 6 mg/kg of intra-arterial prourokinase at the site of occlusion.[110] PROACT II subsequently evaluated the effect of 9 mg of intra-arterial prourokinase in 180 patients with acute ischaemic stroke of less than six hours duration caused by angiographically proven middle cerebral artery occlusion and whilst there was again no difference in mortality and an increased rate of symptomatic ICH (10% versus 2%) and recanalisation (66% versus 18%), outcome measures showed 40% of prourokinase-treated patients have mild or no disability at 90 days compared to 25% of controls ($p = 0.04$).[111] Patients and controls in both PROACT trials also received intravenous heparin infusions.

On the basis of PROACT II, intra-arterial thrombolysis has been recommended as an option for treatment of selected patients who have major stroke of less than six hours duration due to occlusion of the middle cerebral artery and who are not otherwise candidates for intravenous rt-PA.[45] This is particularly relevant to patients who have contraindications to the use of intravenous thrombolysis, such as recent surgery. However, clinical benefit may be counterbalanced by delays to initiating treatment with the intra-arterial approach and treatment requires the patient to be at an experienced stroke centre with immediate access to cerebral angiography and qualified interventionalists.[45] The availability of intra-arterial thrombolysis should generally not preclude the intravenous administration of rt-PA in otherwise eligible patients and time to treatment is just as important in intra-arterial thrombolysis as it is in intravenous thrombolysis.[112] The concept of combining the advantages of intravenous rt-PA (speed of and certainty of initiation of therapy as well as widespread availability) and intra-arterial recanalisation therapy when possible (titrated dosing, mechanical aids to recanalisation, and possibly superior and earlier recanalisation) has been evaluated in pilot trials and advocated as an optimal treatment for patients with angiographically proven large vessel occlusion.[106] Furthermore, pilot studies have demonstrated the feasibility of rescue localised intra-arterial thrombolysis for acute ischaemic stroke patients after early non-responsive intravenous rt-PA therapy.[113]

Adjuncts to Thrombolysis

Perfusion imaging

Despite the evidence for thrombolytic treatement for acute ischaemic stroke, thrombolysis is utilised in a disappointingly low percentage of patients. It has been reported that less than 1% of patients in the United Kingdom actually receive this recommended therapy.[11] In addition to poor public awareness about stroke symptoms and fear of iatrogenic haemorrhage among clinicians, the primary reason for this statistic is the narrow therapeutic time window for thrombolysis.

Salvaging the penumbral tissue surrounding the ischaemic core is a fundamental concept in the treatment of acute ischaemic stroke with thrombolysis. The amount of brain tissue that can be saved progressively diminishes with time but the exact rate and amount of viable tissue remaining is unknown. It is therefore difficult to know reliably and accurately the ratio of ischaemic tissue to infarcted tissue simply on the basis of time alone. Perfusion imaging allows direct visualisation of the brain *in vivo* that enables accurate delineation of potentially salvageable tissue from irreversibly infarcted tissue.[114] This has the potential to improve the ability to select patients who may benefit from reperfusion therapy and allow treatment decisions to be based on individual brain pathophysiology rather than arbitrary time windows (Fig. 4).[115] DEFUSE (DWI in Evolution For Understanding Stroke Etiology) and EPITHET (Echoplanar Imaging THrombolytic Evaluation Trial) are the two largest international multicentre clinical trials that have utilised perfusion imaging in identifying patients with acute ischaemic stroke most likely to benefit from reperfusion therapy.[116,117] Both examined thrombolysis in the 3- to 6-hour time

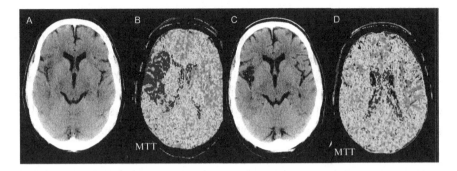

Figure 4. (A) Admission CT brain scan demonstrating minimal early subcortical ischaemic change within the right middle cerebral artery (MCA) territory. (B) Perfusion CT scan on admission showing reduced perfusion in the entire MCA territory. (C) Plain CT scan 24 hours after thrombolysis showing maturation of early changes but no further infarction. (D) Perfusion CT scan 24 hours after thrombolysis showing restoration of blood flow.

window, confirmed that early reperfusion was associated with a more beneficial clinical response in patients with a perfusion mismatch profile compared with those without a mismatch profile and advocated further phase III randomised controlled studies. The DIAS I and II (Desmoteplase In Acute Stroke) and DEDAS (Dose Escalation of Desmoteplase for Acute ischaemic Stroke) trials have investigated extension of the thrombolytic time window to nine hours with the novel thrombolytic agent desmoteplase.[118–120] Whilst DIAS I and DEDAS initially showed promising results, the larger DIAS II randomised controlled trial subsequently demonstrated no benefit of thrombolysis with desmoteplase in the 3- to 9-hour time window. The authors suggested that a high response rate in the placebo group may have been explained by the mild strokes recorded with low baseline NIHSS scores and small ischaemic core lesions, and small mismatch volumes that were associated with no vessel occlusions.[120]

Ultrasound-enhanced thrombolysis

In experimental studies, the use of transcranial Doppler ultrasound (TCD) has been shown to increase fibrinolytic activity with putative mechanisms including improved drug transport, reversible alteration of the fibrin structure, and increased binding of rt-PA to fibrin.[121–123] The CLOTBUST I and II trials (Combined Lysis Of Thrombus in Brain ischaemia with transcranial Ultrasound and Systemic TPA) sought to investigate this *in vivo*. CLOTBUST I was a phase I non-randomised, non-blinded trial in stroke patients, with proximal arterial occlusion receiving intravenous rt-PA within three hours of symptom onset, who were monitored with portable diagnostic TCD equipment.[124] Complete recanalisation (associated with better recovery) on TCD within two hours after rt-PA bolus was found in 20 of 55 patients (36%) and overall symptomatic haemorrhage rate was 5.5%. The CLOTBUST II trial was a prospective, randomised, multicentre clinical trial studying 126 patients with acute ischaemic stroke due to occlusion of the middle cerebral artery who received intravenous rt-PA within three hours after the onset of symptoms. Complete recanalisation or dramatic clinical recovery within two hours after the administration of an rt-PA bolus occurred in 49% of the patients assigned to receive continuous 2-MHz TCD compared with 30% in the control group ($p = 0.03$). However, outcomes at 24 hours and three months were not significantly different between the groups.[125] Symptomatic ICH occurred in three of 63 patients in each of the target and control groups.

Experimental studies have shown that ultrasound-enhanced thrombolysis may be improved by intravenous or intra-arterial administration of microbubbles (small air- or gas-filled microspheres with specific acoustic properties).[126–130] One clinical trial demonstrated 2-hour recanalisation rate and 24-hour clinical improvement (defined as an increase of > 4 points in the NIHSS score) to be greater in patients treated with rt-PA, TCD and microbubbles ($n = 38$, 55%) compared with rt-PA plus TCD ($n = 38$, 41%) and rt-PA alone ($n = 36$, 24%).[131]

Endovascular mechanical thrombolysis

The limitations of intravenous and intra-arterial thrombolysis as well as the desire to demonstrate improved recanalisation rates and long-term outcomes prompted the development of interventional endovascular strategies that include mechanical thrombectomy with the MERCI device and the Penumbra system, in addition to intracranial angioplasty and stent placement.[132] The

MERCI device consists of a flexible tapered wire with five helical loops that can be embedded within the thrombus for retrieval whilst the Penumbra system is a device by which a thromboembolic clot can be removed from large intracranial vessels via aspiration, mechanical disruption, and extraction. Non-randomised clinical studies have demonstrated both devices to achieve successful recanalisation within eight hours of symptom onset in patients with large vessel occlusive acute ischaemic stroke.[133–135]

Antiplatelet agents

As detailed in earlier chapters, randomised trial data has demonstrated the beneficial effect of antiplatelet agents in the secondary prevention of ischaemic stroke. The IST and CAST trials showed aspirin use to reduce significantly the risk of recurrent ischaemic stroke, with benefit being greater in patients receiving aspirin within the first three hours of stroke.[136,137] Where patients are aspirin intolerant, alternative antiplatelet agents such as clopidogrel or dipyridamole may be used and the combination of aspirin with each of these agents has been shown to be beneficial in certain circumstances.[138,139]

Anticoagulation

Twenty-four randomised trials involving 23,748 participants have compared early anticoagulant therapy (started within two weeks of stroke onset) with control in patients with acute ischaemic stroke. Anticoagulants tested include unfractionated heparin, low-molecular-weight heparin, heparinoids, oral anticoagulants and thrombin inhibitors. Meta-analysis of data from these trials has demonstrated no evidence that anticoagulant therapy reduces the odds of death (OR: 1.05; 95% CI: 0.98–1.12) or death or dependency (OR: 0.99; 95% CI: 0.93–1.04). Although anticoagulant therapy is associated with fewer recurrent ischaemic strokes (OR: 0.76; 95% CI: 0.65–0.88), it is also associated with a significant increase in symptomatic ICH (OR: 2.55; 95% CI: 1.95–3.33).[140] Over 15,000 patients have been involved in randomised controlled trials comparing the effectiveness of anticoagulants (unfractionated heparin and low-molecular-weight heparin) with antiplatelet agents in acute ischaemic stroke (started within two weeks of stroke onset). These studies showed that anticoagulants offered no net advantages over antiplatelet agents but were associated with increased risk of symptomatic intracranial haemorrhage.[141,142] Based on these data, current guidelines do not support the routine use of anticoagulant treatment for acute ischaemic stroke.

Management of Intracerebral Haemorrhage

Introduction

ICH is the leading cause of disability and mortality from all stroke subtypes with only one-fifth of survivors left independent at six months.[143] However, there is still uncertainty surrounding its optimal treatment. The lack of evidence of pharmacological interventions for this condition may explain wide variations in practice and also differences in both recent American and European guidelines.[69,70] Development of therapeutic strategies should reflect advances in the understanding of pathophysiological mechanisms of neuronal damage following ICH, whether due to primary causes (microaneursymal disease secondary to hypertension or amyloid angiopathy) or secondary causes (trauma, large vessel aneurysm, arterio-venous malformation or coagulopathy). Pathophysiological mechanisms include: (1) direct compression of surrounding brain parenchyma by the enlarging haematoma over several hours and surrounding oedema leading to neuronal death; (2) compromise of cerebral perfusion pressure (CPP) as a result of elevated ICP resulting in local cytotoxic oedema; (3) disruption of the blood brain barrier leading to subsequent vasogenic oedema; and (4) release of vasoactive substances from the haematoma resulting in perihaematoma ischaemia.[144,145] Potential options available for acute medical therapy include strategies to normalise ICP, maintain physiological homeostasis (such as BP management), haemostatic therapy intervention, measures to limit perihaematomal injury and reversal of coagulopathy (Table 2).[69,146,147]

Investigations

ICH can be quickly identified using CT; however, small haemorrhages can disappear after one week of onset thus mimicking infarction. In cases

Table 2.   Rationale and evidence for early acute medical interventions for ICH

Intervention	Rationale	Level of evidence from randomised trials
Osmotherapy	Increase serum osmolality thereby reducing ICP using mannitol and glycerol.	Level of Evidence B
Haemostatic therapy	To reduce haematoma growth with rFVIIa. Haematoma growth associated with poor outcome.	Level of Evidence B
Corticosteroids	To reduce perihaematoma oedema using dexamethasone. Perihaematoma vasogenic oedema associated with neurological deterioration.	Level of Evidence B
Anti-inflammatory agents	Inflammatory mediators and cytokines release after ICH may be associated with poor outcome, e.g. MMP.	Experimental
Blood pressure lowering	High blood pressure associated with haematoma growth and poor outcome.	Level of Evidence C
Insulin	Hyperglycaemia and diabetes associated with poor outcome.	Level of Evidence C
Temperature reduction	Raised temperature associated with poor outcome.	Level of Evidence C
Anticoagulation reversal	Reversal of INR using vitamin K, PCC, FFP and rFVIIa associated with reduction in haematoma growth.	Level of Evidence C
Prophylactic anticonvulsant therapy	Reduces risk of early seizure occurrence.	Level of Evidence C

Level of Evidence A: Data derived from multiple randomised controlled trials
Level of Evidence B: Data derived from a single randomised controlled trial
Level of Evidence C: Consensus opinion of experts

of delayed presentation, MRI with gradient echo sequence can reliably differentiate between haemorrhage and infarction. MRI is also useful in delineating vascular flow voids indicative of arterio-venous malformations and amyloid angiopathy in the presence of microbleeds distributed in lobar regions of the brain on gradient echo sequence.[148] The age of the patient and location of the ICH is likely to guide further imaging modality. For example, Zhu *et al.* showed that in patients over the age of 45 years with a history of hypertension with ICH affecting the basal ganglia, catheter angiography did not reveal any vascular abnormality; however, angiography was more likely to reveal vascular abnormalities in patients with lobar, non-hypertensive ICH.[149] CT angiography, which is a quick, safe and available alternative to catheter angiography, is a useful modality to investigate younger patients for an underlying large vessel aneurysm, arterio-venous malformation or arterio-venous fistula, particularly if there is no other risk factor identified.

Prognosis

A useful scale which may be of prognostic significance includes five elements of clinical parameters.[150] They include low Glasgow coma scale (< 4/15), raised ICH volume (≥ 30 ml), increasing age (≥ 80 years), presence of intraventricular haemorrhage and infratentorial location. The presence of all five parameters predicts a 30-day mortality of 100% (95% CI: 61–100).

Specific Management Strategies

Management of intracranial pressure

A rise in ICP (defined as > 20 mmHg for five minutes or longer) is frequently seen in patients after ICH and is associated with neurological deterioration.[151,152] This is thought to be secondary to a reduction in CPP and thus CBF leading to further neuronal ischaemia and/or cell necrosis.[153] There is no trial evidence that monitoring of raised ICP after ICH is associated with improved outcome; however, guidelines suggest maintaining CPP > 70 mmHg.[69,70] Which patients to monitor invasively and by which route depends upon the clinical status of the patient, location and volume of haematoma, along with the possible coexistent need for ventriculostomy to manage raised ICP.[154] General strategies to reduce ICP include head elevation, osmotic therapy, hyperventilation and sedation.

General measures to combat raised ICP

Head positioning

Following ICH, cerebral autoregulation may be impaired, thereby risking cerebral hypoperfusion upon overt head elevation.[155] Traditionally, patients with a large hemispheric stroke have been managed with moderate head elevation between 30° and 45° in order to reduce raised ICP,[156] a practice generalised from clinical experience with head trauma patients despite clear differences in pathophysiology.[157] Until evidence specifically confirms these findings in patients with ICH, it is recommended that head positioning to 30° may be adopted if raised ICP is problematic. However positioning should be tailored to the individual's pathophysiological situation depending on BP, CBF, oxygenation and ICP.[158]

Osmotherapy

Theoretically osmotic diuretics reduce ICP by increasing serum osmolarity, thus extracting water from tissues and reducing blood volume by vasoconstriction.[159] Mannitol may also have additional pleotrophic actions improving CPP by either decreasing blood viscosity or by altering red cell morphology, thus increasing tissue oxygenation.[160] There are only two randomised controlled trials evaluating the effects of mannitol in ICH.[161,162] One randomised trial involving 36 patients receiving mannitol showed no beneficial effects of such treatment but it was unclear as to the proportion of haemorrhagic strokes in the study group as no CT criteria were performed.[161] Misra and colleagues demonstrated no benefit in one-month mortality and three-month functional outcome in a randomised trial involving 65 study patients receiving mannitol for six days post-ICH and 63 control patients.[162] Potential adverse effects in humans include 'rebound phenomena' which may result in increased cerebral oedema on its discontinuation as well as electrolyte imbalance.[163]

Only two randomised controlled studies have reported the effects of glycerol in ICH.[164,165] Yu *et al.* demonstrated in a randomised, double-blind, placebo-controlled study of 216 patients after ICH that intravenous glycerol (400 mls of 10% glycerol over four hours for six days) had no additional benefit upon mortality or functional outcome at six months compared to placebo.[165] Mathew *et al.* also demonstrated no benefit in this treatment in eight patients with ICH.[164] A Cochrane review of the use of glycerol in acute stroke (which included patients with ICH) found a favourable but minimal effect of glycerol in the short term and a paucity of evidence of improved outcome in the long term.[166] Currently neither hypertonic saline nor haemodilution have evidence to support their use to reduce ICP.[167]

Hyperventilation

Cerebral vasoconstriction reduces ICP and this may be induced by lowering serum pCO_2 via hyperventilation.[168] Target serum pCO_2 levels of 4.0–4.7 kPa are recommended but current advice warns against prolonged hyperventilation leading to excess vasoconstriction and subsequent ischaemia.[70]

Sedation

Barbiturate anaesthetic agents phenobarbitone and thiopentone may reduce vasospasm and ultimately ICP.[169] Only one published non-randomised study has been undertaken using barbiturate coma in non-traumatic brain injury patients with raised ICP. In 15 patients treated (three had ICH), only those who demonstrated a sustainable reduction in ICP survived.[170] There are no randomised controlled trials using barbiturate coma for the reduction of ICP in ICH and its use may currently only be supported anecdotally.

Measures to combat perihaematoma growth

The volume of haematoma, along with its location is one of the most important prognostic indicators in ICH dictating mortality and functional outcome.[171] Imaging studies have demonstrated that haematoma expansion occurs in 40% of cases within three hours and is a common cause of neurological deterioration acutely (Fig. 5).[147] Therefore haematoma growth is an exciting proposition for targeting with haemostatic therapy in order to limit growth and improve outcome. There are only five randomised trials that have studied haemostatic therapy after acute ICH.[172–177]

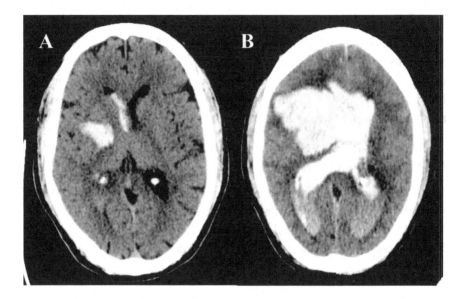

Figure 5. (A) Right basal ganglia haemorrhage with extension into right lateral ventricle. (B) Follow-up scan two hours later after neurologic deterioration shows extension of haemorrhage into right parietal and frontal lobes, occupying third and lateral ventricles and associated midline shift.

Mayer *et al.* conducted a phase IIB dose-ranging, proof-of-concept study evaluating the ability of rFVIIa to reduce haematoma expansion within 24 hours and subsequent mortality and dependency at 90 days when administered within four hours.[175] Patients were assigned to one of three single intravenous doses of rFVIIa (40 μg/kg, 80 μg/kg, 160 μg/kg) or placebo. All doses demonstrated a significant decrease in haematoma volume expansion (40 μg/kg: −16%, 80 μg/kg: −14%, 160 μg/kg: −11% vs. placebo: 29%) and a reduction in poor outcome at three months (40 μg/kg: −55%, 80 μg/kg: −49%, 160 μg/kg: −54% vs. placebo: 69%). Combining the treatment groups demonstrated an absolute risk reduction of 16% for mortality or severe disability at three months. A significant side effect of haemostatic therapy with rFVIIa was the additional risk of thromboembolic events such as myocardial infarction and cerebral infarction (7% treatment vs. 2% placebo).

To confirm these findings, a larger randomised controlled phase III trial with rFVIIa was undertaken involving 841 patients testing 20 μg/kg and 80 μg/kg against placebo within four hours of onset.[176,178] Data suggested that although a reduction of haematoma growth was observed, there were no significant differences in mortality or poor outcome at three months. Whether further trials need to be undertaken to examine the effects of rFVIIa is now debatable.

Measures to combat perihaematoma oedema formation

Corticosteroids have been used anecdotally in the hope of reducing vasogenic oedema which occurs three hours after the initial onset of cytotoxic oedema post-ICH and peaks within 24 hours.[179] The Cochrane Collaboration review of five small randomised controlled trials concluded no evidence of a beneficial effect of dexamethasone on mortality after ICH.[180-185] The largest study by Poungvarin *et al.* demonstrated little benefit in survival and widespread complications in their use of dexamethasone in 93 patients following supratentorial ICH.[181] The potential benefits of corticosteroids of reducing perihaematomal oedema, ICP and strengthening the blood brain barrier has to be tempered with the deleterious effects of hyperglycaemia, relative immunodeficiency and gastrointestinal haemorrhage.[186]

Blood pressure management

The premise of treating acute hypertension after ICH is to prevent haematoma expansion,[187] which is a common cause of neurological deterioration acutely. Systolic BP readings greater than 200 mmHg have been associated with haematoma enlargement post-ICH.[188] A multicentre prospective study examined the safety of aggressive BP lowering therapy in ICH within the first 24 hours of ictus to achieve target systolic BP levels of less than 160 mmHg by using labetalol, hydralazine and nitroprusside as boluses. The results demonstrated a reduction in haematoma expansion and a decline in neurological deterioration.[189] The greatest benefits were observed when treatment was initiated within six hours of ictus. Qureshi *et al.* demonstrated a high rate of tolerability of lowering of mean arterial BP below 130 mmHg using nicardipine within 24 hours of ICH.[190] What is unclear at present is whether active lowering of BP post-ICH leads to reduced haematoma expansion and improved outcome. The pilot randomised controlled INTERACT (INTEnsive blood pressure Reduction in Acute Cerebral haemorrhage Trial) trial demonstrated that BP lowering within six hours of onset to target systolic BP levels of 140 mmHg led to a significant reduction of haematoma growth compared with alternative systolic BP targets of 180 mmHg.[191] The randomised multicentre ATACH (Antihypertensive Treatment in Acute Cerebral Haemorrhage) trial aimed to assess the safety and the rate of neurological deterioration in patients presenting within 24 hours with systolic BP greater than 200 mmHg using intravenous nicardipine with three different BP systolic goals: (1) 170–200 mmHg; (2) 140–170 mmHg; and (3) 110–140 mmHg.[192] Preliminary results demonstrated no major safety issues and no differences in mortality at three months.

At present, there is insufficient evidence for acute BP reduction in haemorrhagic stroke. This has led to different recommendations between the AHA guidelines (treat if systolic BP > 180 mmHg or mean arterial BP > 130 mmHg and keep CPP between 60–80 mmHg if raised ICP present),[70] the European guidelines (treat if systolic BP > 160 mmHg and diastolic BP > 95 mmHg),[69] and United Kingdom guidelines (treat if systolic BP > 200 mmHg).[29] Target BP considered is 160/90 mmHg with no more than 20% reduction of BP at 24 hours. The choice of antihypertensive agent is also still unclear. Potential therapies used include nitroprusside, labetalol, nicardipine, esmolol, enalapril and hydralazine as either a bolus or an infusion.

Measures to combat perihaematomal brain injury

Inflammatory mediators such as interleukin-6, interleukin-1, tumour necrosis factor and intercellular adhesion molecule-1 are released in response to ICH within 48 hours, leading to damage to the blood brain barrier, subsequent vasogenic oedema and perihaematoma ischaemia.[193] Thrombin release at high concentrations from the haematoma initiating an inflammatory cascade has also been postulated, resulting in leucocyte recruitment, expression of adhesion molecules and further cytokine release.[194] Following these findings, direct thrombin inhibitor argatroban has been shown to reduce oedema volume in animal models if administered within six hours of ICH.[195] Erythropoietin, a pleotrophic cytokine, has also been shown to be neuroprotective in the rat model by preventing apoptosis.[196] Overexpression of matrix metalloproteinases (MMPs), in particular MMP-9, have also been described post-ICH resulting in apoptosis, vasogenic oedema and increased mortality.[197] MMPs appear to promote extracellular matrix proteolysis, attack the basal lamina, and degrade cellular fibronectin, a glycoprotein which is important for homeostasis.[198] New Qingkailing injection (NQKLI) has been shown in the rat model to reduce serum MMP-9 48 hours after induced-ICH[199]; however, many of the neuroprotective agents that have been studied in animal models have failed to demonstrate benefits in human studies.

Reversal of Anticoagulation-Associated Intracerebral Haemorrhage

Outcome of anticoagulation-associated ICH tends to be worse than spontaneous ICH and haematoma expansion tends to occur longer (up to 48 hours), thus providing a real opportunity for interventions to reverse anticoagulation.[200] Factors associated with anticoagulation-induced ICH include increasing age, presence of cerebral amyloid angiopathy and leukoaraiosis.[201] Most ICH occurs when the international normalised ratio is within the therapeutic range.[202] Interventions such as vitamin K, fresh frozen plasma, prothrombin complex concentrates and rFVIIa are current treatment options but data is available only from retrospective observational studies.[203] None have been evaluated in randomised controlled trials. Vitamin K tends to achieve its response after more than 24 hours.[204] Fresh frozen plasma tends to rely on large volumes due to unconcentrated forms of coagulation factors.[205] Prothrombin complex has high levels of vitamin K-dependent factors and works faster and reduces haematoma volume compared with fresh frozen plasma,[206] but caution needs to be applied with its thrombotic complications. Although rFVIIa (10 μg/kg to 90 μg/kg) works faster (within minutes) than fresh frozen plasma,[207] concerns remain over its safety profile. Large randomised controlled trials are required to test the efficacy of fresh frozen plasma, prothrombin complex in combination with vitamin K and rFVIIa in patients with ICH. Patients who have had ICH induced by heparin (unfractionated or low molecular weight) should have protamine sulphate for reversal.

Surgery

There is uncertainty whether early surgical evacuation is beneficial for all patients with spontaneous lobar supratentorial ICH. Surgery is generally considered for patients with hydrocephalus if they were previously fit.[208] A systematic review examining the effects of evacuation of spontaneous supratentorial ICH revealed that neurosurgical intervention reduced death and dependence at follow-up.[209] The STICH trial (Surgical Trial in lobar IntraCerebral Haemorrhage) including 1033 patients with supratentorial ICH demonstrated that early craniotomy within 72 hours compared with initial conservative medical treatment did not improve outcome at six months. However, a subgroup analysis did reveal that for patients with haematoma < 1 cm from the cortical surface, early evacuation was more favourable.[210] STICH II aims to evaluate the benefits of surgical evacuation of supratentorial, lobar ICH, < 1 cm from the cortical surface in 600 patients within 48 hours of ictus. Patients in which the neurosurgeon is uncertain about the benefits of surgery will be recruited to the trial. There is consensus opinion that surgical evacuation of infratentorial ICH is merited in patients whose conscious level is deteriorating in the presence of brainstem compression or hydrocephalus such that a randomised controlled trial is unlikely to be undertaken. Trials evaluating other procedures such as mechanical aspiration of haematoma or thrombolytic therapy for intraventricular haemorrhage are also being evaluated in randomised controlled trials.

References

1. Wade DT, Langton Hewer R. Hospital admission for acute stroke: who, for how long, and to what effect? *J Epidemiol Community Health* 1985; 39: 347–352.
2. Kalra L, Evans A, Perez I, Knapp M, Donaldson N, Swift CG. Alternative strategies for stroke care: a prospective randomised controlled trial. *Lancet* 200; 356: 894–899.

3. Hacke W. A late step in the right direction of stroke care. *Lancet* 2000; 356: 869–870.
4. Wardlaw JM, Kier SL, Dennis MS. The impact of delays in computed tomography of the brain on the accuracy of diagnosis and subsequent management in patients with minor stroke. *J Neurol Neurosurg Psychiatry* 2003; 74: 77–81.
5. Evans A, Perez I, Harraf F, Melbourn A, Steadman J, Donaldson N, Kalra L. Can differences in management processes explain different outcomes between stroke unit and stroke-team care? *Lancet* 2001; 358: 1586–1592.
6. National Institute of Neurological Disorders and Stroke (NINDS). rt-PA Stroke Study Group. Tissue Plasminogen activator for acute stroke. *NEJM* 1995; 333: 1581–1587.
7. Stone S. Stroke units. *BMJ* 2002; 325: 291–292.
8. Harbison J, Hossain O, Jenkinson D, Davis J, Louw SJ, Ford GA. Diagnostic accuracy of stroke referrals from primary care, emergency room physicians, and ambulance staff using the face arm speech test. *Stroke* 2003; 34: 71–76.
9. Nor AM, Davis J, Sen B, Shipsey D, Louw SJ, Dyker AG, Davis M, Ford GA. The Recognition of Stroke in the Emergency Room (ROSIER) scale: development and validation of a stroke recognition instrument. *Lancet Neurol* 2005; 4: 727–734.
10. Nor AM, McAllister C, Louw SJ, Dyker AG, Davis M, Jenkinson D, Ford GA. Agreement between ambulance paramedic- and physician-recorded neurological signs with Face Arm Speech Test (FAST) in acute stroke patients. *Stroke* 2004; 35: 1355–1359.
11. Department of Health. National Stroke Strategy. 2007.
12. Birns J, Fitzpatrick M. Thrombolysis for acute ischaemic stroke and the role of the nurse. *BJN* 2004; 13: 1170–1174.
13. Kasner SE. Clinical interpretation and use of stroke scales. *Lancet Neurol* 2006; 5: 603–612.
14. Grotta JC, Chiu D, Lu M, Patel S, Levine SR, Tilley BC, Brott TG, Haley EC Jr, Lyden PD, Kothari R, Frankel M, Lewandowski CA, Libman R, Kwiatkowski T, Broderick JP, Marler JR, Corrigan J, Huff S, Mitsias P, Talati S, Tanne D. Agreement and variability in the interpretation of early CT changes in stroke patients qualifying for intravenous rtPA therapy. *Stroke* 1999; 30: 1528–1533.
15. Kalafut MA, Schriger DL, Saver JL, Starkman S. Detection of early CT signs of > 1/3 middle cerebral artery infarctions: interrater reliability and sensitivity

of CT interpretation by physicians involved in acute stroke care. *Stroke* 2000; 31: 1667–1671.

16. Barber PA, Demchuk AM, Zhang J, Buchan AM. Validity and reliability of a quantitative computed tomography score in predicting outcome of hyperacute stroke before thrombolytic therapy. ASPECTS Study Group. Alberta Stroke Programme Early CT Score. *Lancet* 2000; 355: 1670–1674.

17. Barber PA, Davis SM. Limitations of current brain imaging in stroke. Chapter 2. *Magnetic Resonance Imaging in Stroke.* Davis S, Fisher M, Warach S. (Eds.) Cambridge University Press, 2003.

18. Indredavik B, Bakke RPT, Slordahl SA, Rokseth R, Haheim LL. Treatment in a combined acute and rehabilitation stroke unit. Which aspects are most important? *Stroke* 1999; 30: 917–923.

19. Ronning OM, Guldvog B, Stavem K. The benefit of an acute stroke unit in patients with intracranial haemorrhage: a controlled trial. *J Neurol Neurosurg Psychiatry* 2001; 70: 631–634.

20. Ronning OM, Guldvog B. Stroke unit versus medical wards, II: Neurological deficits and activities of daily living. A quasi randomised controlled trial. *Stroke* 1998; 29: 586–590.

21. Davis M, Hollyman C, McGiven M, Chambers I, Egbuji J, Barer D. Physiological monitoring in acute stroke. *Age Ageing* 1999; 28(Suppl): P45.

22. Cavallini A, Micieli G, Marcheselli S, Quaglini S. Role of monitoring in management of acute ischaemic stroke patients. *Stroke* 2003; 34: 2599–2603.

23. Fisher M. Characterising the target of acute stroke therapy. *Stroke* 1997; 28: 866–872.

24. Guidelines for Management of Ischaemic Stroke and Transient Ischaemic Attack: The European Stroke Organisation (ESO) Executive Committee and the ESO Writing Committee. *Cerebrovasc Dis* 2008; 25: 457–507.

25. Rocco A, Pasquini M, Cecconi E, Sirimarco G, Ricciardi MC, Vicenzini E, Altieri M, Di Piero V, Lenzi GL. Monitoring after the acute stage of stroke: a prospective study. *Stroke* 2007; 38: 1225–1228.

26. Walshaw MJ, Pearson MG. Hypoxia in patients with acute hemiplegia. *Br Med J* 1984; 228: 15–17.

27. Elizabeth J, Singarayar J, Ellul J, Barer D, Lye M. Arterial oxygen saturation and posture in acute stroke. *Age Ageing* 1993; 22: 269–272.

28. Bhalla A, Pomeroy VM, Tallis RC. The effects of positioning after stroke on physiological homeostasis: a review. *Age Ageing* 2005; 34: 401–406.

29. Royal College of Physicians Intercollegiate Stroke Working Party. *National Clinical Guidelines on the Management of People of Stroke.* 3rd Edn. 2008.
30. Mickel HS, Vaishnav YN, Kempski O, von Lubitz D, Weiss JF, Feuertein G. Breathing 100% oxygen after global brain ischaemia in Mongolian gerbils results in increased lipid peroxidation and increased mortality. *Stroke* 1987; 18: 426–430.
31. Ronning OM, Guldvog B. Should stroke victims routinely receive supplemental oxygen? A quasi randomised controlled trial. *Stroke* 1999; 30: 2033–2037.
32. Roffe C. The Stroke Oxygen Pilot Study; a multicentre prospective randomised open, blinded endpoint study of routine oxygen treatment in the first 72 hours after a stroke (SO_2S). http://www.so2s.co.uk
33. Harrison MJG. The influence of haematocrit in the cerebral circulation. *Cerebrovasc Brain Metab Rev* 1989; 1: 55–67.
34. Bhalla A, Sankaralingam S, Dundas R, Swaminathan R, Wolfe CDA, Rudd AG. The influence of raised plasma osmolality on clinical outcome after stroke. *Stroke* 2000; 31: 2043–2048.
35. Asplund K, Israelsson K, Schampi I. Haemodilution for acute ischaemic stroke. *Cochrane Database Syst Rev* 2000; 2: CD000103.
36. Weir JW, Murria GD, Dyker AG, Lees KR. Is hyperglycaemia an independent predictor of poor outcome after stroke? Results of a long term follow-up study. *BMJ* 1997; 314: 1303–1306.
37. Jørgensen H, Nakayama H, Raaschou HO, Olsen TS. Stroke in patients with diabetes. The Copenhagen Stroke Study. *Stroke* 1994; 25: 1977–1984.
38. Helgason CM. Blood glucose and stroke. *Stroke* 1988; 19: 1049–1053.
39. Lindsberg PJ, Roine RO. Hyperglycemia in acute stroke. *Stroke* 2004; 35: 363–364.
40. Fogelholm R, Murros K, Rissanen A, Avikainen S. Admission blood glucose and short term survival in primary intracerebral haemorrhage: A population based study. *J Neurol Neurosurg Psychiatry* 2005; 76: 349–353.
41. Kiers L, Davis SM, Larkins R, Hopper J, Tress B, Rossiter SC, Carlin J, Ratnaike S. Stroke topography and outcome in relation to hyperglycaemia and diabetes. *J Neurol Neurosurg Psychiatry* 1992; 55: 263–270.
42. Fuentes B, Castillo J, San José B, Leira R, Serena J, Vivancos J, Dávalos A, Gil Nuñez A, Egido J, Díez-Tejedor E. The prognostic value of capillary glucose levels in acute stroke: The GLycemia In Acute Stroke (GLIAS) Study. *Stroke* 2009; 40: 562–568.

43. Gray CS, Hildreth AJ, Sandercock PA, O'Connell JE, Johnston DE, Cartlidge NEF, Bamford JM, James OF, Alberti GMM, for the GIST Trialists Collaboration. Glucose–potassium–insulin infusions in the management of post-stroke hyperglycaemia: the UK Glucose Insulin in Stroke Trial (GIST-UK). *Lancet Neurol* 2007; 6: 397–406.

44. Bruno A, Kent TA, Coull BM, Shankar RR, Saha C, Becker KJ, Kissela BM, Williams LS. Treatment of Hyperglycemia in Ischemic Stroke (THIS). A randomised pilot trial. *Stroke* 2008; 39: 384–389.

45. Adams HP Jr, del Zoppo G, Alberts MJ, Bhatt DL, Brass L, Furlan A, Grubb RL, Higashida RT, Jauch EC, Kidwell C, Lyden PD, Morgenstern LB, Qureshi AI, Rosenwasser RH, Scott PA, Wijdicks EF. Guidelines for the early management of adults with ischemic stroke: a guideline from the American Heart Association/American Stroke Association Stroke Council, Clinical Cardiology Council, Cardiovascular Radiology and Intervention Council, and the Atherosclerotic Peripheral Vascular Disease and Quality of Care Outcomes in Research Interdisciplinary Working Groups: the American Academy of Neurology affirms the value of this guideline as an educational tool for neurologists. *Stroke* 2007; 38: 1655–1711.

46. Oppenheimer S, Hachinski V. Complications of acute stroke. *Lancet* 1992; 339: 721–724.

47. Britton M, Carlsson A, De Faire U. Blood pressure course in patients with acute stroke and matched controls. *Stroke* 1986; 17: 861–864.

48. Britton M, Carlsson A. Very high blood pressure in acute stroke. *J Intern Med* 1990; 228: 611–615.

49. Robinson T, Waddington A, Ward-Close S, Taub N, Potter J. The predictive role of 24-hour compared to casual blood pressure levels on outcome following acute stroke. *Cerebrovasc Dis* 1997; 7: 264–272.

50. Leonardi-Bee J, Bath PM, Phillips SJ, Sandercock PA: IST Collaborative Group. Blood pressure and clinical outcomes in the International Stroke Trial. *Stroke* 2002; 23: 1315–1320.

51. Fischberg GM, Lozano E, Rajamani K, Ameriso S, Fisher MJ. Stroke precipitated by moderate blood pressure reduction. *J Emerg Med* 2000; 19: 339–346.

52. Schrader J, Luders S, Kulschewski A, Berger J, Zidek W, Treib J, Einhaupl K, Diener HC, Dominiak P. The ACCESS Study: evaluation of Acute Candesartan Ciliexetil Therapy in Stroke Survivors. *Stroke* 2003; 34: 1699–1703.

53. Potter JF, Robinson TG, Ford GA, Mistri A, James M, Chernova J, Jagger C. Controlling hypertension and hypotension immediately postsroke (CHHIPS): a randomised placebo controlled double blind pilot trials. *Lancet Neurol* 2009; 8: 48–56.

54. COSSACS Trial Group. COSSACS (Continue or Stop post-Stroke Antihypertensives Collaborative Study): rationale and design. *J Hypertens* 2005; 23: 455–458.

55. Wise G, Sutter R, Burkholder J. The treatment of brain ischaemia with vasopressor drugs. *Stroke* 1972; 3: 135–140.

56. Rodorf G, Cranmer SC, Efird JT, Schwamm LH, Buonanno F, Koroshetz WJ. Pharmacological elevation of blood pressure in acute stroke. *Stroke* 1997; 28: 2133–2138.

57. Martino R, Foley N, Bhogal S, Diamant N, Speechley M, Teasell R. Dysphagia after stroke: incidence, diagnosis and pulmonary complications. *Stroke* 2005; 36: 2756–2763.

58. Axlesson K, Asplund K, Norberg A, Alafuzoff I. Nutritional status in patients with acute stroke. *Acta Med Scand* 1988; 224: 217–224.

59. Dennis MS, Lewis SC, Warlow C. Effect of timing and method of enteral tube feeding for dysphagic stroke patients (FOOD): a multicentre randomised controlled trial. *Lancet* 2005; 365: 764–772.

60. Hajat C, Hajat S, Sharma P. Effects of post stroke pyrexia on stroke outcome. A meta-analysis of studies in patients. *Stroke* 2000; 31: 410–414.

61. Deogaonkar A, De Georgia, Bae C *et al.* Fever is associated with third ventricular shift after intracerebral haemorrhage: pathophysiologic implications. *Neurol India* 2005; 53: 202–206.

62. Leira R, Dávalos A, Silva Y, Gil-Peralta A, Tejada J, Garcia M, Castillo J, Stroke Project, Cerebrovascular Diseases Group of the Spanish Neurological Society. Early neurologic deterioration in intracerebral haemorrhage: predictors and associated factors. *Neurology* 2004; 63: 461–467.

63. Schwab S, Schwarz S, Spranger M, Keller E, Bertram M, Hacke W. Moderate hypothermia in the treatment of patients with severe middle cerebral artery infarction. *Stroke* 1998; 29: 2461–2466.

64. Thomas LH, Barrett J, Cross S, French B, Leathley M, Sutton C, Watkins C. Prevention and treatment of urinary incontinence after stroke in adults. *Cochrane Database Syst Rev* 2005; 3: CD004462.

65. Kelly J, Hunt BJ, Lewis RR, Rudd AG. Anticoagulation or inferior vena cava filter placement with primary intracerebral haemorrhage developing venous thromboembolism. *Stroke* 2003; 34: 2999–3005.

66. Kelly J, Rudd A, Lewis R, Hunt BJ. Venous thromboembolism after acute stroke. *Stroke* 2001; 32: 262–267.

67. Bailey RD, Hart RG, Benavente O, Pearce LA. Recurrent brain haemorrhage is more frequent than ischaemic stroke after intracerebral haemorrhage. *Neurology* 2001; 56: 773–777.

68. Gubitz G, Sandercock P, Counsell C. Anticoagulation for acute ischaemic stroke. *Cochrane Database Syst Rev* 2004; 2: CD000024.

69. Steiner T, Kaste M, Forsting M *et al.* Recommendations for the management of intracranial haemorrhage — part I: spontaneous intracerebral haemorrhage. The European Stroke Initiative Writing Committee and the Writing Committee for the EUSI Executive Committee. *Cerebrovasc Dis* 2006; 22: 294–316.

70. Broderick J, Connolly S, Feldman E *et al.* Guidelines for the management of spontaneous intracerebral haemorrhage in adults 2007 update: a guideline from the American Heart Association/American Stroke Association Stroke Council, High Blood Pressure Research Council, and the Quality of Care and Outcomes in Research Interdisciplinary Working Group. *Stroke* 2007; 38: 2001–2023.

71. CLOTS Trials Collaboration, Dennis M, Sandercock PA, Reid J, Graham C, Murray G, Venables G, Rudd A, Bowler G. Effectiveness of thigh-length graduated compression stockings to reduce the risk of deep vein thrombosis after stroke (CLOTS trial 1): a multicentre, randomised controlled trial. *Lancet* 2009; 373: 1958–1965.

72. Passero S, Rocchi R, Rossi S, Ulivelli M, Vatti G. Seizures after spontaneous supratentorial haemorrhage. *Epilepsia* 2002; 43: 1175–1180.

73. Vespa PM, O'Phelan K, Shah M *et al.* Acute seizures after intracerebral haemorrhage: a factor in progressive midline shift and outcome. *Neurology* 2003; 60: 1441–1446.

74. Meyer BC, Raman R, Hemmen T, Obler R, Zivin JA, Rao R, Thomas RG, Lyden PD. Efficacy of site-independent telemedicine in the STRokE DOC trial: a randomised, blinded, prospective study. *Lancet Neurol* 2008; 7: 787–795.

75. Schwamm LH, Holloway RG, Amarenco P, Audebert HJ, Bakas T, Chumbler NR, Handschu R, Jauch EC, Knight WA 4th, Levine SR,

Mayberg M, Meyer BC, Meyers PM, Skalabrin E, Wechsler LR, American Heart Association Stroke Council; Interdisciplinary Council on Peripheral Vascular Disease. A review of the evidence for the use of telemedicine within stroke systems of care: a scientific statement from the American Heart Association/American Stroke Association. *Stroke* 2009; 40: 2616–2634.

76. Schwamm LH, Audebert HJ, Amarenco P, Chumbler NR, Frankel MR, George MG, Gorelick PB, Horton KB, Kaste M, Lackland DT, Levine SR, Meyer BC, Meyers PM, Patterson V, Stranne SK, White CJ, American Heart Association Stroke Council; Council on Epidemiology and Prevention; Interdisciplinary Council on Peripheral Vascular Disease; Council on Cardiovascular Radiology and Intervention. Recommendations for the implementation of telemedicine within stroke systems of care: a policy statement from the American Heart Association. *Stroke* 2009; 40: 2635–2660.

77. LaMonte MP, Bahouth MN, Hu P, Pathan MY, Yarbrough KL, Gunawardane R, Crarey P, Page W. Telemedicine for acute stroke: triumphs and pitfalls. *Stroke* 2003; 34: 725–728.

78. Wiborg A, Widder B. Telemedicine in Stroke in Swabia Project. Teleneurology to improve stroke care in rural areas: The Telemedicine in Stroke in Swabia (TESS) Project. *Stroke* 2003; 34: 2951–2956.

79. Wang S, Gross H, Lee SB, Pardue C, Waller J, Nichols FT 3rd, Adams RJ, Hess DC. Remote evaluation of acute ischemic stroke in rural community hospitals in Georgia. *Stroke* 2004; 35: 1763–1768.

80. Audebert HJ, Kukla C, Clarmann von Claranau S, Kühn J, Vatankhah B, Schenkel J, Ickenstein GW, Haberl RL, Horn M, TEMPiS Group. Telemedicine for safe and extended use of thrombolysis in stroke: the Telemedic Pilot Project for Integrative Stroke Care (TEMPiS) in Bavaria. *Stroke* 2005; 36: 287–291.

81. Switzer JA, Hall C, Gross H, Waller J, Nichols FT, Wang S, Adams RJ, Hess DC. A web-based telestroke system facilitates rapid treatment of acute ischemic stroke patients in rural emergency departments. *J Emerg Med* 2009; 36: 12–18.

82. Miley ML, Bobrow BJ, Demaerschalk BM. Stroke Telemedicine for Arizona Rural Residents (STARR). *Cerebrovasc Dis* 2008; 25(Suppl 2): 101.

83. Audebert H. Telestroke: effective networking. *Lancet Neurol* 2006; 5: 279–282.

84. Demaerschalk BM, Miley ML, Kiernan TE, Bobrow BJ, Corday DA, Wellik KE, Aguilar MI, Ingall TJ, Dodick DW, Brazdys K, Koch TC, Ward MP, Richemont PC; STARR Coinvestigators. Stroke telemedicine. *Mayo Clin Proc* 2009; 84: 53–64.

85. Multicentre Acute Stroke Trial-Italy Group. Randomised controlled trial of streptokinase, aspirin, and combination of both in treatment of acute ischemic stroke. *Lancet* 1995; 346: 1509–1514.

86. The Multicenter Acute Stroke Trial-Europe Study Group.Thrombolytic therapy with streptokinase in acute ischemic stroke. *NEJM* 1996; 335: 145–150.

87. Donnan GA, Davis SM, Chambers BR, Gates PC, Hankey GJ, McNeil JJ, Rosen D, Stewart-Wynne EG, Tuck RR. Streptokinase for acute ischemic stroke with relationship to time of administration: Australian Streptokinase Trial Study Group. *JAMA* 1996; 276: 961–966.

88. Blakeley JO, Llinas RH. Thrombolytic therapy for acute ischemic stroke. *J Neurol Sci* 2007; 261(1–2): 55–62.

89. Saver JL. Number needed to treat estimates incorporating effects over the entire range of clinical outcomes: novel derivation method and application to thrombolytic therapy for acute stroke. *Arch Neurol* 2004; 61: 1066–1070.

90. The NINDS t-PA Stroke Study Group, Generalized efficacy of t-PA for acute ischemic stroke. Subgroup analysis of the NINDS t-PA Stroke Trial. *Stroke* 1997; 28: 2119–2125.

91. Fagan SC, Morgenstern LB, Petitta A, Ward RE, Tilley BC, Marler JR, Levine SR, Broderick JP, Kwiatkowski TG, Frankel M, Brott TG, Walker MD. Cost-effectiveness of tissue plasminogen activator for acute ischemic stroke. NINDS rt-PA Stroke Study Group. *Neurology* 1998; 50: 883–890.

92. Kwiatkowski TG, Libman RB, Frankel M, Kwiatkowski TG, Libman RB, Frankel. Effects of tissue plasminogen activator for acute ischemic stroke at one year. National Institute of Neurological Disorders and Stroke Recombinant Tissue Plasminogen Activator Stroke Study Group. *NEJM* 1999; 340: 1781–1787.

93. Hacke W, Kaste M, Fieschi C, Toni D, Lesaffre E, von Kummer R, Boysen G, Bluhmki E, Höxter G, Mahagne MH *et al.* Intravenous thrombolysis with recombinant tissue plasminogen activator for acute hemispheric stroke: the European Cooperative Acute Stroke Study (ECASS). *JAMA* 1995; 274: 1017–1025.

94. Hacke W, Kaste M, Fieschi C, von Kummer R, Davalos A, Meier D, Larrue V, Bluhmki E, Davis S, Donnan G, Schneider D, Diez-Tejedor E, Trouillas P. Randomised double-blind placebo-controlled trial of thrombolytic therapy with intravenous alteplase in acute ischaemic stroke (ECASS II). *Lancet* 1998; 352: 1245–1251.

95. Clark WM, Wissman S, Albers GW, Jhamandas JH, Madden KP, Hamilton S. Recombinant tissue-type plasminogen activator (alteplase) for ischemic stroke 3 to 5 hours after symptom onset — the ATLANTIS Study: a randomized controlled trial. *JAMA* 1999; 282: 2019–2026.

96. Hacke W, Donnan G, Fieschi C, Kaste M, von Kummer R, Broderick JP, Brott T, Frankel M, Grotta JC, Haley EC Jr, Kwiatkowski T, Levine SR, Lewandowski C, Lu M, Lyden P, Marler JR, Patel S, Tilley BC, Albers G, Bluhmki E, Wilhelm M, Hamilton S; ATLANTIS Trials Investigators, ECASS Trials Investigators, NINDS rt-PA Study Group Investigators. Association of outcome with early stroke treatment: pooled analysis of ATLANTIS, ECASS, and NINDS rt-PA stroke trials. *Lancet* 2004; 363: 768–774.

97. Hacke W, Kaste M, Bluhmki E, Brozman M, Dávalos A, Guidetti D, Larrue V, Lees KR, Medeghri Z, Machnig T, Schneider D, von Kummer R, Wahlgren N, Toni D, ECASS Investigators. Thrombolysis with alteplase 3 to 4.5 hours after acute ischemic stroke. *NEJM* 2008; 359: 1317–1329.

98. Sylaja PN, Cote R, Buchan AM, Hill MD. Thrombolysis in patients older than 80 years with acute ischaemic stroke: Canadian Alteplase for Stroke Effectiveness Study. *J Neurol Neurosurg Psychiatry* 2006; 77: 826–829.

99. Wahlgren N, Ahmed N, Dávalos A, Ford GA, Grond M, Hacke W, Hennerici MG, Kaste M, Kuelkens S, Larrue V, Lees KR, Roine RO, Soinne L, Toni D, Vanhooren G, SITS-MOST investigators. Thrombolysis with alteplase for acute ischaemic stroke in the Safe Implementation of Thrombolysis in Stroke-Monitoring Study (SITS-MOST): an observational study. *Lancet* 2007; 369: 275–282.

100. Lees KR, Ford GA, Muir KW, Ahmed N, Dyker AG, Atula S, Kalra L, Warburton EA, Baron JC, Jenkinson DF, Wahlgren NG, Walters MR, SITS-UK Group. Thrombolytic therapy for acute stroke in the United Kingdom: experience from the safe implementation of thrombolysis in stroke (SITS) register. *QJM* 2008; 101: 863–869.

101. Albers GW, Bates VE, Clark WM, Bell R, Verro P, Hamilton SA. Intravenous tissue-type plasminogen activator for treatment of acute stroke: the Standard Treatment with Alteplase to reverse Stroke (STARS) study. *JAMA* 2000; 283: 1145–1150.

102. Carroll M. Advance nursing practice. *Nursing Standard* 2002; 16: 33–35.

103. Cucchiara B, Tanne D, Levine SR, Demchuk AM, Kasner S. A risk score to predict intracranial hemorrhage after recombinant tissue plasminogen activator for acute ischemic stroke. *J Stroke Cerebrovasc Dis* 2008; 17: 331–333.

104. Larrue V, von Kummer R, Müller A, Bluhmki E. Risk factors for severe hemorrhagic transformation in ischemic stroke patients treated with recombinant tissue plasminogen activator. A secondary analysis of the European-Australasian Acute Stroke Study (ECASS II). *Stroke* 2001; 32: 438–441.

105. Tanne D, Kasner SE, Demchuk AM, Koren-Morag N, Hanson S, Grond M, Levine SR. Markers of increased risk of intracerebral hemorrhage after intravenous recombinant tissue plasminogen activator therapy for acute ischemic stroke in clinical practice. *Circulation* 2002; 105: 1679–1685.

106. The IMS II Investigators. The Interventional Management of Stroke (IMS) II Study. *Stroke* 2007; 38: 2127–2135.

107. Qureshi AI. Endovascular treatment of cerebrovascular diseases and intracranial neoplasms. *Lancet* 2004; 363: 804–813.

108. Ducrocq X, Bracard S, Taillandier L, Anxionnat R, Lacour JC, Guillemin F, Debouverie M, Bollaert PE. Comparison of intravenous and intra-arterial urokinase thrombolysis for acute ischaemic stroke. *J Neuroradiol* 2005; 32: 26–32.

109. Macleod MR, Davis SM, Mitchell PJ, Gerraty RP, Fitt G, Hankey GJ, Stewart-Wynne EG, Rosen D, McNeil JJ, Bladin CF, Chambers BR, Herkes GK, Young D, Donnan GA. Results of a multicentre, randomised controlled trial of intra-arterial urokinase in the treatment of acute posterior circulation ischaemic stroke. *Cerebrovascular Dis* 2005; 20: 12–17.

110. del Zoppo GJ, Higashida RT, Furlan AJ, Pessin MS, Rowley HA, Gent M. PROACT: a phase II randomized trial of recombinant pro-urokinase by direct arterial delivery in acute middle cerebral artery stroke. PROACT Investigators. Prolyse in acute cerebral thromboembolism. *Stroke* 1998; 29: 4–11.

111. Furlan A, Higashida R, Wechsler L, Gent M, Rowley H, Kase C, Pessin M, Ahuja A, Callahan F, Clark WM, Silver F, Rivera F. Intra-arterial prourokinase for acute ischemic stroke. The PROACT II study: a randomized controlled trial. Prolyse in acute cerebral thromboembolism. *JAMA* 1999; 282: 2003–2011.

112. Bourekas EC, Slivka A, Shah R, Mohammad Y, Slone HW, Kehagias DT, Suarez J, Sunshine J, Zaidat OO, Tarr R, Landis DM, Suri MF, Qureshi AI. Intra-arterial thrombolysis within three hours of stroke onset in middle cerebral artery strokes. *Neurocrit Care* 2009; 11: 217–222.

113. Kim DJ, Kim DI, Kim SH, Lee KY, Heo JH, Han SW. Rescue localized intra-arterial thrombolysis for hyperacute MCA ischemic stroke patients after early non-responsive intravenous tissue plasminogen activator therapy. *Neuroradiology* 2005; 47: 616–621.

114. Muir KW, Buchan A, von Kummer R, Rother J, Baron JC. Imaging of acute stroke. *Lancet Neurol* 2006; 5: 755–768.

115. Stemer A, Prabhakaran S. Perfusion imaging in acute ischaemic stroke: time may be on our side. Chapter 5. Brain Hypoxia Ischemia Research Progress. Nova Science Publishers; 2008.

116. Albers GW, Thijs VN, Wechsler L, Kemp S, Schlaug G, Skalabrin E, Bammer R, Kakuda W, Lansberg MG, Shuaib A, Coplin W, Hamilton S, Moseley M, Marks MP; DEFUSE Investigators. Magnetic resonance imaging profiles predict clinical response to early reperfusion: the diffusion and perfusion imaging evaluation for understanding stroke evolution (DEFUSE) study. *Ann Neurol* 2006; 60: 508–517.

117. Davis SM, Donnan GA, Parsons MW, Levi C, Butcher KS, Peeters A, Barber PA, Bladin C, De Silva DA, Byrnes G, Chalk JB, Fink JN, Kimber TE, Schultz D, Hand PJ, Frayne J, Hankey G, Muir K, Gerraty R, Tress BM, Desmond PM, EPITHET investigators. Effects of alteplase beyond 3 h after stroke in the Echoplanar Imaging Thrombolytic Evaluation Trial (EPITHET): a placebo-controlled randomised trial. *Lancet Neurol* 2008; 7: 299–309.

118. Hacke W, Albers G, Al-Rawi Y, Bogousslavsky J, Davalos A, Eliasziw M, Fischer M, Furlan A, Kaste M, Lees KR, Soehngen M, Warach S, DIAS Study Group. The Desmoteplase in Acute Ischemic Stroke Trial (DIAS): a phase II MRI-based 9-hour window acute stroke thrombolysis trial with intravenous desmoteplase. *Stroke* 2005; 36: 66–73.

119. Furlan AJ, Eyding D, Albers GW, Al-Rawi Y, Lees KR, Rowley HA, Sachara C, Soehngen M, Warach S, Hacke W, DEDAS Investigators. Dose Escalation of Desmoteplase for Acute Ischemic Stroke (DEDAS): evidence of safety and efficacy 3 to 9 hours after stroke onset. *Stroke* 2006; 37: 1227–1231.

120. Hacke W, Furlan AJ, Al-Rawi Y, Davalos A, Fiebach JB, Gruber F, Kaste M, Lipka LJ, Pedraza S, Ringleb PA, Rowley HA, Schneider D, Schwamm LH, Leal JS, Söhngen M, Teal PA, Wilhelm-Ogunbiyi K, Wintermark M, Warach S. Intravenous desmoteplase in patients with acute ischaemic stroke selected by MRI perfusion-diffusion weighted imaging or perfusion CT (DIAS-2): a prospective, randomised, double-blind, placebo-controlled study. *Lancet Neurol* 2009; 8: 141–150.

121. Francis CW, Blinc A, Lee S, Cox C. Ultrasound accelerates transport of recombinant tissue plasminogen activator into clots. *Ultrasound Med Biol* 1995; 21: 419–424.

122. Blinc A, Kennedy SD, Bryant RG, Marder VJ, Francis CW. Flow through clots determines the rate and pattern of fibrinolysis. *Thromb Haemost* 1994; 71: 230–235.

123. Lauer CG, Burge R, Tang DB, Bass BG, Gomez ER, Alving BM. Effect of ultrasound on tissue-type plasminogen activator-induced thrombolysis. *Circulation* 1992; 86: 1257–1264.

124. Alexandrov AV, Demchuk AM, Burgin WS, Robinson DJ, Grotta JC, CLOT-BUST Investigators. Ultrasound-enhanced thrombolysis for acute ischemic stroke: phase I. Findings of the CLOTBUST trial. *J Neuroimaging* 2004; 14: 113–117.

125. Alexandrov AV, Molina CA, Grotta JC, Garami Z, Ford SR, Alvarez-Sabin J, Montaner J, Saqqur M, Demchuk AM, Moyé LA, Hill MD, Wojner AW for the CLOTBUST Investigators. Ultrasound-Enhanced Systemic Thrombolysis for Acute Ischemic Stroke. *NEJM* 2004; 351: 2170–2178.

126. Tachibana K, Tachibana S. Albumin microbubble echo-contrast material as an enhancer for ultrasound accelerated thrombolysis. *Circulation* 1995; 92: 1148–1150.

127. Mizushige K, Kondo I, Ohmori K, Hirao K, Matsuo H. Enhancement of ultrasound-accelerated thrombolysis by echo-contrast agents: dependence on microbubble structure. *Ultrasound Med Biol* 1999; 25: 1431–1477.

128. Cintas P, Nguyen F, Boneu B, Larrue V. Enhancement of enzymatic fibrinolysis with 2-MHz ultrasound and microbubbles. *J Thromb Haemost* 2004; 2: 1163–1166.

129. Culp WC, Porter TR, Lowery J, Xie F, Robertson PK, Marky L. Intracranial clot lysis with intravenous microbubbles and transcranial ultrasound in swine. *Stroke* 2004; 35: 2407–2411.
130. Ribo M, Molina CA, Alvarez B, Rubiera M, Alvarez-Sabin J, Matas M. Intra-arterial administration of microbubbles and continuous 2-MHz ultrasound insonation to enhance intra-arterial thrombolysis. *J Neuroimaging* 2009 [Epub ahead of print].
131. Molina CA, Ribo M, Rubiera M, Montaner J, Santamarina E, Delgado-Mederos R, Arenillas JF, Huertas R, Purroy F, Delgado P, Alvarez-Sabin J. Microbubble administration accelerates clot lysis during continuous 2-MHz ultrasound monitoring in stroke patients treated with intravenous tissue plasminogen activator. *Stroke* 2006; 37: 425–429.
132. Gandhi CD, Christiano LD, Prestigiacomo CJ. Endovascular management of acute ischemic stroke. *Neurosurg Focus* 2009; 26: E2.
133. Gobin YP, Starkman S, Duckwiler GR, Grobelny T, Kidwell CS, Jahan R, Pile-Spellman J, Segal A, Vinuela F, Saver JL. MERCI 1: A phase 1 study of Mechanical Embolus Removal in Cerebral Ischemia. *Stroke* 2004; 35: 2848–2854.
134. Smith WS, Sung G, Saver J, Budzik R, Duckwiler G, Liebeskind DS, Lutsep HL, Rymer MM, Higashida RT, Starkman S, Gobin YP, Multi MERCI Investigators, Frei D, Grobelny T, Hellinger F, Huddle D, Kidwell C, Koroshetz W, Marks M, Nesbit G, Silverman IE. Mechanical thrombectomy for acute ischemic stroke: final results of the Multi MERCI trial. *Stroke* 2008; 39: 1205–1212.
135. Bose A, Henkes H, Alfke K, Mayer TE, Berlis A, Branca V, Po Sit S: The Penumbra System: a mechanical device for the treatment of acute stroke due to thromboembolism. *AJNR Am J Neuroradiol* 2008; 29: 1409–1413.
136. IST Collaborative Group. *Lancet* 1997; 349: 1569–1581.
137. CAST Collaborative Group. *Lancet* 1997; 349: 1641–1649.
138. Markus HS, Droste DW, Kaps M, Larrue V, Lees KR, Siebler M, Ringelstein EB. Dual antiplatelet therapy with clopidogrel and aspirin in symptomatic carotid stenosis evaluated using doppler embolic signal detection: the Clopidogrel and Aspirin for Reduction of Emboli in Symptomatic Carotid Stenosis (CARESS) trial. *Circulation* 2005; 111: 2233–2240.
139. ESPRIT Study Group, Halkes PH, van Gijn J, Kappelle LJ, Koudstaal PJ, Algra A. Aspirin plus dipyridamole versus aspirin alone after cerebral

ischaemia of arterial origin (ESPRIT): randomised controlled trial. *Lancet* 2006; 367: 1665–1673.

140. Sandercock PA, Counsell C, Kamal AK. Anticoagulants for acute ischaemic stroke. *Cochrane Database Syst Rev* 2008; 4: CD000024.

141. Berge E, Sandercock P. Anticoagulants versus antiplatelet agents for acute ischaemic stroke. *Cochrane Database Syst Rev* 2002; 4 CD003242.

142. Wong KS, Chen C, Ng PW, Tsoi TH, Li HL, Fong WC, Yeung J, Wong CK, Yip KK, Gao H, Wong HB; FISS-tris Study Investigators. Low-molecular-weight heparin compared with aspirin for the treatment of acute ischaemic stroke in Asian patients with large artery occlusive disease: a randomised study. *Lancet Neurol* 2007; 6: 407–413.

143. Flaherty ML, Haverbusch M, Sekar P *et al.* Long-term mortality after intracerebral haemorrhage. *Neurology* 2006; 66: 1182–1186.

144. Castillo J, Davalos A, Alvarez-Sabin *et al.* Molecular signatures of brain injury after intracerebral haemorrhage. *Neurology* 2002; 58: 624–629.

145. Xi G, Keep RF, Hoff JT. Mechanisms of brain injury after intracerebral haemorrhage. *Lancet Neurol* 2006; 5: 53–63.

146. Rincon F, Mayer SA. Novel therapies for intracerebral haemorrhage. *Curr Opin Crit Care* 2004; 10: 94–100.

147. Broderick JP, Diringer MN, Hill MD *et al.* Determinants of intracerebral haemorrhage growth: an exploratory analysis. *Stroke* 2007; 38: 1072–1075.

148. Viswanathan A, Chabriat H. Cerebral microhemorrhage. *Stroke* 2006; 37: 550–555.

149. Zhu XL, Chan MS, Poon WS. Spontaneous intracranial haemorrhage: which patients need diagnostic cerebral angiography? A prospective study of 206 cases and review of the literature. *Stroke* 1997; 28: 1406–1409.

150. Hemphill JC 3rd, Bonovich DC, Besmertis L, Manley GT, Johnston SC. The ICH score: a simple, reliable grading scale for intracerebral haemorrhage. *Stroke* 2001; 32: 891–897.

151. Holtmannspotter M, Schoch A, Baethmann A, Reulen HJ, Uhl E. Intracranial hypertension influences the resolution of vasogenic brain oedema following intracerebral haemorrhage. *Acta Neurochir Suppl* 2000; 76: 497–499.

152. Sacco C, Marini C, Carolei A. Medical treatment of intracerebral haemorrhage. *Neurol Sci* 2004; 25(Suppl 1): S6–S9.

153. Mayer SA, Chong J. Critical care management of raised intracranial pressure. *J Intensive Care Med* 2000; 17: 55–67.

154. The Brain Trauma Foundation, The American Association of Neurological Surgeons, The Joint Section on Neurotrauma and Critical Care. Guidelines for the management of traumatic brain injury. *J Neurotrauma* 2000; 17: 457–549.

155. Porchet F, Bruder N, Boulard G, Archer DP, Ravussin P. The effect of position on intracranial pressure. *Ann Fr Anesth Reanim* 1998; 17: 149–156.

156. Feldman Z, Kanter MJ, Robertson CS *et al.* Effect of head elevation on intracranial pressure, cerebral perfusion pressure, and cerebral blood flow in head-injured patients. *J Neurosurg* 1992; 76: 207–211.

157. Rosner MJ, Rosner SD, Johnson AH. Cerebral perfusion pressure: management protocol and clinical results. *J Neurosurg* 1995: 83: 949–962.

158. Bhalla A, Tallis RC, Pomeroy VM. The effects of positioning after stroke on physiological homeostasis: a review. *Age Ageing* 2005; 34: 401–406.

159. Winkler SR, Munoz-Ruiz L. Mechanism of action of mannitol. *Surg Neurol* 1995; 43: 59.

160. Andrews RJ, Bringas RS, Muto RP. Effects of mannitol on cerebral blood flow, blood pressure, blood viscosity, haematocrit, sodium, and potassium. *Surg Neurol* 1993; 39: 218–222.

161. Bereczki D, Liu M, do Prado GF, Fekete I. Mannitol for acute stroke. *Cochrane Database Syst Rev* 2001; 1: CD001153.

162. Misra UK, Kalita J, Ranjan P, Mandal SK. Mannitol in intracerebral hemorrhage: a randomized controlled study. *J Neurol Sci* 2005; 234: 41–45.

163. Dziedzic T, Szczudlik A, Klimkowicz A, Rog TM, Slowik A. Is mannitol safe for patients with intracerebral hemorrhages? Renal considerations. *Clin Neurol Neurosurg* 2003; 105: 87–89.

164. Mathew NT, Rivera VM, Meyer JS *et al.* Double blind evaluation of glycerol therapy in acute cerebral infarction. *Lancet* 1972; 2: 1327–1329.

165. Yu YL, Kumana CR, Lauder IJ, Cheung YK, Chan FL, Kou M, Chang CM, Cheung RT, Fong KY. Treatment of acute cerebral haemorrhage with intravenous glycerol. A double-blind, placebo-controlled, randomised trial. *Stroke* 1992; 23: 967–971.

166. Righetti E, Grazia C, Cantisani TA *et al.* Glycerol for acute stroke. *Stroke* 2004; 36: 171–172.

167. Qureshi AI, Suarez JI. Use of hypertonic saline solutions in treatment of cerebral oedema and intracranial hypertension. *Crit Care Med* 2000; 28: 3301–3313.

168. Diringer MN. Intracerebral haemorrhage: pathophysiology and management. *Crit Care Med* 1993; 21: 1591–1603.
169. Cordato DJ, Herkes GK, Mather LE *et al.* Barbiturates for acute neurological and neurosurgical emergencies — do they still have a role? *J Clin Neurosci* 2003; 10: 283–288.
170. Woodcock J, Ropper AH, Kennedy SK. High dose barbiturates in nontraumatic brain swelling: ICP reduction and effect on outcome. *Stroke* 1982; 13: 785–787.
171. Davis SM, Broderick J, Hennerici M, Brun NC, Diringer MN, Mayer SA, Begtrup K, Steiner T; Recombinant Activated Factor VII Intracerebral Hemorrhage Trial Investigators. Haematoma growth is a determinant of mortality and poor outcome after intracerebral hemorrhage. *Neurology* 2006; 66: 1175–1181.
172. Piriyawat P, Morgenstern LB, Yawn DH, Hall CE, Grotta JC. Treatment of acute intracerebral haemorrhage with epsilon aminocaproic acid: a pilot study. *Neurocrit Care* 2004; 1: 47–52.
173. Mayer SA, Brun NC, Begtrup K, Broderick J, Davis S, Diringer MN, Skolnick BE, Steiner T, Recombinant Activated VII Intracerebral Haemorrhage Trial Investigators. Recombinant activated factor VII for acute intracerebral haemorrhage. *NEJM* 2005; 352: 777–785.
174. Mayer SA, Brun NC, Broderick J, Davis S, Diringer MN, Skolnick BE, Steiner T; Europe/AustralAsia NovoSeven ICH Trial Investigators. Safety and feasibility of recombinant factor VIIa for acute cerebral haemorrhage. *Stroke* 2005; 36: 74–79.
175. Mayer SA, Brun NC, Broderick J, Davis SM, Diringer MN, Skolnick BE, Steiner T, United States NovoSeven ICH Trial Investigators. Recombinant factor VIIa for acute intracerebral haemorrhage: US phase IIa trial. *Neurocrit Care* 2006; 4: 206–214.
176. Mayer SA, Brun NC, Begtrup K *et al.* Randomised placebo controlled double blind phase III study to assess rFVIIa efficacy in acute intracerebral haemorrhage: The FAST Trial. *Cerebrovasc Dis* 2007; 23(Suppl 2) 10.
177. Al Shahi R, You H. Haemostatic drug therapies for acute, non traumatic intracerebral haemorrhage. *Stroke* 2007; 38: 204.
178. Al-Shahi Salman R, You H. Haemostatic drug therapies for acute spontaneous intracerebral haemorrhage. *Cochrane Database Syst Rev* 2009; 4: CD005951 (in press).

179. Inaji M, Tomita H, Tone O, Tamaki M, Suzuki R, Ohno K. Chronological changes of perihematomal oedema of human intracerebral hematoma. *Acta Neurochir Suppl* 2003; 86: 445–448.

180. Tellez H, Bauer RB. Dexamethasone as treatment in cerebrovascular disease. A controlled study in intracerebral haemorrhage. *Stroke* 1973; 4: 541–546.

181. Poungvarin N, Bhoopat W, Viriyavejakul A, Rodprasert P, Buranasiri P, Sukondhabhant S, Hensley MJ, Strom BL. Effects of dexamethasone in primary supratentorial intracerebral hemorrhage. *NEJM* 1987; 316: 1229–1233.

182. Kumar N, Jain S, Mehashwari MC. Role of dexamethasone in the outcome from acute stroke. *J Assoc Physicians India* 1989; 37: 315–317.

183. Desai P, Prasad K. Dexamethasone is not necessarily unsafe in primary supratentorial intracerebral haemorrhage. *J Neurol Neurosurg Psychiatry* 1998; 65: 799–801.

184. Ogun SA, Odusote KA. Effectiveness of high dose dexamethasone in the treatment of acute stroke. *West Afr J Med* 2001; 20: 1–6.

185. Feigin VL, Anderson N, Rinkel GJ, Algra A, van Gijn J, Bennett DA. Corticosteroids for aneurysmal subarachnoid haemorrhage and primary intracerebral haemorrhage. *Cochrane Database Syst Rev* 2005; 3: CD004583.

186. Poungvarin N. Steroids have no role in stroke therapy. *Stroke* 2004; 35: 229–230.

187. Fujii Y, Takeuchi S, Sasaki O, Minakawa T, Tanaka R. Multivariate analysis of predictors of haematoma enlargement in spontaneous intracerebral hemorrhage. *Stroke* 1998; 29: 1160–1166.

188. Kazui S, Minematsu K, Yamamoto H, Sawada T, Yamaguchi T. Predisposing factors to enlargement of spontaneous intracerebral haematoma. *Stroke* 1997; 28: 2370–2375.

189. Qureshi A, Mohammad YM, Yahia AM *et al.* A prospective multicentre study to evaluate the feasibility and safety of aggressive antihypertensive treatment in patients with acute intracerebral haemorrhage. *J Intensive Care Med* 2005; 20: 34–42.

190. Qureshi AI, Harris-Lane P, Kirmani JF, Ahmed S, Jacob M, Zada Y, Divani AA. Treatment of acute hypertension in patients with intracerebral hemorrhage using American Heart Association guidelines. *Crit Care Med* 2006; 34: 1975–1980.

191. Anderson CS, Huang Y, Wang JG, Arima H, Neal B, Peng B, Heeley E,
     Skulina C, Parsons MW, Kim JS, Tao QL, Li YC, Jiang JD, Tai LW, Zhang JL,
     Xu E, Cheng Y, Heritier S, Morgenstern LB, Chalmers J, INTERACT
     Investigators. Intensive blood pressure reduction in acute cerebral haemorrhage
     trial. (INTERACT): a randomised pilot trial. *Lancet Neurol* 2008; 7: 391–399.
192. Qureshi AI. Antihypertensive Treatment of Acute Cerebral Hemorrhage
     (ATACH) trial. Paper presented at: International Stroke Conference 2008;
     February 20–22, 2008; New Orleans, LA.
193. Dziedzic T, Bartus S, Klimkowicz A, Motyl M, Slowik A, Szczudlik A.
     Intracerebral haemorrhage triggers interleukin-6 and interleukin-10 release
     in blood. *Stroke* 2002; 33: 2334–2335.
194. Lee KR, Kawai N, Kim S, Sagher O, Hoff JT. Mechanisms of oedema
     formation after intracerebral haemorrhage: effects of thrombin on cerebral
     blood flow, blood-brain barrier permeability, and cell survival in a rat
     model. *J Neurosurg* 1997; 86: 272–278.
195. Kitaoka T, Hua Y, Xi G, Hoff JT, Keep RF. Delayed argatroban treatment
     reduces oedema in a rat model of intracerebral hemorrhage. *Stroke* 2002; 33:
     3012–3018.
196. Lee ST, Chu K, Sinn DI, Jung KH, Kim EH, Kim SJ, Kim JM, Ko SY,
     Kim M, Roh JK. Erythropoietin reduces perihematomal inflammation and
     cell death with eNOS and STAT3 activations in experimental intracerebral
     haemorrhage. *J Neurochem* 2006; 96: 728–739.
197. Abilleira S, Montaner J, Molina CA *et al.* Matrix metalloproteinase 9 con-
     centration after spontaeous intracerebral haemorrhage. *J Neurosurg* 2003;
     99: 65–70.
198. Alvarez-Sabin J, Delagado P, Abilleira S, Molina CA, Arenillas J, Ribo M,
     Santamarina E, Quintana M, Monasterio J, Montaner J. Temporal profile of
     matrix metalloproteinases and their inhibitors after spontaneous intracere-
     bral haemorrhage: relationship to clinical and radiological outcome. *Stroke*
     2004; 35: 1316–1322.
199. Liu M, Guo MZ, Li PY, Zhang H, Li L, Li P, Wang Q. Effect of new
     qingkailing injection on cerebral oedema following intracerebral haemor-
     rhage in rats. *Zhongguo Zhong Xi Yi Jie He Za Zhi* 2006; 26: 244–247.
200. Yasaka M, Minematsu K, Naritomi H, Sakata T, Yamaguchi T. Predisposing
     factors for enlargement of intracerebral haemorrhage in patients treated with
     warfarin. *Thromb Haemost* 2003; 89: 278–283.

201. Rosand J, Hylek EM, O'Donnell HC, Greenberg SM. Warfarin associated haemorrhage and cerebral amyloid angiopathy: a genetic and pathologic study. *Neurology* 2000; 55: 947–951.

202. Rosand J, Eckman MH, Knudsen KA, Singer DE, Greenberg SM. The effect of warfarin and intensity of anticoagulation on outcome of intracerebral haemorrhage. *Arch Intern Med* 2004; 164: 880–884.

203. Aguilar MI, Hart RG, Kase CS *et al.* Treatment of warfarin associated intracerebral haemorrhage: literature review and expert opinion. *Mayo Clin Proc* 2007; 82: 82–92.

204. Guidelines on oral anticoagulation: third edition. *Br J Haematol* 1998; 101: 374–387.

205. Pindur G, Mörsdorf S, Schenk JF, Krischek B, Heinrich W, Wenzel E. The overdosed patient and bleedings with oral anticoagulation. *Semin Thromb Hemost* 1999; 25: 85–88.

206. Huttner HB, Schellinger PD, Hartmann M, Köhrmann M, Juettler E, Wikner J, Mueller S, Meyding-Lamade U, Strobl R, Mansmann U, Schwab S, Steiner T. Haematoma growth and outcome in treated neurocritical care patients with intracerebral haemorrhage related to oral anticoagulant therapy: comparison of acute treatment strategies using vitamin K, fresh frozen plasma and prothrombin complex concentrates. *Stroke* 2006; 37: 1465–1470.

207. Freeman WD, Brott TG, Barrett KM, Castillo PR, Deen HG Jr, Czervionke LF, Meschia JF. Recombinant activated factor VII for rapid reversal of warfarin anticoagulation in acute intracranial haemorrhage. *Mayo Clin Proc* 2004; 79: 1495–1500.

208. National Institute for Health and Clinical Excellence (NICE). Stroke: diagnosis and initial management of acute stroke and transient ischaemic attack (TIA). NICE Guidelines, 2008.

209. Prasad K, Mendelow AD, Gregson B. Surgery for primary supratentorial intracerebral haemorrhage. *Cochrane Database Syst Rev* 2008; 4: CD000200.

210. Mendelow AD, Gregson BA, Fernandes HM, Murray GD, Teasdale GM, Hope DT, Karimi A, Shaw MD, Barer DH; STICH investigators. Early surgery versus initial conservative treatment inpatients with spontaneous supratentorial intracerebral haematomas in the International Surgical Trial in Intracerebral Haemorrhage (STICH): a randomised trial. *Lancet* 2005; 365: 387–397.

6   Malignant Stroke Syndrome

Dulka Manawadu*

Chapter Summary

Malignant MCA infarctions result from proximal occlusions of middle cerebral artery (MCA) or the internal carotid artery. They are characterised by severe neurological deficits and decreases in consciousness levels which progress relentlessly to death in the majority of patients. Typically, brain imaging shows ischaemic damage to two-thirds of the MCA territory, accompanied by cerebral oedema and midline shift. Clinical features that predict a poor outcome include younger age, severe baseline neurological impairments, early impairment in conscious levels and pupillary dilatation. Imaging predictors of poor outcome include hypodensity >50% of MCA territory, involvement of other vascular territories and hyperdense MCA artery sign indicating proximal arterial occlusion.

All patients with the potential of malignant stroke syndrome must be managed in highly specialised units and be monitored intensively for hysiological variables and neurological condition. The only proven evidence-based intervention for malignant stroke syndrome is hemicraniectomy, which halves mortality compared with medical treatment for raised intracranial pressure. However, the effects of hemicraniectomy in reducing the composite measure of death or disability remain controversial. Any

*Department of Stroke Medicine, King's College Hospital NHS Foundation Trust, Denmark Hill, London SE5 9PJ, UK

benefit is only seen in post-hoc pooled analyses rather than on pre-specified outcomes in individual trials. Although further trials may be desirable, the ethics of a conservative management arm may be questionable given the significant and consistent mortality reduction seen with surgery.

The difficulties in treatment decisions for hemicraniectomy are reflected in studies of quality of life, regret and retrospective agreement amongst patients and their relatives following the procedure. The acceptable quality of life after surgery appears to be a personal decision, which is only modestly linked with functional recovery and appears not to be influenced by the side of infarct or level of speech disturbance. Stroke survivors tend to assign a higher quality of life score to the state of living with stroke than those in good health, making these decisions further challenging. Hence, hemicraniectomy in patients with malignant infarction is not only about preventing mortality but also concerns the patients' acceptance of residual disability after the procedure. It is the duty of every clinician to support patients and their relatives in making such decisions by providing a factual assessment of expected outcome and the possible level of residual disability following the procedure.

Introduction

Middle cerebral artery (MCA) infarcts are common. In one prospective registry of 2266 computed tomography (CT) proven ischaemic strokes, MCA infarcts amounted to 1376 in number, thereby accounting for 61% of the total recorded over a 15-year-period.[1] In this study, the MCA territory was divided into three parts: deep, anterior superficial and posterior superficial areas. Strokes involving at least two out of these three areas were labelled as large MCA strokes and these totalled 208 or 9.2% of all ischaemic strokes; the mortality was 17% at one month in this group. From this same study, the authors defined complete MCA infarcts as those comprising ≥ 90% of the total MCA territory and these totalled 72 or 3.2% of all strokes; the inpatient mortality in this latter group was 22%. Other series have found higher mortality rates for similar sized infarcts: in a case series of 50 patients with large hemispheric infarcts, defined as involving at least two of the three MCA territories, the overall mortality was 22% at one month. Of these, 26 were categorised as having massive infarctions;

that is, they had infarction of all three MCA territories — or beyond — and in this group, the 30-day mortality in this group was 42.3%.[2] In an earlier, retrospective study, the clinical course of 55 patients with complete MCA infarction was also reviewed and of these, 43 (78%) died of brain herniation within seven days of stroke onset and the mean Rankin score[3] in those who survived was three.[4]

Clinical features of malignant infarction syndrome

Malignant middle cerebral artery (MCA) infarction is characterised by its clinical presentation and relentless progression with typical neuroradiological findings (Fig. 1).

Those at risk of developing this syndrome are relatively young, without a previous history of stroke and present with signs of MCA infarction: hemiparesis with sensory deficits associated with cortical features such as inattention or speech disturbance. Involvement of other territories, including anterior choroidal artery supply,[5] can increase the risk of

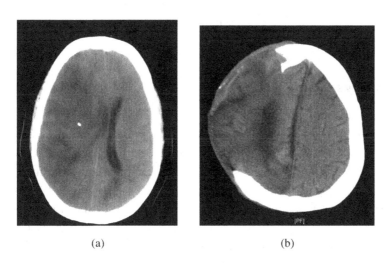

(a)   (b)

Figure 1. CT appearances of the malignant hemisphere infarct syndrome. (a) Day 2 after stroke onset: axial CT brain scan showing extensive infarction of the right MCA territory associated with significant mass effect. (b) Axial CT brain scan of the same patient following hemicraniectomy; this patient died within one month of stroke.

malignant syndrome developing and as such, other neurological deficits may be present. The National Institutes of Health stroke scale (NIHSS) is used most commonly in the hyperacute assessment of stroke patients.[6] An NIH score of > 15 is consistent with the extensive infarction of the MCA territory and has been used as one of the inclusion criteria into the randomised controlled trials of hemicraniectomy for malignant MCA syndrome.[7] As the NIHSS is weighted against patients with speech disorders, higher scores (> 20) will be seen in strokes involving the dominant hemisphere. Patients' level of consciousness will gradually decrease as intracranial pressure rises but drowsiness can be a feature on presentation and those with a score ≥ 1 on part 1a of the NIHSS should be considered early for intervention. In fact, decreased levels of consciousness within a short period of time after stroke onset have been noted as a predictor of early mortality in those with anterior circulation infarcts.[8]

Malignant MCA infarctions are a result of proximal occlusions involving either the internal carotid artery or the proximal MCA. Individuals with congenital abnormalities of the circle of Willis — hypoplasia or atresia/absence of vessels such as the anterior or posterior communicating arteries — may be more susceptible to malignant infarction of the MCA territory.[5]

Pathophysiology

The pathophysiological mechanisms that underlie development of malignant infarction are not fully understood but rapid evolution of cerebral oedema plays a significant role. Brain oedema is harmful because it causes swelling and this situation is further aggravated by the inflexible volume of the skull. The swollen brain displaces surrounding tissues and increases pressure within it; this in itself can cause further ischaemia by compromising blood flow and can lead to damage of previously healthy brain and further oedema,[9] hence the designation of the term, malignant infarction. Classic teaching is that cytotoxic oedema peaks between two and four days after stroke and thereafter decreases over one to two weeks.[10] However, significant oedema can occur even earlier: a case series of neurological deterioration following massive MCA infarction revealed this decline occurred within 24 hours of symptom onset, and by day two in two-thirds of patients.[11] In this retrospective study, the highest frequency of deaths was observed on day three, similar to that seen in a previous study.[4]

Imaging in Malignant Infarct Syndrome

Brain CT is the most widely used modality for the diagnosis and monitoring of patients with malignant MCA infarction. Indeed, plain CT with or without cerebral blood flow studies[12] was used in almost all of the case series that contributed to a systematic review of 138 patients who underwent surgical hemicraniectomy for malignant MCA syndrome.[13] Typically, at least two-thirds of the MCA territory is involved in malignant MCA infarction, although more recent literature suggest a high risk of malignant infarction if more than 50% of the MCA territory and the basal ganglia show ischaemic alterations.[14]

What imaging should ideally be performed on those who present with clinically large ischaemic strokes? Can certain imaging parameters predict those who will benefit from hemicraniectomy and if so, can these guide the timing of intervention? Imaging criteria from various centres for referral for hemicraniectomy have been variable: hemispheric involvement was crucial to some series[15,16] but not to others.[17] Imaging had to show midline shift of strict limits (≥ 5 mm) in some studies[17,18] but not others.[16] One study reported on loss of corticomedullary contrast of greater than 50% of the MCA territory to determine the need for hemicraniectomy,[19] and one used cerebral blood flow of < 5ml/100g/min to identify severely ischaemic and non-viable brain.[12]

The imaging criteria for randomised studies of hemicraniectomy were less variable; both decompressive surgery for the treatment of malignant infarction of the middle cerebral artery (DESTINY)[20] and hemicraniectomy after middle cerebral artery infarction with life-threatening edema trial (HAMLET)[21] required CT scan evidence of unilateral MCA infarction of at least two-thirds of the territory and including at least part of the basal ganglia (DESTINY) or formation of space-occupying oedema (HAMLET). DESTINY included patients with or without additional ipsilateral infarction of the anterior or posterior cerebral artery[20] whereas in

HAMLET, ischaemic stroke of the whole cerebral hemisphere — anterior, middle, and posterior cerebral artery territories — was an exclusion criterion.[21] Decompressive craniectomy in malignant middle cerebral artery infarction (DECIMAL) had the most stringent imaging criterion requiring MRI scanning to demonstrate > 145cm^3 of infarcted brain tissue, as measured on the diffusion weighted imaging (DWI) sequence.[22] This study therefore excluded patients with contraindications to MR imaging, which may be a potential limitation as contraindications to MR imaging have been found in 4% to 10% of consecutive acute stroke patients with a further 10% to 11% patients having medical instability barriers to MRI scanning.[23,24]

An interesting question is: can calculation of DWI lesion volume (quantitative measure) alone be used to select patients for surgical intervention? In DECIMAL, the mean infarct volume in the surgical group was 211.5 cm^3 (range 146–381cm^3) and was similar to the medical group at 214.7 cm^3 (range 150–308 cm^3). A subgroup analysis showed that DWI infarct volume at inclusion correlated positively and significantly with outcome (modified Rankin Scale (mRS) score)[3] at six months in those treated *without* surgery. Indeed, no patient with a volume > 210 cm^3 at inclusion survived without craniectomy; conversely, the 8 people screened but excluded from this trial due to infarct volumes <145 cm^3, all survived. A similar analysis in the surgical arm of DECIMAL also showed a trend towards worse outcome in patients with higher infarct volumes though this did not reach a significance level. This threshold of 145 cm^3 DWI infarct volume has previously been demonstrated to be an accurate predictor for the development of malignant infarction in 28 patients presenting within 14 hours of MCA stroke and persistent arterial occlusion.[25] However, no study to date has confirmed this relationship between infarct volume and functional outcome following hemicraniectomy. If the trend seen in DECIMAL could be established in a future study (i.e. establishing a threshold infarct volume beyond which patients do significantly worse despite surgery) then DWI infarct measurement could be used as an objective decider for surgical decompression. An important issue to consider in such a study would be exactly when this 'deciding' MRI should be performed given that DWI lesions evolve and may exceed the 145 cm^3 barrier with time.[26]

Other radiological features predicting the formation of fatal brain oedema following MCA infarction are as follows:

Hypodensity

Early CT hypodensity involving > 50% of the MCA territory as well as involvement of additional vascular territories (namely anterior and posterior cerebral arteries) is associated with an increased risk of fatal brain oedema.[27]

Corticomedullary contrast

A case-control study that examined CT scans performed within 18 hours of stroke onset showed that loss of grey-white matter differentiation or attenuated corticomedullary contrast (CMC) predicted the development of malignant middle cerebral artery infarct.[28] Neuroradiologists reviewed the initial CT scans, performed within 18 hours of stroke onset in 62 patients with respect to 12 imaging criteria, one of which was attenuated CMC over the entire hemisphere. Half of these patients went on to have a malignant course but the neuroradiologists involved in this study were blinded to this information. Of the 12 criteria, some had high sensitivity for subsequent development of malignant MCA infarction for example, compression of the subarachnoid space (100%) but low specificity (29%) or conversely the high specificity of midline shift (96.7%) but with low sensitivity (19.4%). Attenuated CMC had a sensitivity of 87.1%, specificity of 96.8% and positive predictive value of 96.1% in predicting a malignant course of MCA infarction from the initial CT brain scan.[28]

Single-photon emission CT (SPECT)

This scanning modality can determine the extent of impaired cerebral blood flow following stroke and has also been studied as a prognostic indicator following MCA stroke.[29] One hundred and eight patients were scanned prospectively within six hours of MCA stroke in order to determine the predictive value of SPECT in determining fatal ischaemic oedema, compared with either CT findings or clinical examination alone. An activity deficit of the whole MCA territory was found to be highly accurate — sensitivity 82%, specificity 98% — in predicting death due to malignant MCA infarction.[29] Each SPECT examination lasted less than 30 minutes and in this time, patients had to lie quietly in a dimmed room. Afterwards, visual assessment of the images took a couple of minutes and was done by investigators who were blinded to initial stroke severity and ultimate outcome of the patients. Availability and correct interpretation of scan acquisition, especially if semiquantative measurements are used, are clearly limiting factors to the widespread use of this modality.

In summary, some imaging parameters have shown reasonable predictive value for the development of malignant middle cerebral artery infarction and may assist surgical decision-making. However, the ideal imaging modality — and when to perform it — that would allow optimal patient selection for medical versus surgical treatment in malignant MCA stroke is not yet known. As the authors of the randomised hemicraniectomy trials emphasise and how individual physicians intuitively act, the decision to perform decompressive surgery can only be made on an individual basis for every patient.[7] This decision must consider patient and imaging characteristics but equally relevant, any prior wishes of the patient, social circumstances and their support network. These latter factors have not been examined extensively.

Predictors of Malignant Stroke Syndrome

Reliable prediction to identify those most at risk of developing malignant stroke syndrome has proven challenging. However, some retrospective studies have identified certain features that have been associated with greater morbidity and mortality following MCA infarction (Table 1).

Some of these factors seem intuitive in predicting poorer outcomes, others perhaps less so. Either way, this knowledge has not changed the significant mortality associated with malignant MCA oedema and so perhaps it remains for us to use this information more wisely to identify those at greatest risk and intervene early, either 'aggressively' or otherwise.

Table 1. Predictors of malignant infarction syndrome

Clinical features	Imaging characteristics
History of hypertension[27]	Hypodensity of > 50% MCA territory[27,30,31]
History of heart failure[27]	Involvement of other territories[27]
Younger age[2,5,25]	Hyperdense MCA sign[30]; proximal vessel occlusion[4,5,32]
Pupillary dilatation[2,4]	Vascular abnormality (ipsilateral) of circle of Willis[5]
GCS <10 on day 2[2]	MRI DWI lesion volume > 145 cm^3 [25]
Higher admission NIHSS*[,25,32]	Activity deficit of MCA territory using SPECT[29]
Nausea or vomiting within	Attenuated corticomedullary contrast[28]
24 hours of stroke onset[31]	Low perfusion: diffusion ratio using MR imaging[32]
	Early impairment of peri-infarct autoregulation[33]

*National Institutes of Health Stroke Scale (NIHSS) score[6]

Management of Malignant Strokes

All patients with the potential of malignant stroke syndrome need to be managed in highly specialised stroke or neurocritical care units and be intensively monitored for physiological variables and neurological condition as described in Chapter 5 on hyperacute stroke care. The only proven evidence-based intervention for malignant stroke syndrome is hemicraniectomy. Medical or conservative treatment for raised intracranial pressure in malignant stroke syndromes is widely practiced as a temporary measure but lacks an evidence base and perhaps efficacy. Furthermore, best medical was used as the comparator treatment arm to hemicraniectomy in randomised controlled trials and found to be inferior to surgery for mortality and functional outcomes.[7]

Hemicraniectomy in Malignant Stroke

History

Removal of the skull vault to relieve intracranial pressure in head trauma or toxic insult has been practised for decades. As reviewed by Ivamoto *et al.*,[34] and more recently by others,[35] surgery to remove a portion of skull (craniectomy) and excise necrotic brain tissue in order to prevent fatal brain uncal or diencephalic herniation has been described in case reports and small patient series dating as far back as 1935. Removal of the anterior hemi-cranial vault without concomitant resection of infarcted brain for massive cerebral infarction was first described in 1981; all three patients survived, two with major disability.[36] Prior to surgery, all three patients had received medical 'antiedema' therapy: steroids, mannitol, intubation and hyperventilation in response to signs of raised intracranial pressure, without response. Indeed, this practice of 'conservative' therapy for raised intracranial pressure, as alluded to above, is not supported by a strong evidence base.[37] Surgical intervention appears, therefore, to save lives, but at what cost?[38] The concerns for routine hemicraniectomy in large strokes are based on the longer term outlook for individual patients: would the reduction in early mortality be accompanied by an unacceptable rise in patients surviving in the long term with severe neurological deficits?

The ongoing observations of the natural history of MCA infarctions with its high mortality and limited response to medical therapy[4] led to the report of the largest case series of patients who had undergone surgical decompression for malignant MCA infarction.[18,39] The larger of the two overlapping series consisted of 68 patients and the results showed that hemicraniectomy and duraplasty were associated with a strikingly lower mortality rate (27%) than that occurring during the natural history of malignant MCA infarction (78%); this latter result came from findings observed in 55 contemporaneous patients.[4] Surgical intervention was not only associated with lower mortality, but reasonable functional recovery too. Although left with neurological deficits, none remained permanently wheelchair-dependent and none of the 11 patients with dominant hemisphere strokes remained globally aphasic. This favourable experience renewed interest in decompressive surgery for MCA stroke and additional case series were subsequently reported from around the world.[19,40] A recent systematic review found 12 studies of hemicraniectomy for MCA infarction that were suitable for combined analysis, which in total, included 138 patients.[13] From this, it was found that only a small number (7%) were left independent at four months following surgery, one-third (35%) were mild/moderately disabled and the majority (58%) were severely disabled or dead. Interestingly, dichotomising outcome with respect to age > 50 or ≤ 50 led to a significant difference in outcome: 80% (75 patients) in the former ('older') group compared with 32% (63 patients) in the second were dead or severely disabled following surgery.[13] Certain factors seemed to influence outcome, perhaps age being the most powerful and certainly by now, the stage appeared to be set for randomised trials.

Randomised trials

The first randomised trial of hemicraniectomy for malignant MCA infarction was halted in the United States in 2003 due to slow recruitment — only 26 patients in three years[41] — however, the enrollments in The Hemicraniectomy and Durotomy on Deterioration from Infarction-Related Swelling Trial (HeaDDFIRST) did confirm the theoretical feasibility of recruiting patients into such a trial and no particular disadvantage with surgical intervention.[42] A randomised study from the Philippines Hemicraniectomy for Malignant Middle Cerebral Artery Infarcts (HeMMI)[43] was initiated but the results from this are not known. Three European randomised controlled trials also began, all of which have been reported upon singly[20–22] and in combination.[7]

Decompressive Surgery for the Treatment of Malignant Infarction of the Middle Cerebral Artery (DESTINY) recruited patients between 2004 and 2006. Eligible patients were aged 18 to 60 years with infarcts involving more than two-thirds of the MCA territory that caused hemiplegia and drowsiness but comatose patients (Glasgow Coma Scale < 6) and those with fixed, dilated pupils were excluded.[20] Patients were operated on within 36 hours of symptom onset. Thirty-day mortality was 53% in the medical arm compared to 12% of those who underwent hemicraniectomy and after one year, surgery resulted in a near doubling of the rate of favourable (primary) outcome as defined by a mRS[3] of 3 or less. Only 32 patients were included before the study was terminated due to the large reduction in mortality provided by hemicraniectomy. The inclusion of only 32 patients did not allow a statistically significant difference in the primary end point to be shown, however it was hoped that the planned pooled analysis would have sufficient power to be able to show this difference.

Decompressive Craniectomy in Malignant Middle Cerebral Artery Infarction (DECIMAL) Trial had an upper age limit of 55 years and required diffusion weighted MRI imaging to establish an infarct volume of greater than 145 cm^3 for inclusion into the study; surgery had to be commenced within 30 hours of symptom onset.[22] This trial was also terminated early because of slow recruitment (38 patients between 2001 and 2005), as well as the knowledge that the pre-planned pooled analysis of the three European studies was imminent. DECIMAL showed that hemicraniectomy provided a five-fold increase in patients with minimal disability (mRS ≤ 3) at six months compared with no surgery, although again, small numbers prevented this primary outcome result from being statistically significant.

The third trial, Hemicraniectomy After Middle Cerebral Artery Infarction with Life-threatening Edema Trial (HAMLET) had similar inclusion criteria to DESTINY but was still on going at the time of publication of the pooled analysis and its individual results were only published last year.[21] The major difference in HAMLET was that the time period allowed for randomisation was longer, up to 96 hours from symptom onset. Twenty-three patients recruited in this trial contributed to the pooled analysis.[7] This individual study failed to show that the primary outcome (mRS 0–3) was achieved significantly more by the 32 surgical patients (25%) than the 32 medical patients (25%) randomised at one year. It did however show an absolute reduction in mortality of 38% in favour of surgery.[21]

Pooled analyses

In total, 93 patients from the three preceding European trials were included in a pooled analysis.[7] The primary outcome measure was dichotomised to a favourable (mRS ≤ 4) or unfavourable (mRS 5 and 6) outcome at one year. Secondary outcomes were fatality rates and mRS scores dichotomised between 0–3 and 4–6 at one year, the latter is to examine if surgery can result in survival without severe disability. The combined results from the three studies showed that three times as many people achieved the favourable primary outcome in the decompressive surgery group (75%) than in the conservative treatment group (24%) (Figs. 2 and 3).

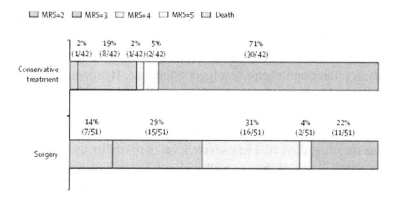

MRS=2   MRS=3   MRS=4   MRS=5   Death

Conservative treatment

2%   19%   2%   5%   71%
(1/42) (8/42) (1/42)(2/42)   (30/42)

Surgery

14%   29%   31%   4%   22%
(7/51)   (15/51)   (16/51)   (2/51)   (11/51)

Figure 2. Range of outcomes at one year from pooled analysis of three trials randomising patients to either best medical therapy with hemicraniectomy (surgery) or without (conservative).[7] Adapted with permission from Elsevier (*The Lancet Neurology*, 2007, 6, 215–222).

	Outcome/patients		ARR (%)	95% CI		OR	95% CI
	Conservative	Surgery					
mRS>4 at 12 months							
DECIMAL	14/18	5/20	52·8	25·8 to 79·8		0·10	0·02–0·43
DESTINY	10/15	4/17	43·1	11·9 to 74·4		0·15	0·03–0·73
HAMLET	8/9	4/14	60·3	29·0 to 91·6		0·05	0·00–0·54
Total	32/42	13/51	51·2	33·9 to 68·5		0·10	0·04–0·27
Significance: p<0·0001							
Heterogeneity: p=0·74							
mRS>3 at 12 months							
DECIMAL	14/18	10/20	27·8	−1·4 to 56·9		0·29	0·07–1·18
DESTINY	11/15	9/17	20·4	−12·2 to 53·0		0·41	0·09–1·81
HAMLET	8/9	10/14	17·5	−13·9 to 48·8		0·31	0·03–3·38
Total	33/42	29/51	22·7	4·6 to 40·9		0·33	0·13–0·86
Significance: p=0·014							
Heterogenity: p=0·89							
Death at 12 months							
DECIMAL	14/18	5/20	52·8	25·8 to 79·8		0·10	0·02–0·43
DESTINY	8/15	3/17	35·7	4·6 to 66·8		0·19	0·04–0·94
HAMLET	8/9	3/14	67·5	37·7 to 97·2		0·03	0·00–0·39
Total	30/42	11/51	50·3	33·3 to 67·4		0·10	0·04–0·27
Significance: p<0·0001							
Heterogenity: p=0·34							

%ARR (95% CI)

Figure 3. Absolute risk differences at one year from pooled analysis of three trials randomising patients to either best medical therapy with hemicraniectomy (surgery) or without (conservative).[7] Adapted with permission from Elsevier (*The Lancet Neurology*, 2007, 6, 215–222).

If the same results could be achieved in 'real-life' practice, then the absolute increase of 51% in achievement of primary outcome would mean that only two patients would need to undergo hemicraniectomy for malignant MCA infarction to achieve a 'good' outcome. Hemicraniectomy also reduced mortality from 71% to 22%, corresponding to an absolute reduction in risk of death of 49% and similarly suggests that in practice, only two patients need to undergo surgery to save one life. The other secondary outcome measure allowed a less severe level of disability as a 'favourable' outcome, that is, the ability to walk independently but requiring help in daily life (mRS 3) would be the 'worst case' scenario as opposed to an mRS of 4 used in the primary outcome, which means that assistance is needed for walking as well as bodily needs. This outcome (mRS 0–3) was achieved in twice the number of patients randomised to surgery (43%) than to conservative treatment (21%), with an absolute increase of 23%, again suggesting that only a few (four) patients need to be operated on to achieve this particular outcome in one.[7]

Since this pooled analysis was reported, there have been two further analyses published which includes more patient data from HAMLET. In the first of these two analyses, the addition of 16 patients, randomised within 48 hours of symptom onset, takes the total 'pool' to 109 patients. This addition did not change the significance of the outcomes of mortality: absolute risk reduction 49.9% (95% CI: 33.9–65.9) or outcome of mRS 0–4: absolute risk reduction 41.9% (95% CI: 25.2–58.6). However, the mRS 0–3 outcome did change in significance with an absolute risk reduction now of 16.3% (95% CI: –0.1 to 33.1).[21] The addition of all 64 patients from HAMLET (including those randomised > 48 hours) to the 38 from DECIMAL and 32 from DESTINY takes the total to 134 patients and forms the basis of the third 'pooled' analysis. This reveals that mortality is still significantly reduced with hemicraniectomy: absolute risk reduction 41% (95% CI: 26–56) but the outcome of mRS 0–3, that is, the originally stated primary outcome in HAMLET,[44] only shows a trend towards significance: absolute risk reduction 13% (95% CI: –0.2 to 28).[45] There is a debate on the interpretation of the results of these analyses. All the results agree that mortality is significantly reduced with hemicraniectomy. However, the outcome of mRS 0–3 (the pre-specified primary outcome of all three individual trials) is not achieved in the latter analyses. On the basis of this, it has been argued that the 'post-hoc' findings are not robust enough to be translated into clinical guidelines and that patients should continue to be randomised.[45] Although further randomisation on the basis of age (older) and duration from symptom onset (over 48 hours) is welcomed, randomising patients into a trial in which 'no hemicraniectomy' was a potential arm may prove ethically difficult given the significant and consistent mortality reduction seen with surgery.

Other limitations in the randomised trials may also be considered: whereas the approach to hemicraniectomy was vastly similar in all three trials included in the pooled anlaysis, the conservative arm was not. There did not appear to be a prescriptive approach to those not randomised to surgical hemicraniectomy and consequently whereas 74% of surgical patients were admitted to the Intensive Care Unit (ICU) in DECIMAL,[22] only 17% of the conservative arm were; these figures were 91% and 16% respectively in HAMLET.[21] Furthermore, 100% of the surgical patients and 61% of the medical patients received mechanical ventilation in DEC-IMAL[22] but only 84% and 16% did so respectively, in HAMLET.[21] Conversely, all patients enrolled into DESTINY[20] were ventilated and treated in an ICU setting.

Clinical Lessons from Hemicraniectomy Trials

Definition of a good outcome

The primary outcome for a 'favourable' result of hemicraniectomy from the pooled analysis was an mRS of 0–4. The functional outcome represented by an mRS of 4 is that of moderately severe disability, meaning that an individual will need help from another person for activities of daily living and for mobility. One step up from this is an mRS of 3, which represents moderate disability, meaning that help will be needed for daily activities but that mobility is independent. An mRS of 3 represented the greatest level of disability as part of the secondary outcomes from the pooled analysis,[7] but was within the primary 'good' outcome (0–3) in the individual trials that contributed to the pooled analysis.[20–22] This contrasts significantly with the definition of a 'favourable' outcome for the trials of intravenous tissue plasminogen activator (tPA) for acute ischaemic stroke, which considered an mRS of 1 as the 'lowest' level of disability allowed for a favourable outcome.[46,47] An mRS of 1 represents an individual who is 'nearly normal', that is, they have no significant disability despite presence of symptoms and remain entirely independent. Clearly, outcomes need to be commensurate with the clinical scenario. It may be unrealistic to expect these 'tPA outcomes' in patients with malignant MCA syndrome, who by inclusion criteria, have extensive infarction and who are already drowsy preoperatively. Indeed, the 'best' functional outcome from the individual trials — and hence the pooled analysis — was an mRS of 2 which represents someone with mild disability; these patients remain independent in daily life but are unable to carry out some previously performed regular activity such as driving, hobbies or employment. Eight people in the pooled analysis achieved an mRS of 2: one (2%) in the conservative arm and seven (14%) in the hemicraniectomy arm.[7] Lastly, it must be noted that 33 people of the 40 (83%) surviving to one year post-hemicraniectomy required some degree of help for activities of daily living.[7] Therefore it is of vital importance to determine the maximum level of dependence that an individual patient or families acting as their advocates will consider acceptable.

Timing of surgery

Is earlier intervention associated with better outcome? The largest cohort study in the systematic review described above,[13] included 63 patients who underwent decompressive hemicraniectomy. Surgery was performed either early (< 24 hours of stroke onset with deterioration from baseline; mean time to surgery 21 hours) or late (> 24 hours after first reversible features of herniation; mean time to surgery 39 hours). The overall mortality was 25%: 16% (5/31) with early and 34% (11/32) with late surgery. The length of neurocritical ICU stay was also shorter in the first group (7 days) compared with the latter (13 days). Other studies have also suggested that earlier surgical times lead to better outcome: ultra-early intervention within six hours of stroke onset was associated with very low mortality rates (8.3%) and better functional outcomes than those with later intervention (mean time to surgery of 68 hours from stroke onset, mortality rate of 36.7%).[48] This study did not, however, have controlled entry into either early or late surgery and both groups had similar baseline stroke severity (mean NIHSS 26) and with similar proportions showing signs of herniation, despite the significant difference in time to hemicraniectomy. Taking a look at the randomised studies, the mean time (and range) to surgery in the DECIMAL, DESTINY and HAMLET studies were 20.5 (7–43) hours, 24.4 (13.5–36) hours, and 41 (29–50) hours (to randomisation), respectively. The longer time allowed to randomisation following stroke onset in HAMLET allowed an insight into the benefits of 'quick' or 'slow' surgery. Twenty-five patients (39%) in HAMLET were randomised > 48 hours after stroke onset and the results are presented in Table 2.

The surgical group did not significantly achieve the primary favourable outcome (mRS 0–3) at one year, regardless of time to randomization. Surgical decompression however, did have a significant benefit over conservative treatment with respect to the secondary outcomes of mRS 5/6 or 6 alone (death) if randomisation occurred < 48 hours. This was not the case for those randomised after 48 hours but because this later group only included 25 patients, the results form this particular sub-analysis may not reflect a true effect of time to randomisation.

Table 2. Results of surgery and best medical therapy with respect to time to randomisation in HAMLET.[21] Adapted with permission from Elsevier (*The Lancet Neurology*, 2007, 8, 326–333)

Randomisation	Surgery	Medical	ARR (%)
<48 hours (39)			
mRS 4–6	76%	78%	2% (−25 to 28)
mRS 5 or 6	48%	78%	30% (1 to 59)
Death	19%	78%	59% (33 to 84)
>48 hours (25)			
mRS 4–6	73%	71%	−1% (−37 to 34)
mRS 5 or 6	27%	36%	8% (−28 to 45)
Death	27%	36%	8% (−28 to 45)

ARR: Absolute risk reduction

Table 3. Achievement of the primary outcome (mRS 0–4) at one year with respect to time to randomisation from the pooled analysis.[7] Adapted with permission from Elsevier (*The Lancet Neurology*, 2007, 6, 215–222)

Time to randomisation (hours)	Surgery	Medicine	ARR
< 24	9/29 = 31%	21/26 = 81%	50%
≥ 24	4/22 = 18%	11/16 = 69%	51%

ARR: Absolute risk reduction

Again, the pooled analysis[7] allows us to see the effect of time to randomisation on outcome, but this time with a 24-hour cut off. The primary outcome (mRS 0–4) at 12 months from both surgical and medical groups is represented in Table 3. No additional benefit was observed for patients randomised to surgery within 24 hours.

Overall, the pooled analysis showed clearly the benefit of surgical decompression over best medical treatment when patients were randomised within 48 hours of symptom onset.

Age

Greater age per se is a risk factor for mortality after ischaemic stroke.[49] Does age influence outcome following surgical intervention for malignant MCA infarction? The systematic review comprising 138 patients revealed that younger age was associated with a better outcome following hemicraniectomy: 80% of the 75 patients over the age of 50 died or were severely disabled compared to 32% of 63 patients 50 years of age or younger.[13] Returning back to the randomised trials, the upper age limit for trial inclusion and mean age in the surgical groups were: 55 years and mean 43.5 years in DECIMAL, 60 years and mean 43.2 years in DESTINY, 60 years and mean 50.0 years in HAMLET. All the data on post-hemicraniectomy prognosis is therefore derived from those under the age of 60 years. However, subgroup analysis performed on those randomised with respect to a cut-off age of 50 years found the absolute risk reduction with surgery was similar in the 66 patients < 50 years (46.9%) and the 27 patients aged ≥ 50 years (44%).[7] Is there other evidence that age makes a difference? A review of the literature on decompressive craniectomy for malignant infarction was undertaken with respect to outcomes in those aged over 60 and those 60 years or younger.[50] Overall, 19 studies were reviewed, ten of which included patients aged > 60 and in total, 273 patients were analysed, 73 (26.7%) of whom were aged over 60 years. From this review, the older age group had a greater proportion of right hemispheric involvement, fewer were operated on within 24 hours of symptoms and time to follow-up after the operation was shorter. The mortality was significantly higher in those > 60 years old (51.3%) than those ≤ 60 (20.8%) and poor functional outcome, as determined by an mRS > 3 or Barthel Index < 60, was also higher at 81.8% and 33.1% respectively.[50] The significance of these results withstood whether or not the analysis was performed on all 19 studies or only the ten that included older patients. One study (not included in this review) that included 24 patients, 14 of whom were > 60, showed a lower mortality, though non-significant in this age group (29%) than those < 60 (40%).[51] The studies included in the review did not include randomised patients, follow-up time was variable and outcome assessment was limited to physical functioning: quality of life scores or family or caregiver opinions were not sought. While age past a strict cut off of 60 years should not absolutely contraindicate decompression surgery, it should be borne in mind that the results from the pooled analysis favouring surgery over medical therapy in malignant MCA infarction, cannot necessarily be extrapolated to those over the age of 60 years.

Hemisphere involved

The majority of patients selected for hemicraniectomy in malignant MCA infarction were those with strokes affecting the non-dominant hemisphere. This was because of concerns that if the patient survived, their residuel disability and quality of life would be adversely influenced by persistent aphasia.[15] This is reflected in the 138 patients included in the systematic review described above, 111 (80%) had malignant strokes involving the right hemisphere.[13] Indeed, some institutions held policies that offered hemicraniectomies only to those with non-dominant hemisphere involvement.[52] There was no such distinction in some series[51] nor in the randomised trials,[20-22] in which language deficit was not an exclusion criterion. Whether or not this played a part in the referring physicians' decisions to enroll a particular patient in trial in the first place, is unknown. Within the pooled analysis, 53 patients (57%) who displayed some form of language disturbance were included; this subgroup benefited equally from surgery when compared to those with no aphasia.[7] This mirrors results found in the systematic review of individual trials in which there were similar amounts of severe disability found in those with either left (33%) or right (34%) sided involvement.[13] Furthermore, there is evidence that following hemicraniectomy, speech function can improve, especially comprehension[53] and that over time most patients show a better ability to communicate.[54] Infarction of the speech-dominant hemisphere therefore, does not preclude significant recovery and should not in itself, contraindicate surgical decompression.

Adverse Effects of Decompressive Surgery

Early complications following surgery are common, and occurred in 62% of the 20 surgical patients enrolled in DECIMAL by one month.[22] The commonest adverse effect was aspiration pneumonia, which occurred in 25% at one week and 16% at one month. This was followed in frequency by venothromboembolic events and these affected 5% at one week and 21% at one month. Late complications in this surgical group were seizures (40%) and neuroalgodystrophy (26%); depression occurred in 20% in this group at one year and in 63% of the 32 surgical patients at this timeline in HAMLET.[21] Other surgical complications have been documented for example, epidural/subdural haematomas occurred in four patients (69%) in one case series of hemicraniectomy, while three (5%) developed space-occupying subarachnoid hygroma over the trepanation site; none led to an additional neurological deficit. Other complications of decompressive hemicraniectomy and durotomy are collection of cerebrospinal fluid (CSF) under the scalp, CSF collection within the brain, hydrocephalus, local infection (empyema and cerebral abscess), extradural haemorrhage, intracerebral haemorrhage and CSF hypotension.[55]

Medical Management of Raised Intracranial Pressure

The medical treatment for raised intracranial pressure (ICP) lacks a robust evidence base but nonetheless is used widely. Although shown to be inferior to hemicraniectomy for malignant syndromes in the pooled analysis of the randomised trials described above,[7] it has a role to play in settings where access to neurosurgery may be limited, or in buying time prior to hemicraniectomy.

Osmotherapy

Osmotic agents such as mannitol, glycerol, starch and hypertonic saline are most widely available and used. In theory, the creation of an osmotic gradient allows water to be drawn from within brain cells into the intravascular space. Guidelines suggest that they can be used to treat raised ICP, despite not only the lack of efficacy on outcome[56] but also with the potential that they can further aggravate pressure differentials by fluid shifts from the healthy hemisphere.[57] These substances are however first-line agents when clinical or radiological signs of space-occupying oedema occur and it is recommended that osmotherapy be used to treat elevated ICP prior to considered surgical decompression.[58]

Mannitol

Mannitol reduces ICP by extracting water from the extracellular compartment of the brain and may improve microvascular cerebral blood flow by haemodilution, thereby reducing blood volume and ICP through vasoconstriction.[37] Mannitol may also have additional pleotrophic actions by altering red cell morphology, thus increasing tissue oxygenation.[59] Animal experiments have shown benefits of mannitol with respect to infarct size, oedema formation and elevated ICP. There is lack of robust evidence in humans and a conclusion of favourable outcome with mannitol in unselected stroke patients cannot be made[60]; some evidence even suggests harm.[61] With respect to raised ICP following acute stroke — not particularly accompanied by malignant oedema — a one-off mannitol infusion (40 g over 15 minutes) has been shown to reduce ICP, albeight temporarily (4 hours).[62] In DESTINY, the dose recommended was 0.5 g/kg four times a day with a maximum daily dose of 2.5 g/kg, to target a serum osmolality of 315 to 320 mOsm.[20]

Glycerol

Unlike mannitol, glycerol has been widely assessed in stroke trials. A review of its use in definite or probable ischaemic stroke showed that risk of death was reduced during the treatment period. A significant detractor from these results was that brain imaging was not commonly used to determine either stroke type or the presence of significant oedema.[63] Glycerol was however, well tolerated and has a theoretical advantage over mannitol in that it is metabolised by the brain on crossing the blood brain barrier (BBB), thus reducing the risk of rebound oedema.[37] Again however, no randomised trial has specifically addressed the effect of glycerol on functional outcome and mortality in patients with massive oedema secondary to large hemispheric infarction. The dosing regime proposed in DESTINY was 250 ml of 10% glycerol solution, four times per day.[20]

Hydroxyethyl starch

In one study that included nine patients with elevated ICP due to massive oedema following hemispheric stroke, a bolus of 100 ml of 7.5% saline plus hydroxyethyl starch solution or mannitol was used prospectively to evaluate a protocol. The starch solution was administered over 15 minutes and significantly lowered ICP in all episodes that were characterised by an ICP rise > 25 mmHg and/or a new pupillary abnormality. Starch has a greater and faster effect than mannitol.[62] Serum osmolality and sodium levels were greater following both infusions but more so in the starch group. The dosing regime proposed in DESTINY was 6% hetastarch in 0.9% NaCl injection, 100–250 ml every eight hours to a maximum daily dose of 750 ml.

Intubation, mechanical ventilation and hyperventilation

The indication for intubation in stroke is for airway protection in cases where there is a depressed ventilatory drive. Patients should be intubated when the Glasgow Coma Scale (GCS) falls to less than 8 or in respiratory failure: partial pressure of oxygen [pO_2] < 60 mmHg or partial pressure of carbon dioxide [pCO_2] > 48 mmHg.[57] In DESTINY, ventilation mode was left to the discretion of the treating physician but target gas parameters in raised intracranial pressure were pO_2 > 100 mmHg and pCO_2 35–40 mmHg. If neurological function deteriorated further despite this, then a target value of pCO_2 28–32 mmHg was aimed for.[20]

Hyperventilation decreases ICP by inducing cerebral vasoconstriction; cerebral blood volume subsequently decreases as does cerebral blood flow. This has been shown mainly in patients with traumatic brain injury and not in those with oedema due to malignant MCA infarction.[64] The disadvantage of this method is that cerebral vasoconstriction may decrease cerebral blood flow to ischaemic levels and rebound vasodilation may occur with the risk of increasing ICP when hyperventilation is discontinued.[37] Hyperventilation is therefore not recommended for first-line therapy and is a short-lived intervention whilst bridging to hemicraniectomy[56]; it may involve increasing the patient's respiratory rate to between 14 and 18 breaths per minute and titrating against pCO_2. Prolonged periods of hyperventilation are discouraged as the effect wears off within three to four hours and cerebral vasoconstriction may further aggravate ischaemic brain injury.[65]

Intracranial pressure monitoring

Invasive measurement of ICP and cerebral perfusion pressure (CPP) in the ipsilateral hemisphere is recommended.[20,57] Monitoring may be helpful in measuring response to ICP lowering strategies and may even predict those with poorer outcomes: none of the 48 patients with clinical signs of increased ICP due to large hemispheric or middle cerebral artery territory infarction in one case series survived, if ICP > 35 mmHg.[66] This intervention was more limited in those with persistently raised ICP in which case monitoring did not help guide future therapy and therefore the ability to predict or influence outcomes.

Sedation

Propofol is recommended during ventilation as a muscle relaxant, though the exact agent used in the randomised trials was left to the discretion of the treating physician. Barbiturates however were specifically discouraged. This agent was investigated in a prospective study of 60 patients with severe brain oedema following MCA/hemispheric infarction, confirmed with CT imaging. A thiopental infusion was used to induce coma after failure of osmotherapy and hyperventilation; ICP and patients were monitored. Following this infusion, ICP dropped in 50 patients but in most, this was short lived. No effect on ICP was found in 17% of patients and furthermore, severe side effects were found in a quarter of patients, which included systemic hypotension with resultant drop in CPP.[67]

Head positioning

Elevation of the head at 15°–30° was recommended in the case of severely increased intracranial pressure or in patients at high risk of infection.[20] Elevating the head is said to decrease ICP by increasing venous outflow. However, it can potentially reduce CPP by lowering systemic blood pressure, which in itself can add to ischaemic injury. In one study of body position in 12 patients with large supratentorial strokes, ICP did decrease mildly from horizontal to 30° positioning; however, with more vertical positioning mean arterial pressure dropped significantly and so did CPP.[68] Experience in one centre states that positioning should be made on an individual basis and that head elevation is reasonable as long as CPP is maintained > 70 mmHg.[37]

Body core temperature

In DESTINY, normothermia was targeted and treatment was advised if temperatures were > 37.5°C with the agent of cooling being left to the discretion of the treating physician.[20]

Hypothermia has been proposed as a neuroprotective agent due to its ability to reduce cerebral metabolic rate, stabilise the BBB, reduce brain oedema and free radical formation, as well as reduce the release of excitatory neurotransmitters.[37]

The ideal use of hypothermia in ischaemic stroke cases is perhaps to preserve penumbral areas for as long as possible in order to gain time until recanalisation therapies can be used to restore blood flow. Initial human studies of hypothermia however, has looked at its effect in space-occupying strokes: early observational studies have collated data on 112 patients with infarction of at least two-thirds of the MCA territory associated with oedema.[37] Methods to reduce core temperature to < 33°C ranged from surface devices — cooling blankets and ice bags[69] — to endovascular methods that used temperature-controlled saline instilled via femoral vein central lines.[70] The time allowed to commence cooling was relatively late, up to 28 hours following stroke onset and mean duration of cooling varied greatly from 55 hours[69] to 19 days.[71] In the case series with the largest number (50) of patients included, there was a mean reduction in ICP of 7.4 mmHg between baseline and steady state hypothermia when body-core temperature ranged between 32°C and 33°C. Measured ICP rose however, during re-warming and this effect appeared to be more pronounced with shorter re-warming times. In this study, 15 patients (30%) died during the re-warming period.[69] Complications of induced hypothermia in this study included low platelet count (70%) and cardiac arrhythmias, including bradycardia (62%) and severe hypotension (4%). Overall, 19 patients (38%) died. However, this is about half the mortality observed in historical controls.[4] There are no randomised trials with respect to cooling alone in treatment of space-occupying infarction, but a small randomised clinical trial has compared the use of moderate hypothermia (35°C) plus hemicraniectomy (12 patients) with hemicraniectomy alone (13 patients) in patients with brain infarction involving more than two-thirds of one hemisphere.[72] The mean age of patients was 49 years in both groups and the mean initial NIHSS score was similar: 19 in the group with hemicraniectomy alone and 18 with additional hypothermia. Hemicraniectomy was performed within 24 hours (mean 15 ± 6 hours) of stroke onset and hypothermia induced immediately afterwards either by external cooling (2 patients) or intravenous cooling methods. At six months, the NIHSS was non-significantly ($p < 0.08$) lower: 10 vs. 11 in those with additional hypothermia; there were no further significant risks, either during cooling, re-warming or during follow-up.

Others

Steroids and diuretics were not recommended in the randomised trials but have been used in clinical practice to reduce ICP in malignant oedema. Given the likely mode of action of steroids, it is possible that patients with vasogenic oedema secondary to large infarction may benefit from such treatment. However, this has not been proven in trials, not even in those involving intracerebral haemorrhage, where one may assume that peri-haematomal oedema is at least partially vasogenic. In fact steroid use in one trial significantly increased the number of sepsis-related and diabetic complications.[73] Steroids are therefore not indicated in raised ICP complicating large ischaemic stroke.[56,58]

Loop diuretics may act by decreasing total body water, increasing blood osmolality and thereby removing water from the brain but neither furosemide nor other diuretics have been evaluated for outcomes after ischaemic stroke. Furthermore, as shown above with other agents that decrease mean arterial pressure, diuretics too may reduce CPP without substantially reducing ICP.[37]

Quality of Life after Hemicraniectomy

All three randomised controlled trials of hemicraniectomy had secondary outcomes which included some form of quality of life measure. The results of these were not pooled but reported separately. The following is a précis of each trial's findings:

In DECIMAL, survivors in the surgical group (15) and medical group (4) at one year underwent questioning of physical and psychosocial functioning using the Stroke Impact Scale 2.0 (SIS) assessing four physical domains (strength, hand function, mobility, and activities of daily living) and four psychosocial domains (emotion, communication, memory and thinking and participation).[74] Only ten surgical patients and two medically treated patients were able to complete the assessment and showed mean physical scores of 33.4 vs. 38.9 respectively; emotional of 57.0 vs. 59.7; communication of 82.5 vs. 100.0 and participation of 32.6 vs. 42.2. Ten of the 15 surgical and two of the four medical group survivors were living at home at one year.[22]

In DESTINY, interviews with surviving patients and their carers were undertaken at one year to assess if they still agreed with treatment. Although complete agreement with the procedure was reported at this time by all 14 surgically treated surviving patients, the opinion of the seven medically treated surviving patients was not reported. Further quality of life measurements and aphasia testing are planned at two and three years to assess further recovery and improvements in language function.[20]

In HAMLET, secondary outcome measures at one year included quality of life measures using the Medical Outcomes Study 36-item short-form health survey (SF-36).[75] For reporting, two summary scores were calculated, one representing physical and the other mental health. The physical score was significantly lower at 29 in the 23 surgical patients compared, to mean score of 36 in the 12 medically treated patients. The mental summary score was not significantly different in the surgical and medically treated groups at 55 and 53 respectively, nor was the quality of life score measured on a visual analogue scale at 12 months. Depression was assessed with the Montgomery and Asberg depression rating scale (MADRS).[76] Mild and severe depression were equally common in the 23 surgically and 12 medically treated patients. Only one out of the 12 medical patients answering was dissatisfied with the treatment received; none of the 20 surgical patients were. Fourteen (44%) surgical and nine (28%) medical patients were living at home at one year; all patients with a mRS score of 5 (severe disability) were residing within a nursing home at this time.[21]

Other studies have looked specifically at quality of life in those who have undergone hemicraniectomy for malignant MCA oedema, and compared findings to age-matched controls. Long-term survivors of those undergoing hemicraniectomy in one series were interviewed by a nurse and physician at a minimum of one year following surgery.[77] Both patients and carers completed the SF-36 to determine the health status of the patient; scores were compared with those from the general population.[78] Fourteen of the 18 patients undergoing hemicraniectomy who survived a minimum of one year were included, of whom 12 (86%) were living at home and two in nursing institutions. All interviewees required help with activities of daily living, mean Barthel Index (BI) score was 64 and ranged from 5 to 100. Two patients had residual language disturbance.

Patients' quality of life scores were significantly lower than those from age-matched controls except on the domains of body pain and emotional role. The domains of physical functioning and physical role were particularly lower in those who had undergone hemicraniectomy than in the general population. Across the group, relatives' scores matched those of the patients.[77] From the results of the life satisfaction questionnaire, five of the 12 interviewed (42%) found their life satisfying or very satisfying; five (42%) found it rather satisfying and two (17%) found their life rather dissatisfying/dissatisfying; the latter compares with 8% finding life dissatisfying from the reference group. The life satisfaction scores did not appear to show any correlation with disability, theorising therefore, that there must be other factors involved, perhaps social and environmental factors or pre-morbid personality that influences 'satisfaction with life', as has been proposed before.[19] Clearly, cortical symptoms of dysphasia and denial of illness may have influenced patients' scores but the fact that they were similar to the scores ascribed by patients' relatives too, probably showed that they had reasonable insight into their circumstances.[77]

What about regret? Asking this question may reveal insights into how content patients are with their current situation. Clearly this is not a 'clean' question as it must be influenced by pre-surgical expectations and current mood. However, a few studies have indeed asked this question, including DESTINY in which no surgical patient regretted their decision, presumably to enter the randomised controlled trial.[20] Others have done the same: 12 of the 18 patients who survived hemicraniectomy in one institution were contacted a minimum of seven months later regarding psychological status and quality of life.[19] Ten of the 12 were living at home and two were placed in nursing homes. With respect to depression, five had no depression, six had mild and one (8%) moderate depression. No patient reported severe depression. Of the five patients with left-sided infarctions alive at seven months, two had good speech, two continued to have reduced speech fluency but with complete understanding and only one patient remained globally aphasic. There was no significant difference in the general quality of life between those with left or right hemispheric infarcts. These observations strengthen the case for hemicraniectomy irrespective of the hemisphere affected as long as the individual, or a family member acting as their advocate, feels that the likely resultant disability, is acceptable. Finally in this study, the patients and their families were asked how they would judge the decision of the operation with hindsight. They were allowed to respond 'yes' or 'no' as to whether they would agree to undergo the surgical procedure again: 11 of the 12 patients and their relatives agreed that on retrospect, the decision to undergo surgery was the correct one. In contrast, relatives of one patient who was severely disabled and aphasic considered that the decision to operate was not the correct one.[19]

Retrospective consent to surgery was also assessed in 18 patients who had undergone hemicraniectomy for non-dominant malignant MCA syndrome and survived one year. Patients were asked whether knowing their present situation before surgery, they would again give their consent to decompressive hemicraniectomy. Patients were divided into groups depending upon functional status and the results are presented in Table 4.

Those who retrospectively agreed had a better functional status (median BI = 75, median mRS = 3) than those who did not agree (median BI = 15, median mRS = 4). Of note, none of those in Group 1 regretted their decision despite the fact that none of the three patients were able to return to their usual vocation.[16]

Finally, from a study population of 48 patients who underwent decompressive hemicraniectomy for malignant MCA, 43 patients were assessed a minimum of three months after the procedure.[79] A quality of life index was calculated based on 11 domains of social living and the results were the same, regardless of the hemisphere involved or presence or absence of aphasia. In contrast to the previous study,[77] dependents of patients rated quality of life significantly lower than patients did. Of the

Table 4. Retrospective agreement to hemicraniectomy in 18 patients[16]

Group	mRS	Number	Regret 'yes'
1	2	3	0
2	3	6	0
3	4	6	1
4	5	3	3

surviving patients and/or dependents, 81% would agree to surgery in the future; that is, 19% regretted this surgical intervention. How this was related to current functional status, is unknown.

These data suggest that factors other than survival alone are important when considering the decision for hemicraniectomy. These areas need to be explored and discussed with patients but more likely their relatives, so that informed decisions to accept or decline hemicraniectomy can be made. The acceptable quality of life or regret after surgery appears to be a personal decision, which is modestly linked with functional recovery and appears not to be influenced by the side of infarct or level of speech disturbance. It is also clear that stroke survivors assign a higher quality of life score, or a 'utility', to the state of living with stroke than those in good health.[80] Many patients who require hemicraniectomy will not have the capacity to give informed consent for hemicraniectomy because of the severity of neurological deficits and alterations in their level of consciousness.[7] Such decisions will therefore fall upon relatives. Some patients may have advance directives or have discussed relevant wishes with family members previously.[81] However, given that malignant MCA syndrome mainly affects younger people, the majority of patients are neither likely to have documented advanced wishes nor discussed acceptable outcomes following a health crisis with those nearest to them. In these situations relatives may find it difficult to make such decisions, particularly because they have had little or no contact with severe disability and may rate its negative impact more so than the patient would, given the same information. Stroke clinicians can support patients and their relatives around decision making by providing facts of expected outcome without surgery, and likely levels of residual disability with survival.

Guidelines

Previously decompressive surgery, which included hemicraniectomy and surgical resection/evacuation, was advised for malignant brain oedema. This procedure attained Class IIa, Level B evidence in some guidelines[56] and Class III in others.[82] In the American Heart Association/American Stroke Association guidelines from 2007, the recommendations state that it is reasonable to perform this procedure and that it may be life-saving but the side of the infarction (dominant versus non-dominant hemisphere) may affect decisions about surgery.[56] More recent guidelines have recommended that surgical decompressive therapy should be undertaken in those with evolving malignant MCA infarcts and this has been upgraded to Class 1 Level A evidence.[58] Other guidelines too have recommended this, as long as patients fulfill the following clinical and neuroimaging criteria[83]:

1. Aged 60 years or younger
2. Examination findings are suggestive of an infarction in the territory of the middle cerebral artery and they have a score on the National Institute of Health Stroke Scale (NIHSS) of > 15
3. The level of consciousness score as measured by item 1a of the NIHSS should be ≥ 1
4. The CT brain scan should show evidence of an infarct of ≥ 50% of the MCA territory, either with or without additional infarction in the territory of the anterior or posterior cerebral artery on the same side, or an infarct volume greater than 145 cm^3 on the diffusion-weighted MRI

These guidelines also recommend that referral should be within 24 hours of symptom onset and that treatment should be performed within a maximum of 48 hours. This latter timeline is also recommended by authors of European guidelines[58]; the American guidelines have yet to be modified based on this recommendation.[56] Clearly, not all centres have the appropriate services to be able to undertake the monitoring and procedures required, thus local services should agree on protocols for transfer of appropriate patients to regional neurosurgical centres.

Future Considerations

Although hemicraniectomy is the treatment of choice for malignant infarction syndrome and it saves lives, further research on functional outcomes and quality of life are required to strengthen its role in the clinical management of such patients. Further research is also required on psychosocial outcomes and social integration in these patients. The upper age limit for surgical intervention remains an unresolved issue. This is particularly relevant given that 75% of all strokes affect those aged over 65.[84]

Although prognosis after hemicraniectomy has been shown to be worse in older people compared with younger patients,[17] baseline differences may have contributed to this finding, as poorer outcomes with conservative therapy were also seen in the older group. In keeping with other acute studies in stroke, the randomised trials excluded patients in the older age category. Taking the example of thrombolysis for acute ischaemic stroke, though functional outcomes were worse and mortality higher in older patients, this may have been due to existing co-morbidities rather than adverse effects of tPA, given that the rates of symptomatic haemorrhage were similar in the two age groups (cut-off, 80 years).[85] This data is derived from observational data only but potential benefits of tPA are being trialled openly in older people and these results are awaited (IST 3).[86] Randomisation of older patients with malignant infarction into hemicraniectomy trials with their consent may be a reasonable future strategy too. This has been planned in the DESTINY-II trial.[87]

The results from HAMLET with respect to early or late hemicraniectomy for malignant infarct syndrome, did not support delayed surgery. However only 25 patients fell into this 'delayed' category and so firm conclusions cannot be drawn.[21] Further studies are needed to determine optimum timing of surgery for best outcomes but trials to investigate this have yet to be registered.

Imaging is another potential area of research that may help predict those who will develop malignant oedema or perhaps identify those who may escape it. Although coupled with some logistical concerns, periodic MR imaging may help track the rate of change of the infarct volume and which may then allow us to identify a threshold at which hemicraniectomy is optimally timed — perhaps even in those who present later than two days after their insult.

Other experimental studies based on reperfusion and inflammatory molecules may help us determine those who will follow a malignant course.[14] Will intracranial pressure reduction methods still be needed in the future? Can we hope that wider uptake and alternative methods of recanalisation, especially in those with proximal occlusion, will reduce the incidence of large middle cerebral artery strokes and concomitant malignant oedema? This is a possibility but perhaps not in the immediate short term.

In the meantime we must aim to promptly recognise those who have incipient malignant oedema and learn to predict more accurately those in whom such oedema is likely to occur. We must have timely and informed discussions with our patients and their relatives so that they can make educated decisions at these times. These efforts, including prompt referral to specialist centres, remain the mainstay for optimum management of patients with malignant infarct syndrome.

References

1. Heinsius T, Bogousslavsky J, Van Melle G. Large infarcts in the middle cerebral artery territory. Etiology and outcome patterns. *Neurology* 1998; 50(2): 341–350.
2. Chen WH, Bai CH, Huang SJ, Chiu HC, Lien LM. Outcome of large hemispheric infarcts: an experience of 50 patients in Taiwan. *Surg Neurol* 2007; 68(Suppl 1): S68–73; discussion S74.
3. van Swieten JC, Koudstaal PJ, Visser MC, Schouten HJ, van Gijn J. Interobserver agreement for the assessment of handicap in stroke patients. *Stroke* 1988; 19(5): 604–607.
4. Hacke W, Schwab S, Horn M, Spranger M, De Georgia M, von Kummer R. 'Malignant' middle cerebral artery territory infarction: clinical course and prognostic signs. *Arch Neurol* 1996; 53(4): 309–315.
5. Jaramillo A, Gongora-Rivera F, Labreuche J, Hauw JJ, Amarenco P. Predictors for malignant middle cerebral artery infarctions: a postmortem analysis. *Neurology* 2006; 66(6): 815–820.
6. Brott T, Adams HP, Jr., Olinger CP, Marler JR, Barsan WG, Biller J *et al.* Measurements of acute cerebral infarction: a clinical examination scale. *Stroke* 1989; 20(7): 864–870.
7. Vahedi K, Hofmeijer J, Juettler E, Vicaut E, George B, Algra A *et al.* Early decompressive surgery in malignant infarction of the middle cerebral artery: a pooled analysis of three randomised controlled trials. *Lancet Neurol* 2007; 6(3): 215–222.
8. Cucchiara BL, Kasner SE, Wolk DA, Lyden PD, Knappertz VA, Ashwood T *et al.* Early impairment in consciousness predicts mortality after hemispheric ischemic stroke. *Crit Care Med* 2004; 32(1): 241–245.

9. Simard JM, Kent TA, Chen M, Tarasov KV, Gerzanich V. Brain oedema in focal ischaemia: molecular pathophysiology and theoretical implications. *Lancet Neurol* 2007; 6(3): 258–268.
10. Specific treatment of acute ischaemic stroke patients. In Warlow CP, Dennis MS, van Gijn J, Hankey GJ, Sandercock PAG, Bamford JM, Wardlaw JM (Eds.). *Stroke: Practical Management.* 3rd Edn. Malden, MA: Blackwell Publishing; 2008, pp. 442–508.
11. Qureshi AI, Suarez JI, Yahia AM, Mohammad Y, Uzun G, Suri MF *et al.* Timing of neurologic deterioration in massive middle cerebral artery infarction: a multicenter review. *Crit Care Med* 2003; 31(1): 272–277.
12. Kalia KK, Yonas H. An aggressive approach to massive middle cerebral artery infarction. *Arch Neurol* 1993; 50(12): 1293–1297.
13. Gupta R, Connolly ES, Mayer S, Elkind MS. Hemicraniectomy for massive middle cerebral artery territory infarction: a systematic review. *Stroke* 2004; 35(2): 539–543.
14. Huttner HB, Schwab S. Malignant middle cerebral artery infarction: clinical characteristics, treatment strategies, and future perspectives. *Lancet Neurol* 2009; 8(10): 949–958.
15. Delashaw JB, Broaddus WC, Kassell NF, Haley EC, Pendleton GA, Vollmer DG *et al.* Treatment of right hemispheric cerebral infarction by hemicraniectomy. *Stroke* 1990; 21(6): 874–881.
16. Leonhardt G, Wilhelm H, Doerfler A, Ehrenfeld CE, Schoch B, Rauhut F *et al.* Clinical outcome and neuropsychological deficits after right decompressive hemicraniectomy in MCA infarction. *J Neurol* 2002; 249(10): 1433–1440.
17. Holtkamp M, Buchheim K, Unterberg A, Hoffmann O, Schielke E, Weber JR *et al.* Hemicraniectomy in elderly patients with space occupying media infarction: improved survival but poor functional outcome. *J Neurol Neurosurg Psychiatry* 2001; 70(2): 226–228.
18. Rieke K, Schwab S, Krieger D, von Kummer R, Aschoff A, Schuchardt V *et al.* Decompressive surgery in space-occupying hemispheric infarction: results of an open, prospective trial. *Crit Care Med* 1995; 23(9): 1576–1587.
19. Walz B, Zimmermann C, Bottger S, Haberl RL. Prognosis of patients after hemicraniectomy in malignant middle cerebral artery infarction. *J Neurol* 2002; 249(9): 1183–1190.
20. Juttler E, Schwab S, Schmiedek P, Unterberg A, Hennerici M, Woitzik J *et al.* Decompressive Surgery for the Treatment of Malignant Infarction of the

Middle Cerebral Artery (DESTINY): a randomized, controlled trial. *Stroke* 2007; 38(9): 2518–2525.

21. Hofmeijer J, Kappelle LJ, Algra A, Amelink GJ, van Gijn J, van der Worp HB. Surgical decompression for space-occupying cerebral infarction (the Hemicraniectomy After Middle Cerebral Artery infarction with Life-threatening Edema Trial [HAMLET]): a multicentre, open, randomised trial. *Lancet Neurol* 2009; 8(4): 326–333.

22. Vahedi K, Vicaut E, Mateo J, Kurtz A, Orabi M, Guichard JP *et al.* Sequential-design, multicenter, randomized, controlled trial of early decompressive craniectomy in malignant middle cerebral artery infarction (DECIMAL Trial). *Stroke* 2007; 38(9): 2506–2517.

23. Hand PJ, Wardlaw JM, Rowat AM, Haisma JA, Lindley RI, Dennis MS. Magnetic resonance brain imaging in patients with acute stroke: feasibility and patient related difficulties. *J Neurol Neurosurg Psychiatry* 2005; 76(11): 1525–1527.

24. Singer OC, Sitzer M, du Mesnil de Rochemont R, Neumann-Haefelin T. Practical limitations of acute stroke MRI due to patient-related problems. *Neurology* 2004; 62(10): 1848–1849.

25. Oppenheim C, Samson Y, Manai R, Lalam T, Vandamme X, Crozier S *et al.* Prediction of malignant middle cerebral artery infarction by diffusion-weighted imaging. *Stroke* 2000; 31(9): 2175–2181.

26. Neumann-Haefelin T, Sitzer M, du Mesnil de Rochemont R, Lanfermann H. Prediction of malignant MCA infarction with DWI: pitfalls in hyperacute stroke. *Stroke* 2001; 32(2): 580–583.

27. Kasner SE, Demchuk AM, Berrouschot J, Schmutzhard E, Harms L, Verro P *et al.* Predictors of fatal brain edema in massive hemispheric ischemic stroke. *Stroke* 2001; 32(9): 2117–2123.

28. Haring HP, Dilitz E, Pallua A, Hessenberger G, Kampfl A, Pfausler B *et al.* Attenuated corticomedullary contrast: an early cerebral computed tomography sign indicating malignant middle cerebral artery infarction. A case-control study. *Stroke* 1999; 30(5): 1076–1082.

29. Berrouschot J, Barthel H, von Kummer R, Knapp WH, Hesse S, Schneider D. 99m technetium-ethyl-cysteinate-dimer single-photon emission CT can predict fatal ischemic brain edema. *Stroke* 1998; 29(12): 2556–2562.

30. Manno EM, Nichols DA, Fulgham JR, Wijdicks EF. Computed tomographic determinants of neurologic deterioration in patients with large middle cerebral artery infarctions. *Mayo Clin Proc* 2003; 78(2): 156–160.

31. Krieger DW, Demchuk AM, Kasner SE, Jauss M, Hantson L. Early clinical and radiological predictors of fatal brain swelling in ischemic stroke. *Stroke* 1999; 30(2): 287–292.

32. Thomalla GJ, Kucinski T, Schoder V, Fiehler J, Knab R, Zeumer H *et al.* Prediction of malignant middle cerebral artery infarction by early perfusion- and diffusion-weighted magnetic resonance imaging. *Stroke* 2003; 34(8): 1892–1899.

33. Dohmen C, Bosche B, Graf R, Reithmeier T, Ernestus RI, Brinker G *et al.* Identification and clinical impact of impaired cerebrovascular autoregulation in patients with malignant middle cerebral artery infarction. *Stroke* 2007; 38(1): 56–61.

34. Ivamoto HS, Numoto M, Donaghy RM. Surgical decompression for cerebral and cerebellar infarcts. *Stroke* 1974; 5(3): 365–370.

35. Robertson SC, Lennarson P, Hasan DM, Traynelis VC. Clinical course and surgical management of massive cerebral infarction. *Neurosurgery* 2004; 55(1): 55–61; discussion 61–62.

36. Rengachary SS, Batnitzky S, Morantz RA, Arjunan K, Jeffries B. Hemicraniectomy for acute massive cerebral infarction. *Neurosurgery* 1981; 8(3): 321–328.

37. Bardutzky J, Schwab S. Antiedema therapy in ischemic stroke. *Stroke* 2007; 38(11): 3084–3094.

38. Donnan GA, Davis SM. Surgical decompression for malignant middle cerebral artery infarction: a challenge to conventional thinking. *Stroke* 2003; 34(9): 2307.

39. Schwab S, Steiner T, Aschoff A, Schwarz S, Steiner HH, Jansen O *et al.* Early hemicraniectomy in patients with complete middle cerebral artery infarction. *Stroke* 1998; 29(9): 1888–1893.

40. Mori K, Aoki A, Yamamoto T, Horinaka N, Maeda M. Aggressive decompressive surgery in patients with massive hemispheric embolic cerebral infarction associated with severe brain swelling. *Acta Neurochir (Wien)* 2001; 143(5): 483–491; discussion 491–492.

41. Frank H, Schobel HP, Heusser K, Geiger H, Fahlbusch R, Naraghi R. Long-term results after microvascular decompression in essential hypertension. *Stroke* 2001; 32(12): 2950–2955.

42. Diringer MN, Kaufmann AM. Heads-up on hemicraniectomy. *Neurology* 2004; 63(11): 1997–1998.

43. http://www.strokecenter.org/trials/browse.aspx?status=4. Accessed October 17th 2009.

44. Hofmeijer J, Amelink GJ, Algra A, van Gijn J, Macleod MR, Kappelle LJ *et al.* Hemicraniectomy after middle cerebral artery infarction with life-threatening Edema trial (HAMLET). Protocol for a randomised controlled trial of decompressive surgery in space-occupying hemispheric infarction. *Trials* 2006; 7: 29.

45. Mitchell P, Gregson BA, Crossman J, Gerber C, Jenkins A, Nicholson C *et al.* Reassessment of the HAMLET study. *Lancet Neurol* 2009; 8(7): 602–603; author reply 603–604.

46. The National Institute of Neurological Disorders and Stroke rt-PA Stroke Study Group. Tissue plasminogen activator for acute ischemic stroke. *N Engl J Med* 1995; 333(24): 1581–1587.

47. Hacke W, Kaste M, Bluhmki E, Brozman M, Davalos A, Guidetti D *et al.* Thrombolysis with alteplase 3 to 4.5 hours after acute ischemic stroke. *N Engl J Med* 2008; 359(13): 1317–1329.

48. Cho DY, Chen TC, Lee HC. Ultra-early decompressive craniectomy for malignant middle cerebral artery infarction. *Surg Neurol* 2003; 60(3): 227–232; discussion 232–233.

49. Carter AM, Catto AJ, Mansfield MW, Bamford JM, Grant PJ. Predictive variables for mortality after acute ischemic stroke. *Stroke* 2007; 38(6): 1873–1880.

50. Arac A, Blanchard V, Lee M, Steinberg GK. Assessment of outcome following decompressive craniectomy for malignant middle cerebral artery infarction in patients older than 60 years of age. *Neurosurg Focus* 2009; 26(6): E3.

51. Sakai K, Iwahashi K, Terada K, Gohda Y, Sakurai M, Matsumoto Y. Outcome after external decompression for massive cerebral infarction. *Neurol Med Chir (Tokyo)* 1998; 38(3): 131–135; discussion 135–136.

52. Carter BS, Ogilvy CS, Candia GJ, Rosas HD, Buonanno F. One-year outcome after decompressive surgery for massive nondominant hemispheric infarction. *Neurosurgery* 1997; 40(6): 1168–1175; discussion 1175–1176.

53. Pranesh MB, Dinesh Nayak S, Mathew V, Prakash B, Natarajan M, Rajmohan V *et al.* Hemicraniectomy for large middle cerebral artery territory infarction: outcome in 19 patients. *J Neurol Neurosurg Psychiatry* 2003; 74(6): 800–802.

54. Kastrau F, Wolter M, Huber W, Block F. Recovery from aphasia after hemicraniectomy for infarction of the speech-dominant hemisphere. *Stroke* 2005; 36(4): 825–829.

55. Vahedi K. Decompressive hemicraniectomy for malignant hemispheric infarction. *Curr Treat Options Neurol* 2009; 11(2): 113–119.

56. Adams HP, Jr., del Zoppo G, Alberts MJ, Bhatt DL, Brass L, Furlan A *et al.* Guidelines for the early management of adults with ischemic stroke: a guideline from the American Heart Association/American Stroke Association Stroke Council, Clinical Cardiology Council, Cardiovascular Radiology and Intervention Council, and the Atherosclerotic Peripheral Vascular Disease and Quality of Care Outcomes in Research Interdisciplinary Working Groups: the American Academy of Neurology affirms the value of this guideline as an educational tool for neurologists. *Stroke* 2007; 38(5): 1655–1711.

57. Juttler E, Schellinger PD, Aschoff A, Zweckberger K, Unterberg A, Hacke W. Clinical review: therapy for refractory intracranial hypertension in ischaemic stroke. *Crit Care* 2007; 11(5): 231.

58. Guidelines for management of ischaemic stroke and transient ischaemic attack 2008. *Cerebrovasc Dis* 2008; 25(5): 457–507.

59. Andrews RJ, Bringas JR, Muto RP. Effects of mannitol on cerebral blood flow, blood pressure, blood viscosity, hematocrit, sodium, and potassium. *Surg Neurol* 1993; 39(3): 218–222.

60. Bereczki D, Liu M, Prado GF, Fekete I. Cochrane report: a systematic review of mannitol therapy for acute ischemic stroke and cerebral parenchymal hemorrhage. *Stroke* 2000; 31(11): 2719–2722.

61. Bereczki D, Mihalka L, Szatmari S, Fekete K, Di Cesar D, Fulesdi B *et al.* Mannitol use in acute stroke: case fatality at 30 days and 1 year. *Stroke* 2003; 34(7): 1730–1735.

62. Schwarz S, Schwab S, Bertram M, Aschoff A, Hacke W. Effects of hypertonic saline hydroxyethyl starch solution and mannitol in patients with increased intracranial pressure after stroke. *Stroke* 1998; 29(8): 1550–1555.

63. Righetti E, Celani MG, Cantisani T, Sterzi R, Boysen G, Ricci S. Glycerol for acute stroke. *Cochrane Database Syst Rev* 2004(2): CD000096.

64. Stocchetti N, Maas AI, Chieregato A, van der Plas AA. Hyperventilation in head injury: a review. *Chest* 2005; 127(5): 1812–1827.

65. Demchuk AM, Krieger DW. Mass effect with cerebral infarction. *Curr Treat Options Neurol* 1999; 1(3): 189–199.

66. Schwab S, Aschoff A, Spranger M, Albert F, Hacke W. The value of intracranial pressure monitoring in acute hemispheric stroke. *Neurology* 1996; 47(2): 393–398.
67. Schwab S, Spranger M, Schwarz S, Hacke W. Barbiturate coma in severe hemispheric stroke: useful or obsolete? *Neurology* 1997; 48(6): 1608–1613.
68. Schwarz S, Georgiadis D, Aschoff A, Schwab S. Effects of body position on intracranial pressure and cerebral perfusion in patients with large hemispheric stroke. *Stroke* 2002; 33(2): 497–501.
69. Schwab S, Georgiadis D, Berrouschot J, Schellinger PD, Graffagnino C, Mayer SA. Feasibility and safety of moderate hypothermia after massive hemispheric infarction. *Stroke* 2001; 32(9): 2033–2035.
70. Georgiadis D, Schwarz S, Kollmar R, Schwab S. Endovascular cooling for moderate hypothermia in patients with acute stroke: first results of a novel approach. *Stroke* 2001; 32(11): 2550–2553.
71. Milhaud D, Thouvenot E, Heroum C, Escuret E. Prolonged moderate hypothermia in massive hemispheric infarction: clinical experience. *J Neurosurg Anesthesiol* 2005; 17(1): 49–53.
72. Els T, Oehm E, Voigt S, Klisch J, Hetzel A, Kassubek J. Safety and therapeutical benefit of hemicraniectomy combined with mild hypothermia in comparison with hemicraniectomy alone in patients with malignant ischemic stroke. *Cerebrovasc Dis* 2006; 21(1–2): 79–85.
73. Poungvarin N, Bhoopat W, Viriyavejakul A, Rodprasert P, Buranasiri P, Sukondhabhant S *et al.* Effects of dexamethasone in primary supratentorial intracerebral hemorrhage. *N Engl J Med* 1987; 316: 1229–1233.
74. Duncan PW, Wallace D, Lai SM, Johnson D, Embretson S, Laster LJ. The stroke impact scale version 2.0. Evaluation of reliability, validity, and sensitivity to change. *Stroke* 1999; 30(10): 2131–2140.
75. Ware J, Jr., Kosinski M, Keller SD. A 12-Item Short-Form Health Survey: construction of scales and preliminary tests of reliability and validity. *Med Care* 1996; 34(3): 220–233.
76. Svanborg P, Asberg M. A comparison between the Beck Depression Inventory (BDI) and the self-rating version of the Montgomery Asberg Depression Rating Scale (MADRS). *J Affect Disord* 2001; 64(2–3): 203–216.
77. Skoglund TS, Eriksson-Ritzen C, Sorbo A, Jensen C, Rydenhag B. Health status and life satisfaction after decompressive craniectomy for malignant middle cerebral artery infarction. *Acta Neurol Scand* 2007; 117(5): 305–310.

78. Jenkinson C, Coulter A, Wright L. Short form 36 (SF36) health survey questionnaire: normative data for adults of working age. *BMJ* 1993; 306(6890): 1437–1440.

79. Woertgen C, Erban P, Rothoerl RD, Bein T, Horn M, Brawanski A. Quality of life after decompressive craniectomy in patients suffering from supratentorial brain ischemia. *Acta Neurochir (Wien)* 2004; 146(7): 691–695.

80. Post PN, Stiggelbout AM, Wakker PP. The utility of health states after stroke: a systematic review of the literature. *Stroke* 2001; 32(6): 1425–1429.

81. Siminoff LA, Gordon N, Hewlett J, Arnold RM. Factors influencing families' consent for donation of solid organs for transplantation. *JAMA* 2001; 286(1): 71–77.

82. Olsen TS, Langhorne P, Diener HC, Hennerici M, Ferro J, Sivenius J *et al.* European Stroke Initiative Recommendations for Stroke Management-update 2003. *Cerebrovasc Dis* 2003; 16(4): 311–337.

83. NICE National Collaborating Centre for Chronic C. Stroke: national clinical guideline for diagnosis and initial management of acute stroke and transient ischaemic attack (TIA). Royal College of Physicians, London; 2008.

84. www.statistics.gov.uk/. Accessed October 2009.

85. Engelter ST, Bonati LH, Lyrer PA. Intravenous thrombolysis in stroke patients of ≥ 80 versus < 80 years of age — a systematic review across cohort studies. *Age Ageing* 2006; 35(6): 572–580.

86. www.dcn.ed.ac.uk/ist3/. Accessed September 2009.

87. http://strokecenter.info/trials/trialDetail.aspx?tid=1015&search_string= destiny. Accessed October 11th 2009.

7 Stroke Unit Care

Ian Wellwood* and Peter Langhorne[†]

Chapter Summary

The evidence base supporting organised inpatient (stroke unit) care has been established over the last 15 years[1] and stroke unit care is now recognised as the most widely applicable and broadly effective stroke treatment,[2] as well as being the only one to significantly reduce case fatality. Although there are encouraging examples of successful implementation, there remain many challenges before stroke unit care is universally available as routine care for all stroke patients. In this chapter, we consider the stroke unit as one (key) component of an overall or comprehensive stroke service. Although most of the information relates to stroke unit care in the UK context, a broader international perspective is taken where possible. The various terms used to describe stroke unit care are defined and an outline of the typical structures and processes seen in stroke units is provided. We provide an updated summary of the best available evidence, drawing not only on the Stroke Unit Trialists' Collaboration overview of stroke unit effectiveness,[3] but also including

*King's College London, Division of Health and Social Care Research, Guy's Campus, 7th Floor Capital House, 42 Weston Street, London SE1 3QD, UK
[†]University of Glasgow, Academic Section of Geriatric Medicine, 3rd Floor, University Block, Glasgow Royal Infirmary, Alexandra Parade, Glasgow G31 2ER, UK

evaluations of early supported discharge and economic evaluations. We then discuss the ways in which this evidence has been interpreted in different models of stroke unit care.

Stroke unit care has been implemented in a variety of ways and the chapter identifies and discusses some practical issues in implementing stroke policy and strategy. It goes on to provide two examples of how stroke unit care has been evaluated at a national (UK Royal College of Physicians Sentinel stroke audit[4]) and international (European Registries of Stroke (EROS) study[5]) level. Such evaluations may help to provide new insights into the nature of stroke care provision and differences in outcomes. Finally, this chapter points to the direction in which stroke units might develop in the future, including stroke unit research and the methods to evaluate them. Until we have the results of such research, clinicians and service planners should direct their efforts towards ensuring that the key basic systems of stroke unit care are implemented for as many patients with stroke as possible.

Introduction

The evidence base for stroke unit care has been established over the last 15 years[1] and is now recognised as the most broadly effective stroke treatment.[2] However, a great deal of work needs to be done before stroke unit care is available and delivered universally to all stroke patients. Aiming to highlight the delivery of high quality stroke services, this chapter describes and discusses the ways in which the best available evidence has been interpreted in different stroke unit models and the variety of ways in which 'stroke unit care' has been implemented and evaluated. We provide an updated summary of the best available evidence and provide an overview of how it might develop in the future.

This chapter may therefore be of interest to those implementing evidence-based stroke care and stroke strategies, developing or reviewing the quality of care in stroke units or those involved in commissioning care. It may also indicate to researchers where evidence is lacking and the strengths and weaknesses of the current evidence base on which clinical guidelines, policy and purchasing decisions are currently based. Finally, it may be of interest to those tracking the translation of research into practice and the evolution of service delivery.

In this chapter, we consider the stroke unit as one (key) part of an overall or comprehensive stroke service and discuss services in relation to the general needs of the majority of patients as opposed to the consideration required when dealing with individual patients with specific and unique needs. Much of the information in this chapter relates to stroke unit care in the UK context, however, a broader international perspective is taken where possible.

Defining Organised Inpatient Stroke Unit Care

The terminology used to describe organised inpatient stroke unit care can be confusing and make comparison and evaluation difficult. One useful working definition describes organised inpatient stroke unit care as that of a service delivering 'coordinated multidisciplinary care, usually in a geographically discrete area such as a stroke ward'. The multidisciplinary team typically consists of medical, nursing, physiotherapy, occupational therapy, speech and language therapy and social work staff that meets regularly to coordinate their care. In this section, some of the terms used to describe organised inpatient stroke unit care are defined and examples provided. These are largely drawn from the updated definitions of stroke unit care given in the Stroke Unit Trialist' Collaboration (SUTC) review.[3]

1. **Stroke unit:** A multidisciplinary team including specialist nursing staff based in a discrete ward caring exclusively for stroke patients. This category included the following subdivisions:

    (a) *acute stroke units* which accept patients acutely but discharge early (usually within seven days). These appear to fall into three broad subcategories:

    (i) 'intensive' model of care with continuous monitoring, high nurse staffing levels and the potential for life support;
    (ii) 'semi-intensive' with continuous monitoring, high nurse staffing but no life support facilities; and

(iii) 'non-intensive' with none of the above.

In acute stroke units, patients are rapidly admitted to the stroke unit where interventions are given to correct any physiological abnormalities and maintain their physiological function within normal limits.

These types of stroke units are common features of stroke care in parts of North America and Germany.

(b) *rehabilitation stroke units* that accept patients after a delay, usually of seven days or more, and focus on rehabilitation; and

(c) *comprehensive* (that is, combined acute and rehabilitation) *stroke units* which accept patients acutely but also provide rehabilitation for at least several weeks if necessary.

Both the rehabilitation unit and comprehensive unit models offered prolonged periods of rehabilitation. The comprehensive stroke unit is perhaps the most successfully implemented unit and this model is common in the Scandinavian countries and in some parts of Europe. Rehabilitation can start as early as possible and many patients can be discharged directly home.

2. **Mixed rehabilitation ward:** A multidisciplinary team including specialist nursing staff in a ward providing a generic rehabilitation service but not exclusively caring for stroke patients. Patients are usually admitted to these units early after having a stroke and remain there while they have rehabilitation needs.

The service descriptions are given in Table 1. There are some other terms often associated with stroke unit care and worth defining for our consideration of stroke unit care.[3,6]

Stroke service

This describes the overall organisation for delivering care to individuals with transient ischaemic attacks and strokes. A stroke service should include a stroke unit, but is more than just a stroke unit.

Table 1. Definitions relating to stroke units

Term	Definition
Stroke unit	A multidisciplinary team including specialist nursing staff based in a discrete ward caring exclusively for stroke patients.
Acute stroke unit	In acute stroke units patients are rapidly admitted to the stroke unit where interventions are given to correct any physiological abnormalities and maintain within normal limits. Patients are discharged early (usually within seven days).
(i) Intensive stroke unit	These units feature an 'intensive' model of care with continuous monitoring, high nurse staffing levels and the potential for life support.
(ii) Semi-intensive stroke unit	The 'semi-intensive' model typically provides continuous monitoring, high nurse staffing but no life support facilities.
(iii) Non-intensive stroke unit	The 'non-intensive' model features none of the above.
Rehabilitation stroke unit	Stroke units that accept patients after a delay, usually of seven days or more, and focus on rehabilitation which may be offered for prolonged periods.
Comprehensive stroke unit (i.e. combined acute and rehabilitation)	These are stroke units which accept patients acutely but also provide rehabilitation for at least several weeks if necessary. Rehabilitation can start as early as possible and many patients can be discharged directly home.
Mixed rehabilitation ward	A multidisciplinary team including specialist nursing staff in a ward providing a generic rehabilitation service but not exclusively caring for stroke patients Patients are usually admitted to these units early after after having a stroke and remain there while they have rehabilitation needs.

Mobile stroke teams

These are multidisciplinary teams (usually excluding specialist nursing staff) providing care in a variety of settings,[3] i.e. not based in a discrete ward. This model suffers from practical problems of coordinating care and often lack of involvement of specialist nursing staff. Mobile stroke teams appear to be less effective than geographically discrete stroke units.[7]

Early supported discharge

Early supported discharge (ESD) services have been defined as those aiming to accelerate discharge from hospital with the provision of rehabilitation and support (regular assistance) in a community setting.[8] ESD services often start in a stroke unit and extend out into the patient's home.

From these definitions, we can see that the key features vary around the time of admission, the type of patients admitted, the function of the unit and which members of staff are involved in delivering which aspects of care. The models do however have a number of common features in their structures and processes of care.[9]

Structures and Processes of Care

Structures

All the stroke units included in the SUTC review had a ward base with a geographically discrete location and featured dedicated nursing staff. Other specialist staff with a special interest and level of expertise in stroke care were present and participated in the multidisciplinary teamwork (MDT) of the units.

MDT working was considered to be occurring if a formal meeting of staff members occurred at least once per week at which there was discussion and planning of the management of individual patient's care. Other key structures were the presence of formal structures for the education and training of staff members and that information on both stroke and the available services were provided for both patients and their carers.

Process

Care processes in the SUTC trials typically involved a period of assessment, stroke management, discharge planning and post-discharge care.[9] See Fig. 1.

1. Assessment

This typically involves relevant members of the MDT with each patient having a full clinical assessment, including evaluation of any neurological impairment, routine blood biochemistry and haematology and a CT scan

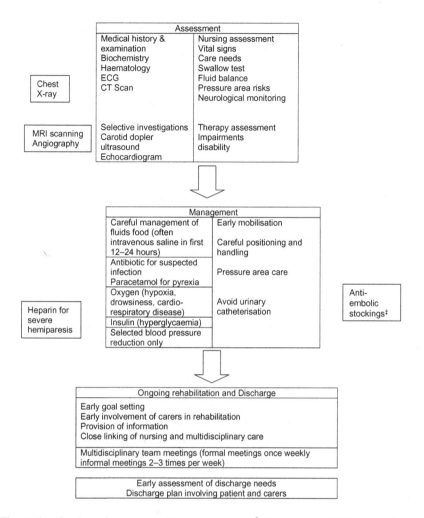

Figure 1. Outline of processes of stroke unit care.[9] Central part of figure represents processes reported in the majority of trials in SUTC while those in the peripheral boxes were reported in the minority of units in the SUTC.

of the brain. Investigations such as MRI scanning, carotid doppler ultrasound, and echocardiography are usually targeted at selected patients. Within the first few days of being admitted, nurses and therapists carry out assessments to identify the patients' general care needs, any swallowing

‡The CLOTS trial now indicates this strategy is ineffective.[10]

abnormalities, and to assess risk of developing pressure sores along with an evaluation of impairment and disability.

2. Management

In the acute phase, patients were typically managed with the use of intravenous fluids to prevent and treat dehydration, the early use of antibiotics and antipyretics in cases of infection, monitoring for hypoxia and treating with insulin therapy to correct hyperglycaemia.[11] There is some evidence that patients in stroke units are more closely monitored and receive a greater number of interventions aimed at maintaining key homeostatic physiological variables.[12] Such interventions may improve functional outcome by reducing the risk of further neurological deterioration.[13–15]

To minimise the risk of complications associated with immobility such as venous thromboembolism, interventions such as the use of compression stockings[‡], early mobilisation and careful positioning are employed. Nursing management involves careful attention to the patients' posture and positioning, appropriate moving and handling during care, and monitoring of key variables (e.g. swallowing problems, continence, skin integrity and nutritional status).

Therapists have an early contact with the patient, with nurses having a key role in the link between therapy staff and patients, incorporating and encouraging recommended practices in everyday handling and care of the patient. The use of intravenous fluids and nasogastric supplements are usually considered in those with impaired swallowing.

The ongoing management of the patients' rehabilitation involves the regular re-assessment of impairments and disabilities and the setting (and regular review) of multidisciplinary goals with the patient and their carers where this is feasible.

3. Discharge planning and post-discharge support

Stroke patient care typically involves a period in hospital with discharge planning being started at or before the time the patient has made some recovery and has a reasonable prospect of returning home either alone or with the support of a carer.

[‡]The CLOTS trial now indicates this strategy is ineffective.[10]

Early supported discharge schemes are a feature of a number of stroke services (31% of trusts surveyed in the Royal College of Physicians (RCP) UK National Sentinel Audit of Stroke 2008[16]) and may be particularly suited to stroke patients with moderate levels of disability.[8] Information on post-discharge support services is limited and although the RCP Sentinel Audit of Stroke found that 70% of hospital trusts in the UK have specialist community stroke teams, specific information about their structures and processes was limited.

Many of these structures and processes have been incorporated into the recommendations made in clinical guidelines on stroke care, e.g. Scottish Intercollegiate Guidelines Network (SIGN), Guideline on management of patients with stroke: Rehabilitation, Prevention and Management of Complications, and Discharge Planning (SIGN 64),[17] the Royal College of Physicians (RCP) National (UK) Clinical Guidelines for stroke,[18] European Stroke Organisation guidelines.[19] These were further validated by a series of consensus-based statements from a variety of government and professional bodies concerned with stroke care, e.g. the Helsingborg declarations.[20]

Evidence for the Effectiveness of Stroke Units

In 1993, the first systematic review of stroke unit care was published in *Lancet*,[1] which formed the basis of subsequent Cochrane reviews, and the work of the Stroke Unit Trialists' Collaboration (SUTC). It analysed the outcomes of organised inpatient (stroke unit) care versus conventional care usually provided in general wards. The analysis demonstrated benefits of organised stroke unit care in terms of reducing the numbers of patients who died, remained dependent, or required institutional care at one year follow-up after stroke. These benefits appeared to apply to all patients with stroke, regardless of age, clinical subtype or severity.[21]

The apparent benefits were observed in all types of stroke unit which were able to provide a period of care lasting several weeks if necessary (comprehensive stroke units or rehabilitation stroke units). Effective units were housed in a variety of departments, including general medicine, geriatric medicine, neurology and rehabilitation medicine, but all had similar processes of care (see above).

The most recent Cochrane review of organised inpatient (stroke unit) care (including trials up to April 2006) refined this question to accommodate the varying models of stroke care delivery being evaluated, by initially comparing stroke unit care to 'alternative forms of care' (which included general wards, mixed rehabilitation units and mobile stroke teams). Thirty-one trials were included, involving 6936 participants, and again found that more organised care was consistently associated with improved outcomes. Stroke unit care showed reductions in the odds of death recorded at final (median one year) follow-up (odds ratio (OR) 0.86; 95% confidence interval (CI: 0.76–0.98; p = 0.02), the odds of death or institutionalised care (OR 0.82; 95% CI: 0.73–0.92; p = 0.0006) and death or dependency (OR 0.82; 95% CI: 0.73–0.92; p = 0.001). Sensitivity analyses indicated that the observed benefits remained when the analysis was restricted to the most methodologically robust trials (that used formal randomisation procedures with blinded outcome assessment). There was no indication that organised stroke unit care resulted in a longer hospital stay.[3] Outcomes from the Cochrane review expressed in absolute terms are summarised in Table 2.

The benefit of organised stroke unit care appears to differ according to the severity of stroke. An analysis of pooled randomised controlled trails (RCT) data for patients stratified according to severity of stroke demonstrated a treatment effect of 1 death prevented per 100 patients

Table 2. Summary of systematic review of organised stroke unit care[3]

Outcomes at median 12 months	Number of trials (n)	Comparison group	Weighted event rates	OR (95% CI)	NNT (95% CI)
Death	31 (6936)	All alternative care	21% v 24%	0.86 (0.76 to 0.98)	29 (19 to 67)
Institutional care or death	30 (6884)	All alternative care	37% v 42%	0.81 (0.74 to 0.90)	20 (15 to 40)
Dependency or death	28 (5960)	All alternative care	52% v 58%	0.79 (0.71 to 0.88)	18 (12 to 32)

CI = Confidence interval, OR = Odds ratio, NNT = Number needed to treat treated (95% CI: 2 to 3 deaths) in mild stroke, 3 deaths prevented per 100 patients treated (95% CI: 1 to 6 deaths) in moderate stroke and 9 deaths prevented per 100 patients treated (95% CI: 4 to 14 deaths) in severe stroke.[22]

Full results and tables from the comparisons in the review of organised inpatient (stroke unit) care versus alternative care, organised inpatient (stroke unit) care versus general medical ward and comparisons of different forms of organised inpatient (stroke unit) care are available from: http://www.cochrane.org/reviews/en/ab000197.html

The review has acknowledged some limitations in terms of the number of trials available for subgroup analyses and the availability of outcomes and limited data on the long-term follow-up of patients. It does, however, continue to provide strong evidence that confirms organised stroke unit care as the most widely applicable and effective intervention after stroke that is currently available.

Evidence Supporting Early Supported Discharge (ESD)

Recently, there has been increased interest in reducing the length of hospital stay for patients with a number of conditions, including stroke. The concept of earlier discharge from hospital with augmented level of rehabilitation input at home has been proposed and investigated. When this form of early supported discharge has been evaluated in a systematic review using individual patient data,[8] it indicated that these systems of care can shorten length of stay and there is a trend to improved functional outcomes in the longer term. Some studies have also reported reduced costs.[23,24] This particular type of intervention is likely to be of benefit to patients with moderate levels of disability.

Evaluating the Economical Impact of Stroke Unit Care

The important issue of financial evaluation of stroke unit and stroke service provision is covered in a later chapter. Reducing hospital length of stay is an important component of cost is reductions since the greatest proportion of care costs is associated with nursing care and hospital overheads.[6] Costs in the longer term are attributable to the care of dependent individuals in hospitals or nursing homes[6] and so are likely to be sensitive to the number of patients left with long-term disability after stroke. It is possible that stroke unit care could be considered as potentially more cost effective than conventional care. In the SUTC review, there was no systematic increase in length of hospital stay associated with stroke unit care.[3] Some formal economic analyses suggest that stroke unit care is likely to save resources or provide improved outcomes for a modest increase in cost (based on studies in France, Germany and New Zealand), though a recent UK-based analysis found stroke unit care when combined with early supported discharge to be cost effective.[24]

It is also important that stroke services consider methods of evaluating personal cost to patients and their carers to avoid simply shifting the burden of care. However, the improved quality of life demonstrated for stroke unit patients[11,25] suggest that the reduction in disability seen with stroke unit care also reduces overall burden. Further careful economic analyses of stroke unit care in a variety of settings are likely to be important in providing information that might assist decisions on implementation.[26]

Implementation of Stroke Unit Care

The demonstration of the effectiveness of stroke units in randomised trials should encourage wide implementation. However, concerns have been raised that the benefits of stroke unit care may not be fully translated in routine care. Observational studies and audit offer methods complimentary to clinical trials and meta-analysis[27] and are useful, particularly when experimental methods may be inadequate to allow generalisability of results.

Particular examples of such studies include the national quality register on stroke care in Sweden, a system organised to describe and monitor quality of healthcare delivery and provide local and national data for those involved in healthcare delivery and planning. This register started in 1994 and since 1998 has collected data for approximately 20,000 stroke events every year from all 85 Swedish hospitals admitting patients with stroke.[28] The register is able to demonstrate variations in stroke service provision and consistently shows the benefits of stroke unit care in terms of improved death and functional outcomes and reduced institutionalisation compared to those treated in general wards. So the benefits of stroke unit care appear to be present not just in the academic centres carrying out RCTs but also seen in routine care.

Another recent example of a pre-intervention–post-intervention design observational study comes from a state-wide government funded clinician-led health system redesign programme set in New South Wales, Australia.[29] This study used retrospective case notes audit of more than 1500 cases sampled from 15 hospitals and examined on predetermined process indicators. The authors found significant improvements in the majority of process indicators, including improved access to CT scanning and stroke unit care (with a 22-fold increase in access) and significant increases in inpatient independence at discharge observed after the implementation of the redesign programme.

These results were included in a meta-analysis[30] of all the available observational studies of stroke unit care that largely confirmed the stroke unit benefits seen in the randomised trials, with stroke unit care being associated with significantly decreased odds of death (OR 0.79, 95% CI: 0.73–0.86; $p < 0.00001$) and odds of death or poor outcome (OR 0.87, 95% CI: 0.80–0.95; $p = 0.002$).

Access to Stroke Unit Care

Despite the available trial and observational evidence, uptake and dissemination of stroke unit care varied across countries, with stroke units a feature of only 38% of hospitals in a US survey[31] and 31% of stroke patients receiving stroke unit care in a Canadian network study.[32] In contrast, the Scandinavian countries are relatively successful in implementing stroke unit care and > 80% of stroke patients in Sweden are offered stroke unit care.[33] Progress in other parts of Europe is variable. Access to a stroke unit is generally good in Norway but variable in France, Hungary, Italy, Poland, and Portugal, while countries such as Germany and Austria have tended to develop and implement a different model of stroke unit care.[34] These findings are supported by recent European surveys[5,35,36] demonstrating variation in structures and processes in a number of aspects of stroke care.

Not only are the proportions of patients accessing 'organised stroke unit care' different, but the components of stroke unit care appear to differ between and within countries. To illustrate this further, we present examples from both the RCP Sentinel Audit of Stroke care in the UK[16] and an international comparison of stroke services carried out in conjunction with community-based stroke registers being run in a number of sites across Europe.[5]

The RCP Sentinel Stroke Audit

The background and details of the successful repeated cycles of this national audit project in the UK are described elsewhere in this book (See Chapter 11). Essentially, the RCP Sentinel Stroke Audit[16] has monitored the availability of structures and processes related to the provision of quality stroke care in all hospitals treating patients with stroke in England, Wales, Northern Ireland and the Channel Islands ($n = 224$ hospital sites in 2008). Compliance with evidence-based guidelines from the RCP is monitored based on self-reported questionnaire and by review of a sample of cases from each site. Key variables such as the availability of stroke unit care are steadily improving from 73% of hospitals in the audit in 2002 to 92% in 2008. On the day of audit in 2008, there were 6177 patients across all the sites audited, and 5816 stroke unit beds available (an overall ratio of 0.94 beds per stroke patient with a median stroke unit ratio per site of 1.0, up from 0.77 in 2004). The audit also focused on the presence of important structures and processes: the presence of staff with a specialist interest in stroke; routine involvement of carers in the rehabilitation process; coordinated multidisciplinary team care incorporating meetings at least once per week; information provided to patients and carers and regular programmes of education and training. Year by year there has been steady improvement in the proportion of stroke units featuring these key elements; however, implementation is far from universal and some concerns remain about the adequacy of resources and expertise.[4]

The EROS Study

This study set up concurrent population-based stroke registers in six different European study centres (in UK, France, Spain, Italy, Lithuania, and Poland)[5] using standardised methods of data collection and inclusion criteria with overlapping sources of notification. The registers gathered data on all patients of all ages with first ever strokes in the defined populations (with an overall total of 1,087,048 inhabitants) for a minimum period of two years. This allowed the adjusted incidence rates to be compared and for data on the patients' risk factors and management to be gathered and analysed as part of the study.[37]

In addition to the data from the registers, information on the structures and processes of care was gathered by an international, multidisciplinary team of stroke experts carrying out visits to each site over a period of a few days. They administered a quality assessment questionnaire which was largely evidence-based and drawn on structures and processes identified from a comprehensive literature review and the available clinical guidelines. It aimed to cover a broad spectrum of stroke care, including acute hospital care and discharge into the community and long-term follow-up.

The basic structure of the tool began with the Royal College of Physicians' (London) audit tool (see above) which was supplemented with additional questions used in a previous study of stroke in Europe (BIOMED II)[38] in order to gain a broader perspective of the non-UK healthcare systems.

The key recommendations from the evidence base and guidelines were collated and allocated to 11 different domains covering the whole patient pathway: specialist stroke services, management protocols, the multidisciplinary team, carers and family, acute specific medical diagnosis, acute medical and surgical interventions, early disability assessment and management, rehabilitation interventions, transfer back to the community, long-term management, supplementary questions (various non-clinical topics).

There was a wide range in access to stroke unit care between the centres (from 0% of patients to > 80% patients through a stroke unit) and major differences between units in terms of the care provided.[35] This diversity was even more marked during the rehabilitation and later phases of the patient journey. It is not yet known to what extent this diversity of care influences patient outcomes.

How Best to Assess Quality?

Previous chapters have discussed some of the broad differences in clinical stroke outcomes that appear internationally. We need to be cautious when making such comparisons[39] due to heterogeneity in methods used to describe outcomes and processes of care, and there may be obvious reasons for some of these differences in outcome, such as variations in the incidence of stroke or the prevalence of risk factors.[37,40–43] Another possible explanation is variation in healthcare provision. Unfortunately, direct comparison of stroke care across international boundaries is complex due to the national context in which each service operates, e.g. healthcare economy, medical specialties providing stroke care, type of stroke unit, coverage and equity of access and access to other services.

One recent cross-sectional study attempted to examine provision of stroke care in Europe.[33] They selected a random sample of hospitals in Europe that treated patients with stroke and applied a postal questionnaire available in several languages, containing items based on expert consensus statements.[44] This survey indicated limited implementation of stroke unit facilities and limited access to broader stroke services and facilities. Although this self-report study raised some important issues, it was limited to the acute phase of treatment and on structures and processes around the medical management of patients with stroke. The longer patient journey and non-medical aspects of stroke care were not fully covered.

Many of these areas were addressed in the EROS study which largely drew items on its quality assessment questionnaire from the available evidence base and a comprehensive literature review. Its scope went beyond acute medical management of stroke, attempting to cover a broad spectrum of stroke care including acute hospital care and discharge into the community as well as long-term follow-up. The questionnaire was largely conducted in English language with informal translation where necessary. The focus was on the service delivery rather than individual patient journeys, attempting to gain a picture of care for the majority of patients with stroke.[36]

Findings from this cross-sectional study of quality of stroke care were triangulated with direct observational studies using recognised behavioural mapping methods to record aspects of stroke care on a number of the sites.[45] Both these observational studies showed a diversity of stroke care across the study centres; however, there are limitations in each study and further development of assessment tools is required in order to provide practical, valid measures of stroke care quality that might be delivered in future studies.

Practical Implementation of Stroke Policy and Strategy

In this section, we consider factors that may influence service planners and managers when delivering, or planning to deliver stroke services, namely the evidence, patient needs, the available resources, the healthcare system and the views of service users.

The evidence: Ideally we would like to be able to provide any healthcare intervention that has a sound evidence base (e.g. meta-analyses and large randomised clinical trials in populations that reflect those to be served). Despite the evidence outlined above, the number of organised stroke unit trials is still relatively small and interpreting and generalising the results can be difficult. This may lead to some variation in interpretation of the results and implementation in local populations.

The needs of different patient groups: although the majority of patients need a common basic service, a small number may have particular requirements for more specialised components of care. The prevalence of these cases and the availability of alternative service providers may influence decisions on resource allocation.

Stroke unit care should be offered to all patients with stroke, from those with mild disability to those with severe strokes, as even patients with the most severe strokes have been shown to derive significant benefit from stroke unit care.[22]

The availability of resources: With the evidence supporting organisation of stroke units rather than provision of care on general medical wards or by alternative methods, restructuring and reorganising existing resources is likely to contribute to resources required for new services.

The total number of stroke unit beds available should reflect the local stroke incidence and hospital activity. The service is likely to experience fluctuations in stroke patient numbers, stroke severity, length of hospital stay and gender mix and systems should allow flexibility to accommodate demand.

Stroke units require a core multidisciplinary team with medical, nursing, physiotherapy, occupational therapy, speech and language therapy and social work input, though other professionals may be involved in the management of some stroke patients.[9,46]

It can be argued that the available evidence does not advocate a change in the total number of patients being treated in hospital, and that length of hospital stay is not significantly increased in the organised stroke unit trials.[3] Therefore, all that is required is a reorganisation and reconfiguration of existing hospital beds and training of staff to allow care of all stroke patients in a stroke unit.

The local healthcare culture and economy: The existing method of healthcare delivery, funding or reimbursement (e.g. in insurance-led systems) will influence the decisions about service design and provision.

Views of patients and families about how services might be delivered: There is increasing emphasis placed on the views of service users and public consultation in planning of healthcare, encouraged in many settings by service planners (e.g. Department of Health in UK[47]), patient groups and bodies representing the interests of patients. There are however a number of questions around the definition and benefits of user involvement and the methods by which it might be evaluated.[48]

Establishing a Stroke Unit

The key questions outlined in Table 3 may act as a practical starting point for those charged with developing stroke unit care or maintaining and improving quality.

Where does Stroke Unit Research Go Next?

Four key areas have been identified for future work relating to stroke unit research (and development): the search for new interventions, defining and measuring what we should be doing and extending the available knowledge into areas of need.

Table 3. Key issues for those setting up and maintaining stroke unit services

---

- What are the needs of the population?
- Is the available stroke research evidence applicable to the setting?
- Which model of organised stroke unit care would best serve the needs of the local population given the resources available?
- What are the barriers to all patients with stroke receiving appropriate care.
- How are quality criteria defined and measured?
- What systems exist to allow monitoring of activity and outcomes, e.g. clinical audit?
- How can the importance of stroke care be highlighted and maintained on the healthcare agenda?

Define Better What We Should be Doing

We need to further examine the elements of the stroke unit care in order to identify which are the most effective components and to maximise benefit by adjusting these components, e.g. staffing levels or contact time spent by patients with different aspects of the care. For example, one of the recognised stroke unit effects appears to be a reduction in the risk of death mediated through the prevention and treatment of complications, in particular infections.[49] This supports the idea of studying interventions around the prevention and management of recognised complications. Similar gains in information may arise from detailed study and comparison of current organised stroke unit practices (e.g. refs. 50 and 51).

Further development and research might centre around the development of professional roles within the multidisciplinary team, e.g. development of stroke specialist nurses,[52] different staffing levels or patterns of care delivery. The level of skill and the training required by stroke unit staff and how this should best be delivered also need to be explored.

Although in the introduction section we said the focus of this chapter would be on the majority of stroke patients, we recognise that there is scope to look at the management of individuals with particular needs outwith those of the majority, e.g. stroke in the very young people and children, and other individuals who are likely to have different specific service needs.

Measure Better What We Should be Doing

Linked with our understanding of the content of organised stroke unit care is the question of how we best measure quality. Some studies and audit programmes have started to develop stroke specific quality measures, although these may not focus exclusively on the stroke unit element of stroke care. Any measures that are used should have established measurement properties, i.e. they should be valid, reliable, relevant, practical, sensitive, and communicable.[6] Carrying out careful cost effectiveness studies examining stroke unit care in a variety of settings may also prove important in assisting implementation.[26]

The benefits of repeated cycles of audit can be seen from the example of the UK National Sentinel Stroke Audit carried out by the Royal College of Physicians, where year by year there has been steady improvement in access to organised stroke unit care in the greater part of those areas audited. However, such large projects require commitment to maintain the regular monitoring in order to sustain improvements. There may be specific challenges to implementation in areas which are slow to adopt organised stroke unit strategies and little evidence to guide the process of implementation around the use of incentives to ensure evidence is put into practice, e.g. policies around payments or penalties.

Develop New Interventions

New interventions need to be developed and tested, requiring a body of skilled researchers with the capacity to carry out high quality studies. Two good examples of interventions arising out of stroke unit care are early mobilisation and physiological monitoring. The very early rehabilitation trial (AVERT) is an international phase III multicentre RCT of early mobilisation[53] which is developed from the recognition of the importance of early mobilisation in stroke units.[54] It is specifically looking at the effects of mobilisation within the first 48 hours of hospital admission involving therapy and nursing staff to deliver the intervention. A variety of outcome measures will be collected at follow-up as well as monitoring for potential complications or risks associated with the intervention. The other example is a small scale trial of intensive physiological monitoring of patients[55] examining the effect of regular monitoring for treatable complications and early intervention to treat these when they arise. Both these studies have been carefully designed and conducted and have formed the basis of further research or may contribute useful data to future meta-analyses. Further areas of study include nursing procedures, prevention of complications and carer involvement.

Extend into More Resource Limited Settings

Taking a wider perspective, there also remains the challenge of stroke service delivery in developing countries, where different models may need to be adopted and evaluated in order to meet the challenge of changing disease and population profiles.[56] The risk factors and patterns of disease in the low to middle income countries appears to be similar to other regions and the burden of stroke is likely to be significant. The challenges of implementing organised healthcare in these countries may not be unique to stroke. However, implementation of organised stroke care adapted to local needs and practice should be developed urgently.[56,57]

In many respects it is artificial to consider stroke unit research in isolation from the other components of stroke care. Although to some extent, this is what happened in the past, when enthusiasm for stroke care and its research was initiated in stroke units and subsequently spread to other areas along the stroke care pathway.) Obtaining evidence for delivery of care in the community setting after stroke unit care continues to be challenging.[58] However, some of the shift in resources from acute centres like hospitals to community-based centres may facilitate increased research in the community setting.

Conclusion

In conclusion, the evidence base supporting the provision of organised inpatient (stroke unit) care is well established as the most widely applicable effective intervention after stroke and the only one to significantly reduce case fatality.

Though our understanding of the complex nature of organised care remains incomplete, a number of elements of organised stroke unit care have been identified from the clinical trials. The evidence base continues to evolve with examples available of the variety of complimentary research methods such as experimental designs to test effectiveness, meta-analysis to guide decisions on the available evidence, economic analyses to assess economic implications and observational studies and audit to help guide implementation strategies.

Although there are encouraging examples of stroke unit provision, there remains many challenges ahead in implementation of these findings into a variety of settings before stroke unit care is universally available as routine care. Future stroke unit research needs to better define and refine the stroke unit model and the constituent elements of the model need to be explored. Along with this we need to develop methods with which to measure the provision of high quality stroke care, allowing comparisons within and across national boundaries. These might provide new insights into the nature of stroke care provision and differences in outcomes. While this chapter concentrated on stroke units, there is also a need to broaden the research focus from acute care to include community provision and long-term challenges facing those with stroke and their carers. Beyond our national boundaries lies the challenge of global provision of effective stroke care to areas facing significant resource limitation and potentially considerable burden from stroke disease. Until we receive the results of such research, clinicians and service planners should direct efforts towards ensuring that the key basic systems of stroke unit care, whose benefit has been clearly demonstrated, are implemented with as many patients with stroke as possible.

References

1. Langhorne P, Williams B, Gilchrist W, Howie K. Do stroke units save lives? *Lancet* 1993; 342: 395–398.
2. Gilligan A, Thrift A, Sturm J, Dewey H, Macdonell R, Donnan G. Stroke units, tissue plasminogen activator, aspirin and neuroprotection: which stroke intervention could provide the greatest community benefit? *Cerebrovasc Dis* 2005; 20: 239–244.
3. Stroke Unit Trialists' Collaboration overview of stroke unit effectiveness Stroke Unit Trialists' Collaboration. Organised inpatient (stroke unit) care for stroke. *Cochrane Database Syst Rev* 2007, Issue 4. Art. No.: CD000197. DOI: 10.1002/14651858.CD000197.pub2.

4. Rudd AG, Hoffman A, Irwin P *et al*. Stroke units: research and reality. Results from the National Sentinel Audit of Stroke. *Qual Saf Health Care* 2005; 14: 7–12.

5. European Registers of Stroke (EROS) [Online]. 2009 [cited 2009 March 1]. Available from: URL: http://phs.kcl.ac.uk/eros/default.htm.

6. Warlow CP, van Gijn J, Dennis MS, Wardlaw J, Bamford JM, Hankey GJ, *et al*. *Stroke: A Practical Guide to Management*. 3rd Edn. Oxford: Blackwell Science; 2007.

7. Langhorne P, Dey P, Woodman M, Kalra L, Wood-Dauphinee S, Patel N, *et al*. Is stroke care portable? A systematic review of the clinical trials. *Age Ageing* 2005; 34: 324–330.

8. Langhorne P, Taylor G, Murray G, Dennis M, Anderson C, Bautz-Holter E *et al*. Early supported discharge services for stroke patients: a meta-analysis of individual patients' data. *Lancet* 2005; 365: 501–506.

9. Langhorne P, Pollock A, in collaboration with the Stoke Unit Trialists' Collaboration. What are the components of effective stroke unit care? *Age Ageing* 2002; 31: 365–371.

10. The CLOTS Trials Collaboration. Effectiveness of thigh-length graduated compression stockings to reduce the risk of deep vein thrombosis after stroke (CLOTS trial 1): a multicentre, randomised controlled trial. Lancet 2009; 373: 1958–1965.

11. Indredavik B, Bakke F, Slørdahl SA, Rokseth R, Håheim LL. Stroke unit treatment improves long-term quality of life: a randomized controlled trial. *Stroke* 1998; 29: 895–899.

12. Evans A, Perez I, Harraf F, Melbourn A, Steadman J, Donaldson N *et al*. Can differences in management processes explain different outcomes between stroke unit and stroke team care? *Lancet* 2001; 358: 1586–1591.

13. Langhorne P, Li Pak Tong, Stott DJ. Association between physiological homeostasis and early recovery after stroke. *Stroke* 1999; 30: 2526–2527.

14. Indredavik B, Bakke F, Slørdahl SA, Rokseth R, Håheim LL. Treatment in a combined acute and rehabilitation stroke unit: which aspects are most important? *Stroke* 1999; 30: 917–923.

15. Jørgensen HS, Reith J, Nakayama H, Kammersgaard LP, Houth JG, Raaschou HO *et al*. Potentially reversible factors during the very acute phase of stroke and their impact on prognosis: is there a large therapeutic potential to be explored? *Cerebrovascular Dis* 2001; 11: 207–211.

16. Intercollegiate Stroke Working Party. *National Sentinel Stroke Audit Phase I Organizational Audit 2008.* Clinical Effectiveness and Evaluation Unit Royal College of Physicians, London; 2009.

17. Scottish Intercollegiate Guidelines Network (SIGN), Management of patients with Stroke: Rehabilitation, Prevention and Management of Complications, and Discharge Planning (SIGN 64) (updated 2006) Edinburgh, UK; 2006.

18. Intercollegiate Stroke Working Party. National Clinical Guideline for Stroke. 3rd Edn. Royal College of Physicians, London, UK; 2008.

19. European Stroke Organisation (ESO) Executive Committee and the ESO writing committee. Guidelines for management of ischaemic stroke and transient ischaemic attack 2008. *Cerbrovasc Dis* 2008; 25: 457–507.

20. Kjellstrom T, Norrving B, Shatchkute A. Helsingborg Declaration 2006 on European Stroke Strategies. *Cerebrovasc Dis* 2007; 23: 229–241.

21. Stroke Unit Trialists' Collaboration. Organised inpatient (stroke unit) care for stroke. *Cochrane Database Syst Rev* 1997.

22. Langhorne P, for Stroke Unit Trialist Collaboration. The effect of organized inpatient (stroke unit) care on death after stroke. *Cerebrovasc Dis* 2005; 19: (Suppl 2).

23. Fjaertoft H, Indredavik B, Magnussen J, Johnsen R. Early supported discharge for stroke patients improves clinical outcome. Does it also reduce use of health services and costs? *Cerebrovasc Dis* 2005; 19: 376–383.

24. Saka O, Serra V, Samyshkin Y, McGuire A, Wolfe C. Cost-effectiveness of stroke unit care followed by early supported discharge. *Stroke* 2009; 40: 24–29.

25. Patel M, McKevitt C, Lawrence E, Rudd A, Wolfe C. Clinical determinants of long-term quality of life after stroke. *Age Ageing* 2007; 36: 316–322.

26. Indredavik B. Stroke unit care is beneficial both for the patient and for the health service and should be widely implemented. *Stroke* 2009; 40: 1–2.

27. Black N. Why we need observational studies to evaluate the effectiveness of health care. *BMJ* 1996; 312: 1215–1218.

28. Asplund K, Asberg K, Norving B, Stegmayr B, Terent A, Wester P-O for the Riks-Stroke Collaboration. Riks-Stroke — a Swedish National quality register for stroke care. *Cerebrovasc Dis* 2003; 15(Suppl 1): 5–7.

29. Cadilhac D, Pearce D, Levi C, Donnan G, on behalf of Metropolitan Clinical Taskforce and New South Wales Stroke Services Coordinating Committee. Improvements in the quality of care and health outcomes with new stroke

care units following implementation of a clinician led, health system redesign programme in New South Wales, Australia. *Qual Saf Health Care* 2008; 17: 329–333.

30. Seenan P, Long M, Langhorne P. Stroke Units in their natural habitat. Systematic review of observational studies. *Stroke* 2007; 38: 1886–1892.

31. Kidwell C, Shephard T, Ton S, Lawyers B, Murdock M, Koroshetz W *et al.* Establishment of primary stroke centres. A survey of physicians' attitudes and hospital resources. *Neurology* 2003; 60: 452–456.

32. Kapral M, Laupacis A, Phillips S, Silver F, Hill M, Fang J *et al.* for the Investigators of the registry of the Canadian Stroke Network. *Stroke* 2004; 35: 1756–1762.

33. Kaste M, Boysen G, Indredavik B, Norving B. Stroke unit care in Scandinavian countries. *Int J Stroke* 2006; 1: 44.

34. Langhorne P, Dennis M. Stroke units: the next 10 years. *Lancet* 2005; 363: 834–835.

35. Leys D, Ringlestein B, Kaste M, Hacke W for the Executive Committee of the European Stroke Initiative. Facilities available in European hospitals treating stroke. *Stroke* 2007; 38: 2985–2991.

36. Wellwood I, Wu O, Langhorne P, Sayed I, Wolfe C. European Registers of Stroke (EROS) Project: developing measures to estimate quality of stroke care across Europe. *Cerebrovascular Dis* 2009; 27(Suppl 6): 234.

37. European Registers of Stroke (EROS) Investigators. Incidence of stroke in Europe in the 21st Century. *Stroke* 2009; 40: 1557–1563.

38. Bhalla A, Grieve R, Tilling K, Rudd AG, Wolfe CD. BIOMED II European Study of Stroke Care. Older stroke patients in Europe: stroke care and determinants of outcome. *Age Ageing* 2004 Nov; 33(6): 618–624.

39. Walsh K, Gompertz P, Rudd A. Stroke care: how do we measure quality? *Postgrad Med J* 2002; 79: 322–326.

40. Wolfe C, Giroud M, Kolominsky-Rabas P, Dundas R, Lemesle M, Heuschmann P *et al.* for the European Registries of Stroke (EROS) Collaboration. Variations in stroke incidence and survival in 3 areas of Europe. *Stroke* 2000; 31: 2074–2079.

41. Giroud M, Czlonkowska A, Ryglewicz D, Wolfe C. The problem of interpreting variations in health status (morbidity and mortality) in Europe. *Stroke Services, Policy and Practice across Europe.* Wolfe C, McKevitt Rudd A (Eds.). Abingdon, UK: Radcliffe Medical Press; 2002.

42. Wolfe C, Tilling K, Rudd A, Giroud M, Inzitari D. Variations in care and outcome in the first year after stroke: a Western and Central European perspective. *J Neurol Neurosurg Psychiatry* 2004; 75: 1702–1706.

43. Wolfe C, Smeeton C, Coshall C, Tilling K, Rudd A. Survival differences after stroke in a multiethnic population: follow-up study with the south London stroke register. *BMJ* 2005; 331: 431.

44. Leys D, Ringlestein B, Kaste M, Hacke W for the Executive Committee of the European Stroke Initiative. The main components of stroke unit care: results of a European expert survey. *Stroke* 2007; 23: 344–352.

45. Wellwood I, Langhorne P, McKevitt C, Bernhardt J, Rudd A, Wolfe C on behalf of the European Registers of Stroke (EROS) collaborative group. An observational study of acute stroke in four countries: The European Registers of Stroke (EROS) Study. *Cerebrovasc Dis* 2009; 28: 171–176.

46. Dewey H, Sherry L, Collier J. Stroke rehabilitation 2007: what should it be? *Int J Stroke* 2007; 2: 191–200.

47. Department of Health. Creating a patient-led NHS. [Online]. 2005 [cited 2009 March 1]. Available from: www.dh.gov.uk/assetRoot/04/10/65/07/041 06507.pdf.

48. Fudge N, Wolfe C, McKevitt C. Assessing the promise of user involvement in health service development: ethnographic study. *BMJ* 2008; 336: 313–317.

49. Govan L, Langhorne P, Weir C, for the Stroke Unit Trialists' Collaboration. Does the prevention of complications explain the survival benefit of organized inpatient (Stroke Unit) Care? *Stroke* 2007; 38: 2536–2540.

50. De Wit L, Putman K, Lincoln N, Baert I, Berman P, Beyens H *et al.* Stroke rehabilitation in Europe. What do physiotherapists and occupational therapists actually do? *Stroke* 2006; 37: 1483–1489.

51. Bernhardt J, Chitravas N, Meslo IL, Thrift A, Indredavik B. Not all stroke units are the same. A comparison of physical activity patterns in Melbourne, Australia, and Trondheim, Norway. *Stroke* 2008; 39: 2059–2065.

52. Cadilhac D. How should stroke services be organized? *Lancet Neurol* 2002; 1: 63–64.

53. Bernhardt J, Dewey HM, Thrift AG, Collier J, Donnan G. A very early rehabilitation trial for stroke (AVERT): phase II safety and feasibility. *Stroke* 2008; 39: 390–396.

54. Indredavik B, Bakke F, Solberg R, Rokseth R, Haahein LL, Holme I. Benefit of a stroke rehabilitation unit: a randomized controlled trial. *Stroke* 1991; 22: 1026–1031.

55. Sulter G, Elting J, Langedijk M, Maurits N, De Keyser J. Admitting acute ischaemic stroke patients to a stroke care monitoring unit versus a conventional stroke unit: a randomized pilot study. *Stroke* 2003; 34: 101–104.

56. Norving B, Adams R. Organized stroke care. *Stroke* 2006; 37: 326–328.

57. Langhorne P, Sandercock P, Prasad K. Evidence-based practice for stroke. *Lancet Neurol* 2009; 8: 308–309.

58. Outpatient Service Trialists. Therapy-based rehabilitation services for stroke patients at home. *Cochrane Database Syst Rev* 2003, Issue 1. Art. No.: CD002925. DOI: 10.1002/14651858.CD002925.

8 Stroke Rehabilitation

Lalit Kalra* and Ruth Harris[†]

Chapter Summary

The human brain is capable of significant recovery after stroke. It is now clear that multiple circuits in the brain can serve similar functions and the paradigm has shifted from strict cerebral localisation of function to that of cortical plasticity, whereby unaffected areas in the brain can take over the function of areas affected by stroke. Recent research has also shown that neurogenesis plays a key role in recovery and newly generated nerve cells form synaptic contacts which become fully integrated into existing neuronal circuitry. Furthermore, animal experiments suggest that this process can be harnessed by therapy or pharmaceutical interventions to enhance and hasten functional improvements after stroke. Thus, the human brain is capable of significant recovery after stroke, provided that the appropriate treatments and stimuli are applied in adequate amounts and at the right time.

There is consensus that well-organised and well-planned rehabilitation guided by well-defined goals based on adequate assessment and sensitive negotiation with patients and caregivers reduces disability and long-term institutionalisation. A pragmatic functional approach individualised to each

*Professor of Stroke Medicine, Academic Neuroscience Centre, King's College London
[†]Reader Faculty of Health and Social Care Sciences, Kingston University and St. George's, University of London

patient's needs with early, intensive interventions has been recommended and shown to speed recovery in clinical trials. Of the newer approaches, available evidence would favour interventions such as constraint induced movement therapy and motor imagery. Regardless of impairment or techniques, greatest improvements is seen with high-intensity and repetitive task-specific interventions. There is evidence suggesting that early intervention by therapists may speed recovery and hasten discharge from the hospital without increasing the total amount of therapeutic input.

Multidisciplinary team work is considered to be the gold standard for delivering specialist rehabilitation. The characteristics and dynamics of the multidisciplinary team are central to delivery cost-effective quality care. Finally, the chapter discusses some of the challenges facing stroke rehabilitation in a global context.

Introduction

Stroke rehabilitation is based on the concepts of neuroplasticity and reorganisation of cerebral structure and activity after injury. The validity of these long-help theoretical concepts has been reinforced by findings in experimental models of stroke in animals as well as by neuroimaging studies using magnetic resonance (MR) and positron emission tomography (PET) techniques in humans. These studies have also shown the diversity and complexity of reorganisation patterns, suggesting that the process of reorganisation is dynamic and dependent upon the nature of injury, substrates involved and the duration since the initial insult. Hyperacute imaging studies have shown that early rapid recovery of function corresponds with successful reperfusion of the ischaemic penumbra, suggesting that successful thrombolysis and optimisation of collateral flow may be the first step for successful rehabilitation.[1] Despite the proven efficacy of thrombolysis, limitations on its use imposed by strict therapeutic time windows means that it will have only a modest impact on eventual outcome in the vast majority of stroke patients.[2] Early and planned multidisciplinary rehabilitation remains the cornerstone of stroke management because it is applicable to most stroke survivors. Furthermore, 300 randomised controlled trials provide a sound foundation for evidence-based practice in stroke rehabilitation, supplementing and often confirming decades of clinical experience.

Recovery from Stroke

Recovery is of two types; intrinsic, which involves neuronal regeneration and setting up of new axonal connections, and adaptive, in which alternative strategies, usually behavioural changes, are used to overcome disability.[3] The majority of patients show both intrinsic and adaptive recovery, the proportion of each being dependent upon factors such as age, the severity of stroke, cognitive abilities and rehabilitation input after stroke. Intrinsic mechanisms consists of restitution, which include repair of partially damaged pathways and strengthening of existing pathways. These processes are mediated by local changes in blood flow, growth factor release and changes in metabolite or neurotransmitter concentrations, which induce neurogenesis and cell migration. Diaschisis or substitution is the development of new, but functionally related pathways in the unaffected areas of brain to take over the lost function. The degree of recovery due to intrinsic mechanisms is variable and may be incomplete in a significant number of patients. In these circumstances, adaptive recovery that involves re-education in compensatory techniques with specialist input becomes important. These techniques usually involve behavioural adaptations to improve function and reduce the level of disability posed by the impairment, either by changed use of the affected side or retraining of the unaffected side.

New evidence suggests that neurogenesis represents a key factor in plasticity of the normal brain in response to environmental stimuli, and that newly generated nerve cells form synaptic connections which become fully integrated into existing neuronal circuitry.[4] Emerging evidence from animal experiments and autopsy studies shows that these processes play a key role in stroke recovery with evidence of increased neurogenesis and neural progenitor cell migration following acute ischaemic injury to the brain.[5] Stroke-induced neurogenesis takes place in the subventricular zone and ischaemic boundary of adult human brains and has been demonstrated even in elderly patients up to 90 years of age.[6] Increased neurogenesis must be coupled with a strategy that permits recruitment of these 'repair' cells to the site of injury.[5] Ischaemic injury to the brain sets up orchestrated

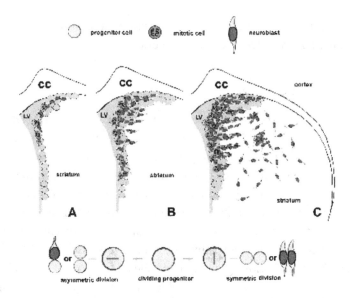

Figure 1. Neurogenesis after focal cerebral ischaemia. (A) Neural progenitor cells (NPC) in the subventricular zone. (B) Ischaemia increases division of NPC and neuroblasts migrate toward ischaemic striatum in a chain-like structure. (C) When migrating neuroblasts reach the ischaemic boundary, they form clusters and later disperse. Reproduced with permission from Zhang RL, Zhang ZG, Chopp M. Neurogenesis in the adult ischaemic brain: generation, migration, survival, and restorative therapy. *Neuroscientist* 2005; 11(5): 408–416.

waves of cellular and molecular events characterised by a reduction in growth-inhibitory molecules and activation of growth-promoting genes by neurons (Fig. 1).

Vascular endothelial growth factor (VEGF) and stromal derived factor (SDF-1) are transcriptionally regulated by hypoxia via the transcriptional activator, hypoxia inducible factor (HIF-1).[7] Angiogenesis is regulated by VEGF and appears to be the first step in regeneration. SDF-1 is also released by regenerating blood vessels and provides a source of chemotactic growth factor to facilitate survival and migration of neural progenitors. Chemokine receptor-4 is a receptor on progenitor cells that when bound with a gradient of stromal derived factor (SDF-1), facilitates homing of progenitors to injury sites. These events interact with other cells such as the astrocytes and oligodendrocytes and other growth factors, creating a microenvironment which promotes neurite outgrowth that repair damaged connections or establish new signalling pathways.[7]

PET and MR studies have helped to demonstrate the processes of reorganisation of neural activity after stroke in human subjects. These studies have shown that motor recovery in stroke patients is associated with activation in the peri-infarct cortex and supplementary areas of the affected side and also in additional regions including the ipsilateral sensorimotor and premotor cortex.[3] The cerebellum, thalamus and prefrontal areas play an important part in restoration of function. The process of reorganisation is dynamic, there is an evolution of changes with time and several different patterns have been described. These include activation of bilateral cerebellar and prefrontal areas, an initial increase followed by a decrease in activation of motor areas and progression from early contralesion activity to late ipsilateral activity.[3] Recent studies in acute recovery have also shown that the integrity of the corticospinal tract system is critical for motor recovery within the first four weeks of stroke, irrespective of involvement of the somatosensory system, providing a physiological explanation for the clinical observation of slower recovery in older people and those with underlying white matter disease.[8]

Another important emerging concept is that of 'mirror neurons' which discharge during the execution of various hand-directed actions and during the observation of the same actions performed by other individuals.[9] The mirror neuron system was first identified in the ventral premotor cortex and the inferior parietal lobule in monkeys, but a similar mirror neuron system has now been identified in humans. This system has also been shown to extend to mouth, and foot-directed actions. Recent studies have shown that this system performs an important role in action understanding, imitation learning of novel complex actions, and internal rehearsal of actions.[10] These studies support the use of motor imagery as a novel approach for the treatment of stroke patients with motor impairments. As interventions through the mirror neuron system may offer an alternate access to motor networks independent of the affected primary motor cortex, motor imagery based interventions may prove particularly beneficial in patients in whom active movement therapies cannot be undertaken.

It is now clear that there are multiple motor circuits in the brain which serve similar functions. Conventional pathways dominate in healthy subjects and inhibit the activity of alternate pathways in other areas of the brain. Disruption of traditional pathways in cerebral ischaemia reduces or eliminates the inhibition normally exerted by these pathways and allows activation of alternate pathways in the premotor areas of the affected side and primary motor areas on the unaffected side.[11] Hence, the paradigm for function has shifted from strict cerebral localisation to that of interactive functioning of diverse cortical areas activated by the constantly changing balance of inhibitory and excitatory impulses.

To summarise, research shows that the human brain is capable of significant recovery after stroke, provided that the appropriate treatments and stimuli are applied in adequate amounts and at the right time. Furthermore, advances in understanding the biology of injury and repair suggest that neurogenesis may be important in stroke recovery and that this process can be harnessed to enhance and hasten functional improvements after stroke. Hence, the stage is set for the focus of rehabilitation broaden from the traditional methods to enhance recovery employed at present to incorporating new innovative strategies that are firmly rooted in the neuroscience of recovery.

Facilitating Recovery from Stroke

The basis of all stroke rehabilitation is the expectation that patients will improve with spontaneous recovery, learning and practice. Plasticity is an important concept in rehabilitation, which implies that it is possible to modulate or facilitate reorganisation of cerebral processes by external inputs. Reorganisation in the brain occurs by recovery and learning but improves significantly in both with practice and increased intensity of therapy inputs. Motor learning mechanisms are operative during spontaneous stroke recovery and interact with rehabilitative training. Studies have shown significant increases in the size and activation of representative cortical motor areas following either constraint therapy or intensive treatment to the affected limb.[12] Absence of adequate external inputs may have a negative effect — primate studies have shown that lack of afferent stimulation, e.g. physical restraint of affected limb in squirrel monkeys

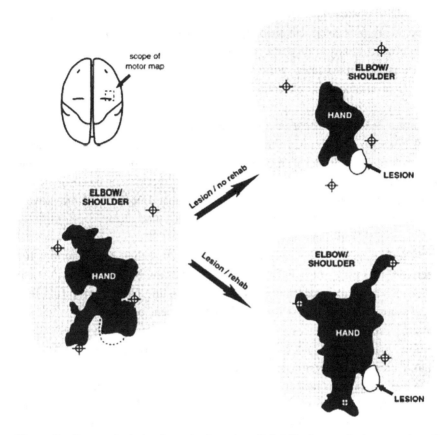

Figure 2. Post-stroke lesion in squirrel monkey. Rehabilitation results in expansion of hand representation on the cortex; no rehabilitation results in contraction. Reprinted with permission from AAAS.[13]

following experimental stroke, impedes recovery in function after induced ischaemic injury to the brain (Fig. 2).[13]

A progressive down-regulation of sensorimotor function with inactivity has also been demonstrated in stroke patients, which is reversed by training.[14] Cerebral activity in response to passive movements was reduced significantly in stroke patients and this activation decreased even further with time in the absence of any rehabilitative activity. On the other hand, daily training for four weeks with repetitive passive and active arm movements increased cortical activation significantly. It may also be possible to up-regulate sensorimotor activation by using the conditioning effects of increased proprioceptive inflow.[15] Repetitive peripheral magnetic stimulation of paralysed muscles that resulted in painless contractions was associated with significantly increased activation of the parieto-premotor network in the affected hemisphere, improved kinematics of finger movements and reduced spasticity after stroke.[15] Retention of motor learning is best accomplished with variable training schedules and, for optimal results, rehabilitation techniques need to be geared towards patients' specific motor deficits.[16] Several promising new rehabilitation approaches have been developed on theories of motor learning and include impairment oriented-training, constraint-induced movement therapy, electromyogram-triggered neuromuscular stimulation, robotic interactive therapy and virtual reality.

Predicting when a stroke patient has reached their full potential for recovery and may not benefit from further therapy inputs is an imprecise science. The traditional view is that recovery is the fastest in the first few weeks after stroke, with a further 5 to 10 percent occurring between six months and one year. About 30 percent of survivors are independent within three weeks, and by six months this proportion rises to 50 percent.[17] Late neurophysiologic recovery can continue for several years but is at a much slower rate and seldom results in dramatic changes in overall functional ability.[18] This view has been challenged by a recent meta-analysis of functional imaging studies, as intervention effects in stroke rehabilitation has shown that cortical reorganisation and clinical improvements occurred even late after injury and after subjects were deemed to have reached a recovery plateau; recovery was significantly influenced by the type of intervention given.[19]

Estimation of the functional capacity for recovery is particularly important for chronic stroke patients (more than one year after stroke), especially as these are the patients most likely to be denied further rehabilitation inputs. Unfortunately, imaging and electrophysiological techniques to aid such predictions have generally proven to be expensive and unhelpful in clinical practice. However, it may be possible to combine these modalities to develop algorithms for patient selection for both research and clinical programmes. A recent example of this was the combined use of Transcranial Magnetic Stimulation (TMS) and MRI to determine the integrity of corticospinal tracts and predict functional recovery potential.[20] The study showed that motor evoked potentials to TMS in the affected limb in the presence of little or no asymmetry in fractional anisotropy map of the internal capsule on MRI (indicative of minimal long tract damage) was associated with a potential for improvement up to three years after stroke.

Selected Techniques to Facilitate Recovery

Enhancing post-stroke regeneration

Regenerative treatment approaches provide a novel intervention strategy that potentially has the capacity not only to modify disease pathology, but also to repair and reverse damage. Preclinical studies show that cell-based and pharmacological therapies can both enhance brain-repair processes substantially and improve functional recovery.[5] Cell-based therapies under investigation include use of bone marrow mesenchymal cells, cord blood cells, foetal cells, and embryonic cells. Pharmacological treatments of interest include already available growth factors such as erythropoietin and granulocyte colony stimulating factor, drugs such as sildenafil, statins, nicotinic acid, minocycline, cholinesterase inhibitors or fluoxetine and novel agents such as cannabinoid CB2 receptor agonists or retinoids. These agents are known to result in a three-fold or greater increase in neurogenesis in rodent models but their potential in humans is not known. Nevertheless, these are extremely attractive candidate of 'regenerative' therapies for stroke, which if proven in animal models can be rapidly progressed to clinical trials and translated into clinical practice.

Translating cellular or pharmacological regenerative treatments proven to be successful in animal models for human use presents several challenges.[5] Although the success of stem cell implantation in experimental studies offers exciting opportunities for stroke repair, safety issues, including tumour formation and immune rejection, as well as ethical and technical challenges have hampered progress of such treatments into clinical practice. Pharmacological treatments to modulate endogenous neurogenesis do not present the same ethical or technical challenges and many are known to be safe as they are already in human use for other indications with known safety or tolerability profiles.[21] Regardless of whether treatments are cellular or pharmacological, their benefit will be significantly modulated by the type and intensity of therapy input during rehabilitation, the environments that patients are treated in (e.g. better outcome on stroke rehabilitation units compared with non-specialist settings[22]) and differences in the home and social environments of patients. It is also likely that improvements in specific impairments using regenerative treatments may be difficult to detect using conventional outcome tools that assess global function or disability. An imaging approach based on non-invasive magnetic resonance studies, which focuses on the restructuring of white matter, angiogenesis, and neurogenesis or synaptic activity may be more appropriate to monitoring responses to regenerative treatments.[23]

Early mobilisation

Early mobilisation is a key rehabilitation strategy associated with good functional outcomes in several observational and controlled studies.[24] Unfortunately, despite several studies over the last 50 years, mobilisation protocols remain poorly defined and vary both with geography and the nature of the unit on which patients are being managed. A review which combined data from observational studies and meta-analyses over the last 55 years was not able to find any positive, unequivocal benefit associated with early mobilisation, independent of other aspects of stroke care.[25] The review concluded that although data were insufficient to prove the beneficial effects of early mobilisation after stroke, it was not harmful for most stroke patients. However, early neurological rehabilitation as part of routine stroke unit care appeared to contribute to good long-term outcome in stroke patients.

Restoration of motor function

Restoration of motor function is a primary objective of stroke rehabilitation and there are several pooled data analyses of studies on various strategies for improving motor performance in stroke patients.[26] A prospective meta-analysis of the effectiveness of bilateral movement training in post-stroke motor rehabilitation showed that bilateral movements alone or in combination with auxiliary sensory feedback were effective in improving functional and mobility outcomes in stroke patients.[27] On the other hand, bilateral standing with visual feedback therapy to improve postural control appears to have no significant benefits over conventional therapy for weight distribution and postural sway, balance and gait performance, and gait speed.[28]

Constraint induced movement therapy (CIMT) has been one of the most important and well-research therapeutic approaches to restoring motor function. CIMT is based on the assumption that immobilisation of the unaffected side to prevent learned 'non-use' and promote use of the affected limb results in faster (and more complete) recovery. The most convincing evidence for CIMT comes from the Extremity Constraint-Induced Therapy Evaluation (EXCITE) Trial.[29] The study showed that CIMT intervention in stroke patients was associated with statistically significant and clinically relevant improvements in arm motor function that persisted for at least one year. In fact, participants' force and torque generation qualities on a kinetic key turning task were similar to those of able-bodied controls. Despite this successful demonstration in a clinical trial, there continue to be doubts on the extent to which individualised CIMT is practical or cost-effective.[30] A meta-analysis has also suggested that recovery with CIMT is proportional to the amount of exercise given to the affected limb and it may be possible to achieve comparable benefits by less hazardous and less frustrating conventional therapy methods.[31]

Neuromuscular stimulation

There is evidence to support a role of peripheral neuromuscular electro-stimulation in stroke rehabilitation as these techniques appear to improve aspects of functional motor ability, motor impairment and normality of movement compared with no treatment, placebo or conventional physical therapy.[32] A review of the use of repetitive transcranial magnetic stimulation (rTMS) in patients with post-stroke motor deficit, visuospatial neglect, or aphasia showed that low frequency rTMS to restore inhibition applied over the unaffected hemisphere or high-frequency rTMS to reactivate hypoactive regions applied over the affected hemisphere were associated with functional recovery.[33] There was great variation regarding the number of rTMS sessions required for a sustained effect and the timing of rTMS application after stroke. In addition, rTMS used as adjuvant to constraint-induced therapy for upper-limb hemiparesis had little effect on motor learning in a group of stroke survivors over and above constraint-induced therapy.[34]

Motor imagery

Recent years have seen several small clinical studies exploring the concept of motor imagery in stroke rehabilitation.[35] All studies have been small and differ in patient characteristics, intervention protocol, and outcome measures. Most tasks involved mentally rehearsing movements of the arm but intervention periods varied from two to six weeks and frequencies ranged from multiple sessions per day to three times a week. The meta-analysis of these studies shows that mental practice has a positive effect on recovery of arm function and may have promising effect for improving leg function after stroke. The effects of motor imagery training appear even greater when combined with a conventional stroke rehabilitation programme in subacute stroke patients.[36]

Spatial neglect

Advanced imaging studies have also provided new insights into the rehabilitation of neglect, shifting the focus from spatial attentional deficits to the treatment of more generalised impairments in attention.[37] This is strengthened by a clinical study showing non-spatial attention training was associated with improvements in neglect, underpinned by changes in cortical activation patterns in areas known to be associated with attention.[38] The clinical implications are that it may be possible to overcome spatial neglect in stroke patients by interventions that improve generalised or sustained attention. The expectation is that these techniques may prove to be more effective and have a sustained effect compared with conventional spatially oriented methods which did not result in sustained improvements in neglect that could be transferred to functional tasks. It is less recognised that neglect may be associated with motor impairments. Many patients with neglect have directional hypokinesia and are slower to initiate a motor response to targets appearing in the left hemispace, even when using their unaffected arm. This has been attributed to relative depletion of dopamine in the nigrostriatal pathway on the same side of the lesion, which potentially may be amenable to intervention.[39] However, there are no studies to date using L-dopa administration as an intervention.

The Process of Rehabilitation

Rehabilitation in stroke is a multidisciplinary problem-solving process focusing on disability and intended to reduce handicap. Rehabilitation begins with documenting and measuring pre-morbid and stroke related impairments, disabilities, and handicaps using simple, valid scales. It is very important that the measures used are familiar to the wider multidisciplinary teams and can be used for communication with outside agencies. The objective of rehabilitation is to maximise independence and minimise learned dependency using a range of therapies, assistive aids and counselling. It is very important to adopt a holistic approach to patients that takes into account their physical and psychosocial background, support mechanisms and environment. Finally, rehabilitation is also about supporting care-givers and helping them to develop physical and psychological skills to provide long-term, sustainable support to stroke patients. Rehabilitation has four important components: assessment, planning, intervention, and evaluation.

Assessment

Assessment is fundamental to ascertaining the precise nature and severity of deficits and defining treatment goals prior to commencement of a rehabilitation programme. It provides a logical basis for treatment and management of stroke patients. The objectives of assessment are to:

- Define unique patient characteristics, the extent of disability, and the potential for recovery and/or responding to intervention (prognostication).

- Identify main areas of difficulty and their underlying causes as well as the expectations of the patient and the family (problem-solving).
- Assess the degree of recovery or residual disability at the end of the rehabilitation process (outcome)
- Monitor the process of rehabilitation (evaluation)

Planning

Planning of rehabilitation involves goal setting between patients, professionals and families. It is quite likely that initial goals will relate to basic personal activities of daily living such as achievement of sitting balance, independent transfers and independence in toileting activities. As patients progress, goals need to be set for higher levels of function that incorporate not only independence in household activities but also the ability to undertake social, leisure and occupational pursuits. It is important that planning takes into account not only the immediate needs of the patients but also their potential needs when they return to their own environment. This often involves adapting rehabilitation to the home setting and addressing the needs of caregivers, many of whom will play an important role in providing ongoing support and management of disability at home. Many of the difficulties ultimately faced in rehabilitation can be traced back to conflicts between the goals of patients and those of the multidisciplinary team. An essential function of the whole rehabilitation team is to identify and modify unrealistically high (and sometimes unjustifiably low) expectations of patients and their families by making them more aware of the nature of residual deficit and expected prognosis as soon as these are reasonably clear.

Intervention

The minimum requirement of any stroke intervention is to provide care necessary to maintain *status quo* and prevent deterioration of the patient's condition or functional ability due to poor management or complications. However, modern rehabilitation aims to achieve more than just that and is aimed at facilitating recovery by reducing impairment, minimising disability and preventing handicap. A major limitation in the translation of therapy research into clinical practice has been the validity and generalisability of the findings of intervention studies because of the small sample sizes, variability in subject selection and differences in interventions or outcome measures. Evidence from the bulk of clinical and functional imaging studies suggest that more intense therapy over a shorter period of time provides a better outcome compared with less intense treatment given over longer durations.[40] In addition to quantity, the quality of interventions is equally important. Evidence suggests that task-specific approaches, especially with stroke motor therapy, can be more efficacious than traditional approaches which focus on impairment.[40]

There is consensus that well-organised and well-planned rehabilitation guided by well-defined goals based on adequate assessment and sensitive negotiation with patients and caregivers reduces disability and long-term institutionalisation.[22] A large number of therapy interventions are used for motor recovery in stroke rehabilitation, depending upon the nature and severity of impairment, patient characteristics and the training, experience or preference of therapists. Although each technique has its supporters, the small size and methodological limitations of individual studies has limited agreement on benefit in clinical practice. Some of the emerging concepts and interventions based in the science of recovery have been reviewed earlier in this chapter. Overall, a pragmatic functional approach individualised for each patient's needs is recommended, and strict adherence to theories with little scientific basis or clinical evidence of effectiveness should be discouraged. Regardless of impairment or techniques, greatest improvement is seen with high-intensity and repetitive task-specific interventions. There is also evidence suggesting that early intervention by therapists may speed recovery and hasten discharge from the hospital without increasing the total amount of therapeutic input.

Evaluation

Evaluation is the process of monitoring a patient's progress (or lack of it) and assessing the effectiveness of the rehabilitation process itself. Objective assessment of effectiveness of stroke rehabilitation has proven difficult for several reasons. These include the confounding effect of spontaneous recovery from stroke, difficulty in defining the extent of need, and perceptions of good outcome, which may vary with the perspective of different observers. The wide variety of impairments and disabilities associated with stroke, as well as the large number of instruments available to measure each impairment and disability, have also contributed significantly to the lack of a common assessment for outcome in stroke rehabilitation. A sensible approach is to use simple assessments more frequently during the rehabilitation process to monitor and adjust the treatment programme.

There is little consensus on the most relevant outcome, the perception of a favourable outcome may vary depending upon professional, patient or carer perspectives and how long after stroke it is assessed. Although it has been recommended that outcomes should be measured at different levels within the World Health Organization International Classification of Impairments, Disabilities, and Handicaps (ICIDH) framework,[41] patients will value their ability to undertake desired activities or participate in social roles more than improvements in specific areas of performance. Even within the ICIDH framework, the rate and extent of change may vary between the different levels and continue over months. Consequently, it is important to consider the timing of any assessments and the influence of factors known to affect the chosen outcome measures. An overview of the ICIDH framework, the various scales used to measure recovery and the contextual factors that influence these measurements is given in Chapter 9.

Multidisciplinary Team Work

Multidisciplinary team work is considered to be the gold standard for delivering specialist rehabilitation to stroke patients being managed on specialist stroke rehabilitation units and by community teams. There is strong evidence that patients who receive care from multidisciplinary specialist teams in organised stroke units are more likely to be alive, independent and living at home one year after stroke.[42] Furthermore, early supported discharge by specialist multidisciplinary stroke teams is associated with improved patient outcome and satisfaction.[43] The work of the multidisciplinary team within these dedicated stroke services is considered to be an important contribution to positive outcomes.[44]

However, it is somewhat surprising that little is known about which aspects of the multidisciplinary team and team working influence patient outcome in stroke care and other healthcare services. Despite extensive literature defining and describing effective team work, there remains a lack of robust evidence of the impact of multidisciplinary team work on patient outcome and a continued need for applied research to inform the management and development of healthcare teams.[45] There is also a lack of literature that explores the effectiveness and impact of multidisciplinary team working on outcomes as patients make transitions from acute care to care closer to home. This lack of evidence is, in part, due to the conceptual and methodological challenges of research on the effect of multidisciplinary teamwork, especially in trying to identify the impact of the other organisational and contextual factors (e.g. level and availability of commissioned services) that will influence outcomes of treatment. In the care of people with a stroke, transitions are made between types of teams: from well-defined and organised hospital-based stroke teams to looser, extended teams in primary care with input from general practitioners, rehabilitation specialists, community matrons and social care, often working out of separate agencies. Research has tended to evaluate team effectiveness on the basis of productive output, team processes, e.g. team cohesion and individual team member outcomes, e.g. staff satisfaction and well-being.[46] However, team effectiveness may be perceived differently by team members, healthcare organisations, patients and their carers[47] and therefore while staff satisfaction and well-being are important, they do not necessarily reflect effective team work. Similarly, patient and carer satisfaction may not indicate team effectiveness as it may be difficult for patients and carers to separate the effect of team work from the effect of clinical intervention. Therefore, it is important to consider a range of perspectives and outcomes in the evaluation of multidisciplinary team effectiveness.

Even though there is a lack of evidence about the impact of multidisciplinary team working on patient outcome, there are a number of reasons why team work is considered important in stroke care. Patients who have had a stroke frequently require multiple treatments from a range of health professionals with different skills and expertise. Good quality patient care depends upon a range of skilled professionals collaborating together in teams since it is very unusual that one professional can deliver a complete episode of care. Although definitions of teams can differ, there is general consensus within the teamwork literature that teams are comprised of a small, manageable number of members, with an appropriate mix of skills and expertise, all committed to a meaningful purpose and have collective responsibility to achieve performance objectives or outcomes. There are several terms that are used to describe clinical teams in stroke care, multidisciplinary (multiprofessional), interdisciplinary (interprofessional) and transdisciplinary (transprofessional), which progressively involve more shared working and flexibility as well as boundary blurring between different professional roles.

Team Effectiveness

Lemieux-Charles and McGuire (2006)[48] have developed a model drawn from healthcare and organisational literature, which describes how teams and effectiveness can be conceptualised in healthcare. This model, the Integrated (Health Care) Team Effectiveness Model (ITEM), describes how task design, team processes and team psycho-social traits influence team outcomes and shows the complex interactions between these elements related to team effectiveness. This model will be used to discuss how multidisciplinary team work may influence patient outcome and experience in stroke care.

Task design

Task design includes team features and team composition and is influenced by organisational context. Within clinical stroke care, the multidisciplinary team is composed of members from a range of health professional groups including doctors, nurses, physiotherapists, occupational therapists, speech and language therapists, dietitians, social workers, psychologists and pharmacists. Each team member should have a distinctive and necessary role.[49] Each member contributes his or her specialist knowledge, skills, experience, resources and networks that enables a more comprehensive understanding and assessment of the patient and their needs. Clear objectives and shared values and vision among team members leads to a consistent approach to care and treatment goals as well as enhances team member morale, motivation and commitment to their work. Team members share responsibility for the team's decisions and their outcomes. It is important that the team includes members of all the professions required for patient care to ensure that the necessary expertise is available to the team.[50] Moreover, where team members are based in close proximity and work at similar times, there are increased opportunities to work together.[51]

Team processes

Team processes include communication, collaboration, conflict, leadership and decision-making. Equitable communication within the multidisciplinary team is important to enable each member to fully participate in discussion about patient assessment, progress and goal planning. It also helps build trust among team members and allows ideas and decisions to be challenged and debated which may help improve care and avoid errors. Teams engage in multidisciplinary team meetings and share patient records and protocols to facilitate communication and collective decision-making.[51] Where communication is not equitable, for example, where one professional dominates, is unwilling to listen to others or is unwilling to share views and information, patient care is likely to be inconsistent and uncoordinated and members of the team may feel resentful and unsupported.[52,53] Where team members from different disciplines fully understand each other's roles and responsibilities, collaboration is enhanced and care delivery is more efficient with less duplication or omission of care and treatment.[54]

Collaboration is one of the most important and challenging aspects of multidisciplinary team work. There is a big risk that the diversity of knowledge, skills, attitudes, working practices, professional priorities and occupational loyalties represented within such teams will result in different professionals working in parallel with no 'added value'. Role blurring, where different professionals share knowledge and skill between team members and can take on some elements of each other's role where needed, is thought to be important to facilitate continuity and consistency of patient care.[54] In particular, in inpatient care, nurses are more likely to take on some of the roles of others, for example, continue the treatment plans of therapy staff at the weekend or in the evenings.[55] This is seen as a way of reinforcing the therapy staff's work in order to maximise the effectiveness of the therapy and to meet client's needs. However, it is important that there is reciprocity among all team members to reinforce team working and to ensure some members do not feel undermined and still have the capacity to fulfil their own professional role. Furthermore, where professionals have strong feelings of occupational autonomy, role blurring can lead to feeling of resentment and anxiety and cause friction within the team. When team members are confident in their own ability and that of others, they are more likely to feel comfortable in sharing some aspects of role.[56] Role blurring can also aid team members' professional development by enabling them to gain a greater range of expertise. However, Rushmer (2005)[57] cautions that blurring the boundaries between professional roles can lead to role ambiguity, inequity, resentment and anxiety. Thus, she recommends that the limits of role sharing are clearly defined and that '*crossed* boundaries working' may be a better terminology.

Team working provides learning opportunities for individuals and the team through sharing of ideas and discussion of clinical and organisational issues. This can help teams become more effective and able to deliver improved patient care. Furthermore, professional development for individuals is promoted through the development of a more comprehensive understanding of patient need and treatment, increased professional confidence as well as improved problem-solving and care delivery skills. West (1996)[58] proposes that task team reflexivity, where teams reflect upon their objectives, strategies, processes and environment and adapt these to their work situations, is an overarching factor that influences team effectiveness. Reflecting on actions and decisions, and giving and receiving feedback can promote greater self-regulation and improve efficiency and quality of care.[59]

The role of the team leader is considered essential for team effectiveness.[60] It is important that the team leader provides direction for team and motivates the team to work together to fulfil team objectives. The leader ensures good communication so that all members are able to participate in the team activities and decision-making. The leader sets the 'tone' or culture of the team[54] and should facilitate a safe environment so that disagreements between team members are constructively resolved.

Team psycho-social traits

The psychosocial traits of the team are thought to interact with team processes to directly influence team outcomes.[48] It is important that team members feel supported, trusted and valued by other members of the team and this facilitates other team processes, for example, communication, reflexivity and a shared team focus. Where the work environment is more sociable and relationships are supportive, staff tend to be more enthusiastic, motivated and committed to the team, which in turn leads to increased productivity, reduced staff burnout and greater staff and patient satisfaction. However, status hierarchy, where the expertise of some professions is considered more important, can cause conflict between team members and restrict team participation.[61] Teams frequently share expectations about how they are expected to work or communicate with each other. These norms can be either explicit or implicit and can lead to difficult consequences for individual team members if they are not followed.[62,63]

The ITEM model[48] offers a useful way of thinking about team effectiveness, although it has not been developed specifically in stroke care. It is important to acknowledge the importance of organisational and service context on team effectiveness and the attributes and influences of individual team members. Furthermore, there has been considerable change recently in the way health and social care is organised and this change will certainly have an impact on the future composition and functioning of teams. Furthermore, multidisciplinary team working is becoming more complex; the nature of multidisciplinary teamwork is developing to accommodate changes in service delivery, the roles of the healthcare workforce and health technologies with increased flexibility and diversity of the structure and process of team working. There is considerable scope for these developments to have a beneficial impact on patient care and experience for patients and their families. The challenge for multidisciplinary teams in stroke care is to further develop the way they work together to maximise these benefits for all stakeholders.

Challenges in Stroke Rehabilitation

There is no doubt that stroke rehabilitation management has changed beyond recognition in terms of the range of stroke services now available to patients or the political and professional willingness to drive the process even further. Another significant achievement has been the improvements in stroke care, especially the increase in the number of specialist units specially dedicated to the care of stroke patients. For example, 79% of hospitals in the UK had specialist stroke rehabilitation units in 2004, which increased to 91% by 2006 and 97% of hospitals by 2008.[64] The number of stroke patients receiving specialist stroke care in the UK has also risen from 46% in 2004 to 67% in 2006 and 74% in 2008. In addition, increasingly higher proportions of patients have gained earlier access to specialist therapy services. Despite these encouraging figures, most studies show that stroke rehabilitation remains sub-optimal in many settings and significant improvements in recovery, patient outcomes and cost-effectiveness of services can be achieved by better organisation of stroke care.

Sub-optimal stroke rehabilitation and poor outcomes are often attributed to reduced availability of rehabilitation resources and lack of investment by healthcare systems. A case study of stroke services in a publicly funded universal healthcare system, such as the National Health Service in the UK, suggests that this may not always be true.[65] A Europe-wide comparison of outcomes in stroke shows higher mortality and dependence in stroke patients in the UK compared with peers such as Germany or France. However, stroke patients in the UK receive 70 hours of multidisciplinary input per week compared with 30 hours in Germany or 43 hours in Switzerland. At three months, 50% of the patients were still receiving physiotherapy and 33% still receiving occupational therapy in UK, compared with 50% and 25% respectively in Germany. The UK spends 6122 euros per patient on each stroke episode, 25% of which is spent on stroke unit care. The comparative spending is 3457 euros (5% on stroke unit care) in Germany and 4337 euros (4% on stroke unit care) in France.

Improving poor outcomes to justify the high investment in stroke is a major challenge for stroke rehabilitation and the failure of organised stroke care to achieve its full potential can be attributed to deficiencies within the processes and practices of providing specialist care. For example, the National Stroke Audit in the UK (Chapter 12) shows that nearly all hospitals in the UK have a stroke unit but only 60% of stroke patients actually receive a significant proportion of their care on such units. More importantly, less than half of these units actually meet the accepted criteria to be a stroke unit and more than a quarter may not even meet the basic standards for rehabilitation care. In other words, simple designation as a specialist unit does not ensure the multidisciplinary expertise required for good outcomes, the effectiveness being further diluted by more than a third of eligible patients not being able to access this care.

Up-to-date and comprehensive guidelines for stroke rehabilitation are published regularly by stroke working groups across the world but many studies show that their implementation and impact on clinical practice, even within stroke rehabilitation units, is limited. The issue of compliance with guidelines is a matter of much debate and depends upon several factors. There are limited opportunities for multidisciplinary education or training on many units and implementation is further hampered by the experience, personal preferences and established practices of individuals within the rehabilitation unit. Other barriers to implementation include professional autonomy of members of the multidisciplinary teams who may reflect specialist views and devolution of accountability to the multidisciplinary team as a whole, whereby no single individual or professional sees themselves as being responsible for their implementation.

The impact of rehabilitation culture on therapy input was elegantly illustrated in the CERISE study,[66] a comparison of stroke rehabilitation units across four settings in Europe. Stroke patients in all settings spent the majority of their time alone and unoccupied: nearly 65% of the therapeutic day was spent sitting, lying or sleeping and patients had greater contact with visitors than with therapists. Even more worrying was the finding that stroke patients received a very small proportion of therapy time allocated to them in face-to-face therapeutic activities, with the vast majority of time being spent on administrative and non-therapeutic activities.

Stroke rehabilitation in clinical practice remains focused on therapist based interventions, which are labour intensive, expensive and limited.

Recent years have seen significant advances in technology to complement therapist input and provide greater intensity of more flexible treatment to patients. Much of this technology is yet to make an impact on therapy practices and there is an urgent need to evaluate their place, cost and benefit in mainstream settings.

The importance of matching professional and patient priorities for improving the effectiveness and efficiency of stroke rehabilitation is becoming increasingly evident in qualitative stroke literature.[67] Patients define recovery in relation to their own social context and their own expectations from rehabilitation, whereas professionals measure recovery in terms of actual gains in function against those expected for the severity of impairment. Furthermore, the goals of the patients are often seen as subordinate to those of professionals, and unrealistic anticipation of the degree of recovery by patients is not managed adequately, resulting in less than desirable outcomes.

One of the key things that stroke survivors complain about is that they do not receive enough rehabilitation after discharge from inpatient rehabilitation. Quite often, there is reluctance in patients to leave the certainty of inpatient therapy input for uncertain rehabilitation in the community.[68] Whether longer rehabilitation within institutional facilities will be appropriate to enhance higher level functions required for community living is not known. Community based studies on rehabilitation interventions that directly address higher level functions in activities of daily living, such as outdoor mobility, shopping and leisure activities have shown benefit,[69] but well-structured and intensive community rehabilitation programmes are not available universally.[70]

Conclusions

The last two decades have seen dramatic advances in stroke rehabilitation from being intuitive practice underpinned by theoretical concepts of recovery to evidence based interventions firmly rooted in the science of recovery. The major contributors to these advances include the significant strides in neurobiology, which have shown that the brain has the capacity to regenerate after stroke and that it may be possible to modulate this regeneration by cellular, pharmacological and therapeutic interventions.

Developments in neuroimaging have made it possible to objectively measure changes taking place in the brain and correlate these to improvements in functional recovery. More importantly, imaging modalities have shown that further recovery with targeted interventions may even occur in stroke patients several months or even years after the initial injury. More recent studies show that imaging can also be used to identify patients who would be most suited for specific interventions.

There has been a plethora of clinical trials on different therapeutic, pharmacological and even cellular interventions to expedite stroke recovery in the last 20 years. Many new treatment concepts have emerged and have been tested in well-designed studies, resulting in new interventions such as treadmill training, constraint induced movement therapy and motor imagery being added to treatments available for stroke patients. It has also become increasingly clear that stroke rehabilitation is a complex intervention requiring high degrees of coordination and multidisciplinary functioning. The exponential rise in the number of studies in service delivery and organisation has helped to provide an insight into the structure, functioning and inter-relationships of complex systems such as the multidisciplinary team and stroke units. This has been strengthened by emerging qualitative research on the expectations and needs of service users.

On the clinical side, there have been dramatic improvements in stroke rehabilitation, underpinned by coherent policies for the management of stroke patients, well-organised services within a framework of guidelines and monitoring of performance to ensure quality of care. However, further work is needed to translate the new and exciting research on regenerative interventions into clinical practice, increase the evidence base for the types and effectiveness of complex rehabilitation interventions, and improve multidisciplinary interactions and communications with patients and their caregivers. Of these, increasing therapy input to make the best use of time that patients spend in rehabilitation settings remains the leading priority.

References

1. Butefisch CM, Kleiser R, Seitz RJ. Post-lesional cerebral reorganisation: evidence from functional neuroimaging and transcranial magnetic stimulation. *J Physiol Paris* 2006; 99(4–6): 437–454.

2. Cadilhac DA, Carter RC, Thrift AG, Dewey HM. Why invest in a national public health program for stroke? An example using Australian data to estimate the potential benefits and cost implications. *Health Policy* 2007; 83(2–3): 287–294.
3. Cramer SC. Repairing the human brain after stroke: I. Mechanisms of spontaneous recovery. *Ann Neurol* 2008; 63: 272–287.
4. Ma DK, Bonaguidi MA, Ming GL, Song H. Adult neural stem cells in the mammalian central nervous system. *Cell Res* 2009; 19(6): 672–682.
5. Zhang ZG, Chopp M. Neurorestorative therapies for stroke: underlying mechanisms and translation to the clinic. *Lancet Neurol* 2009; 8(5): 491–500.
6. Minger SL, Ekonomou A, Carta EM *et al.* Endogenous neurogenesis in the human brain following cerebral infarction. *Regen Med* 2007; 2(1): 69–74.
7. Ratan RR, Siddiq A, Smirnova N *et al.* Harnessing hypoxic adaptation to prevent, treat, and repair stroke. *J Mol Med* 2007; 85: 1331–1338.
8. Sasaki Y, Araki T, Millbrandt J. Stimulation of nicotinamide adenine dinucleotide biosynthetic pathways delays axonal degeneration after axotomy. *J Neurosci* 2006; 26(33): 8484–8491.
9. Buccino G, Solodkin A, Small SL. Functions of the mirror neuron system: implications for neurorehabilitation. *Cogn Behav Neurol* 2006; 19(1): 55–63.
10. Sharma N, Pomeroy VM, Baron JC. Motor imagery: a backdoor to the motor system after stroke? *Stroke* 2006; 37(7): 1941–1952.
11. Ward NS. Mechanisms underlying recovery of motor function after stroke. *Postgrad Med J* 2005; 81(958): 510–514.
12. Johansen-Berg H, Dawes H, Guy C, Smith SM, Wade DT, Matthews PM. Correlation between motor improvements and altered fMRI activity after rehabilitative therapy. *Brain* 2002; 125(Pt 12): 2731–2742.
13. Nudo RJ, Wise BM, SiFuentes F, Millken GW. Neural substrates for the effects of rehabilitative training on motor recovery after ischaemic infarct. *Science* 1996; 272: 1791–1794.
14. Lindberg PG, Schmitz C, Engardt M, Forssberg H, Borg J. Use-dependent up- and down-regulation of sensorimotor brain circuits in stroke patients. *Neurorehabil Neural Repair* 2007; 21(4): 315–326.
15. Struppler A, Binkofski F, Angerer B, Bernhardt M, Spiegel S, Drzezga A, Bartenstein P. A fronto-parietal network is mediating improvement of motor function related to repetitive peripheral magnetic stimulation: A PET-H2O15 study. *Neuroimage* 2007; 36(Suppl 2): T174–186.

16. Krakauer JW. Motor learning: its relevance to stroke recovery and neurore-habilitation. *Curr Opin Neurol* 2006; 19(1): 84–90.

17. Wade DT, Langton Hewer R. Functional abilities after stroke: measurement, natural history and prognosis. *J Neurol Neurosurg Psychiatry* 1987; 50: 177–182.

18. Skilbeck CE, Wade DT, Hewer RL, Wood VA. Recovery after stroke. *J Neurol Neurosurg Psychiatry* 1983; 46: 5–8.

19. Hodics T, Cohen LG, Cramer SC. Functional imaging of intervention effects in stroke motor rehabilitation. *Arch Phys Med Rehabil* 2006; 87(12 Suppl 2): S36–42.

20. Stinear CM, Barber PA, Smale PR, Coxon JP, Fleming MK, Byblow WD. Functional potential in chronic stroke patients depends on corticospinal tract integrity. *Brain* 2007; 130(Pt 1): 170–180.

21. Wang Y, Zhang ZG, Rhodes K, Renzi M, Zhang RL, Kapke A, *et al.* Post-ischemic treatment with erythropoietin or carbamylated erythropoietin reduces infarction and improves neurological outcome in a rat model of focal cerebral ischemia. *Br J Pharmacol* 2007; 151(8): 1377–1384.

22. Kalra L, Langhorne P. Facilitating recovery: Evidence for organised stroke care. *J Rehabil* 2007; 39: 97–102.

23. Carmichael ST. Themes and strategies for studying the biology of stroke recovery in the poststroke epoch. *Stroke* 2008; 39: 1380–1388.

24. Fjaertoft H, Indredavik B, Johnsen R, Lydersen S. Acute stroke unit care combined with early supported discharge. Long-term effects on quality of life. A randomized controlled trial. *Clin Rehabil* 2004; 18(5): 580–586.

25. Diserens K, Michel P, Bogousslavsky J. Early mobilisation after stroke: review of the literature. *Cerebrovasc Dis* 2006; 22(2–3): 183–190.

26. Kalra L, Ratan R. What's new and exciting in stroke regenerative medicine. *Stroke* 2008; 39(2): 273–275.

27. Stewart KC, Cauraugh JH, Summers JJ. Bilateral movement training and stroke rehabilitation: a systematic review and meta-analysis. *J Neurol Sci* 2006; 244(1–2): 89–95.

28. Van Peppen RP, Kortsmit M, Lindeman E, Kwakkel G. Effects of visual feedback therapy on postural control in bilateral standing after stroke: a systematic review. *J Rehabil Med* 2006; 38(1): 3–9.

29. Wolf SL, Winstein CJ, Miller JP *et al.* Effect of constraint-induced movement therapy on upper extremity function 3 to 9 months after stroke: the EXCITE randomized clinical trial. *JAMA* 2006; 296: 2095–2104.

30. Wolf SL. Revisiting constraint-induced movement therapy: are we too smitten with the mitten? Is all nonuse "learned"? and other quandaries. *Phys Ther* 2007; 87(9): 1212–1223.
31. van der Lee JH. Constraint-induced therapy for stroke: more of the same of something completely different? *Curr Opin Neurol* 2001; 14(6): 741–744.
32. Brown JA, Lutsep HL, Weinand M, Cramer SC. Motor cortex stimulation for the enhancement of recovery from stroke: a prospective, multicenter safety study. *Neurosurgery* 2006; 58(3): 464–473.
33. Lefaucheur JP. Stroke recovery can be enhanced by using repetitive transcranial magnetic stimulation (rTMS). *Neurophysiol Clin* 2006; 36(3): 105–115.
34. Malcolm MP, Triggs WJ, Light KE, Gonzalez Rothi LJ, Wu S, Reid K, Nadeau SE. Repetitive transcranial magnetic stimulation as an adjunct to constraint-induced therapy: an exploratory randomized controlled trial. *Am J Phys Med Rehabil* 2007; 86(9): 707–715.
35. Braun SM, Beurskens AJ, Borm PJ, Schack T, Wade DT. The effects of mental practice in stroke rehabilitation: a systematic review. *Arch Phys Med Rehabil* 2006; 87(6): 842–852.
36. Sütbeyaz S, Yavuzer G, Sezer N, Koseoglu BF. Mirror therapy enhances lower-extremity motor recovery and motor functioning after stroke: a randomized controlled trial. *Arch Phys Med Rehabil* 2007; 88(5): 555–559.
37. He BJ, Snyder AZ, Vincent JL, Epstein A, Shulman GL, Corbetta M. Breakdown of functional connectivity in frontoparietal networks underlies behavioral deficits in spatial neglect. *Neuron* 2007; 53: 905–918.
38. Hillis AE. Rehabilitation of unilateral spatial neglect: new insights from magnetic resonance perfusion imaging. *Arch Phys Med Rehabil* 2006; 87(12 Suppl 2): S43–49.
39. Sapir A, Kaplan JB, He BJ, Corbetta M. Anatomical correlates of directional hypokinesia in patients with hemispatial neglect. *J Neurosci* 2007; 27(15): 4045–4051.
40. Kalra L, Ratan, R. Recent advances in stroke rehabilitation 2006. *Stroke* 2007; 38: 235–237.
41. www.cdc.gov/nchs/about/otheract/icd9/icfhome.htm
42. Stroke Unit Trialists' Collaboration. Organised inpatient (stroke unit) care for stroke. *Cochrane Database of Systematic Reviews* 2007, Issue 4. Art. No.: CD000197. DOI: 10.1002/14651858.CD000197.pub2.

43. Early Supported Discharge Trialists. Services for reducing duration of hospital care for acute stroke patients. *Cochrane Database of Systematic Reviews* 2005, Issue 2. Art. No.: CD000443.

44. Fuentes B, Díez-Tejedor E. Stroke units: many questions, some answers. *Int J Stroke* 2009; 4(1): 28–37.

45. Mickan SM, Rodger SA. Effective health care teams: a model of six characteristics developed from shared perceptions. *J Interprof Care* 2005; 19(4): 358–370.

46. Mickan SM. Evaluating the effectiveness of health care teams. *Australian Health Review* 2005; 29(2): 211–217.

47. Lemieux-Charles L, Murray M, Baker GR, Barnsley J, Tasa K, Salahadin AI. The effects of quality improvement practices on team effectiveness: a mediational model. *J Org Behav* 2002; 23: 533–553.

48. Lemieux-Charles L, McGuire WL. What do we know about health care team effectiveness: a review of the literature. *Med Care Res Rev* 2006; 63: 263–300.

49. Mickan S, Rodger S. Characteristics of effective teams: a literature review. *Australian Health Review* 2000; 23(3): 201–208.

50. Kvarnstrom S. Difficulties in collaboration: A critical incident study of interprofessional healthcare teamwork. *J Interprof Care* 2008; 22(2): 191–203.

51. Baxter SK, Brumfitt SM. Once a week is not enough: evaluating current measures of teamworking in stroke. *J Eva Clin Pract* 2008; 14(2): 241–247.

52. Sands RG, Stafford J, McClelland M. "I Beg to Differ". *Soc Work Health Care* 1990; 14: 55–72.

53. Freeman M, Miller C, Ross N. The impact of individual philosophies of teamwork on multi-professional practice and the implications for education. *J Interprof Care* 2000; 14(3): 237–247.

54. Proctor-Childs T, Freeman M, Miller C. Visions of teamwork: the realities of an interdisciplinary approach. *Br J Ther Rehabil* 1998; 5(12): 616.

55. Long AF, Kneafsey R, Ryan J. Rehabilitation practice: challenges to effective team working. *Int J Nursing Stud* 2003; 40(6): 663–673.

56. Molleman E, Broekhuis M, Stoffels R, Jaspers F. How health care complexity leads to cooperation and affects the autonomy of health care professionals. *Health Care Anal* 2008; 16(4): 329–341.

57. Rushmer R. Blurred boundaries damage inter-professional working. *Nurse Researcher* 2005; 12(3): 74–85.

58. West MA. Reflexivity and work group effectiveness: a conceptual integration. *Handbook of Work Group Psychology*. West MA (Ed.) Chichester: John Wiley; 1996; 555–579.

59. Wittenberg-Lyles EM, Oliver DP. The power of interdisciplinary collaboration in hospice. *Prog Palliative Care* 2007; 15(1): 6–12.

60. Zaccaro SJ, Heinen B, Shuffler M. Team leadership and team effectiveness. Team Effectiveness in Complex Organization: Cross-disciplinary Perspectives and Approaches. Salas E, Goodwin GF, Burke S (Eds.) New York: Psychology Press 2009.

61. Coombs M. Power and conflict in intensive care clinical decision making. *Intensive Crit Care Nurs* 2003; 19(3): 125–135.

62. Lingard L, Espin S, Evans C, Hawryluck L. The rules of the game: interprofessional collaboration on the intensive care unit team. *Crit Care* 2004; 8(6): R403–R408.

63. Craigie Jr FC, Hobbs RF. Exploring the organizational culture of exemplary community health center practices. *Family Medicine* 2004; 36(10): 733–738.

64. www.rcplondon.ac.uk/.../Public%20organisational%20report2008.pdf

65. Kalra L, Walker MF. Stroke rehabilitation in the United kingdom. *Top Stroke Rehabil* 2009; 16(1): 27–33.

66. De Wit L, Putman K, Dejaeger E, Baert I, Berman P, Bogaerts K, Brinkmann N, Connell L, Feys H, Jenni W, Kaske C, Lesaffre E, Leys M, Lincoln N, Louckx F, Schuback B, Schupp W, Smith B, De Weerdt W. Use of time by stroke patients: a comparison of four European rehabilitation centers. *Stroke* 2005; 36: 1977–1983.

67. McKevitt C, Redfern J, Mold F, Wolfe C. Qualitative studies of stroke — a systematic review. *Stroke* 2004; 35: 1499–1505.

68. Howell E, Reeves R. Stroke National Service Framework Patient Survey 2004, Picker Institute Europe, July 2005.

69. Walker MF, Leonardi-Bee J, Bath P, Langhorne P, Dewey M, Corr S, Drummond A, Gilbertson L, Gladman JRF, Jongbloed L, Logan P, Parker C. An individual patient data meta-analysis of community occupational therapy trials for stroke patients. *Stroke* 2004; 35: 2226–2232.

70. Mold F, Wolfe C, McKevitt C. Falling through the net of stroke care. *Health Soc Care Community* 2006; 14(4): 349–356.

9 Long-Term Management of Stroke

Kethakie Sumathipala*, Siobhan Crichton*,
Keerthi Mohan*, Charles Wolfe*,†
and Christopher McKevitt*

Chapter Summary

This chapter reviews the long-term needs, outcomes and proven interventions after stroke, using the framework of the International Classification of Functioning, Disability and Health (ICF). It also reviews current services to meet these needs and considers patients' perspectives of need, and identifies variations in how needs are perceived by patients, caregivers, healthcare professionals and service providers.

Despite continuing long-term needs, most stroke specific services concentrate on the acute event and early rehabilitation period. Services for long-term stroke survivors are often provided by charitable organisations and there is a need for more widespread and consistent evidence-based services. Most intervention studies focus on increasing activity and participation in the longer term. However, trials of these interventions which include physiotherapy, leisure, speech, occupational and educational therapy, have shown mixed results.

*King's College London, Division of Health and Social Care Research, London, UK
†NIHR Biomedical Research Centre, Guy's and St Thomas' NHS Foundation Trust and King's College London, London, UK

Long-Term Needs

Following a stroke, patients and their carers often face a multitude of physical, social and psychological challenges. A third of stroke survivors are left with long-term residual disabilities and ongoing challenges that can persist for many years.[1,2] Increasingly, stroke is seen as a chronic condition that requires long-term management. However, evidence of long-term outcomes are poorly estimated and the majority of stroke services available concentrate on the acute event and the early rehabilitation period.

The Royal College of Physicians (RCP) guidelines on stroke describe the long-term as 'over six months', following the period which is usually dominated by support and care,[3] during which maximum recovery is thought to occur. However, the guidelines also note that for younger patients, recovery can continue for a longer time, whilst for others, dependency may increase due to ageing or other developmental disorders.[3]

In this chapter, we present the long-term consequences of stroke using the World Health Organizations (WHO) International Classification of Functioning, Disability and Health.[4]

Classification of Needs and Outcomes

The International Classification of Functioning, Disability and Health (ICF) proposed in 2001 is a revision of the original WHO classification, the International Classification of Impairments, Disabilities and Handicaps (ICIDH), developed in 1980.[5]

The ICF attempts to provide a unified and standard language for defining health and health-related outcomes. It is divided into two parts, which take into account all aspects of an individual's life, including their functional status and ability to participate in day-to-day activities. The first considers the body (previously impairments), activities (previously disability) and participation (previously handicap). The second part considers environmental and personal contextual factors which may act as barriers or facilitators in the areas covered by part 1.[4] In contrast to the ICIDH which was considered to be a more of a 'medical model' concentrating on the consequences and impact of disease, the ICF

Table 1. An overview of the ICF from International Classification of Functioning, Disability and Health[4]

	Part 1: Functioning and Disability		Part 2: Contextual Factors	
Components	Body functions and structures	Activity and participation	Environmental factors	Personal factors
Domains	Body functions Body structures	Life areas (tasks and actions)	External influences on functioning and disability	Internal influences on functioning and disability
Constructs	Change in body functions (physiological)	Capacity executing tasks in a standard environment	Facilitating or hindering impact of features of the physical, social and attitudinal world	Impact of attributes of the person
	Change in body structures (anatomical)	Performance executing tasks in the current environment		
Positive aspects	Functional and structural integrity	Activities and participation	Facilitators	Not applicable
Negative aspects	Functional Impairment	Activity limitation Participation restriction	Barriers/ hindrances	Not applicable

attempts to provide a coherent biopsychosocial view concentrating on components of health (Table 1). The ICF acknowledges that disease and disorder are not solely linked to an individual's functional outcome, and places emphasis on interaction between its four components. For example, a physical impairment of the body such as paralysis, could lead to difficulties in executing activities and restrictions in participation.

ICF Domains

Body

> The body domain is made up of two elements — body structure and body
> function. Body structure includes, for example, limbs, eyes or organs,
> such as the brain or lungs. Body functions are physiological functions
> such as movement, or psychological function, such as cognition.
> Impairments are problems in both body structures and function.[4]

The impact of stroke can vary between individuals, with some experiencing minor or no long lasting effects, whilst others may be left with
permanent debilitating physical or cognitive impairments. Many studies
of stroke survivors attempt to estimate the prevalence of these impairments in order to gain insight into the long-term outcomes after stroke.
Table 2 presents a list of validated scales and measures commonly used to
quantify functioning and a summary of the levels of impairments
observed in stroke survivors using these scales is presented in Table 3.

Deficits in motor functioning are commonly found in patients presenting
with a stroke and for many the impairment persists for months or years
after the stroke.[15] A 2002 review of motor recovery found 35% of patients
who presented with lower limb and 56% with upper limb hemiparesis had
not recovered by follow-up, which was typically between six and
12 months after stroke.[15] Spasticity, an increase in muscle tone, can
interfere with motor functioning. Measuring spasticity can be difficult;
however, there are a number of scales which are used to detect spasticity.[10,11]
In a hospital based sample, the Modified Ashworth Scale and the Tone
Assessment Scale were both utilised in a study by Watkins *et al.*, which
measured the prevalence of spasticity one year after stroke in a hospital
based sample of 106 patients in Liverpool, England. Using the Modified
Ashworth Scale, spasticity was estimated to occur in 27% of survivors
while the Tone Assessment Scale identified spasticity in 36% of
survivors.[16] However, Lundstrom *et al.*, also using the Modified Ashworth
Scale at one year, found spasticity in only 17% of survivors in a cross-
sectional sample from 'Riks-Stroke', the Swedish national stroke register.
Further, they diagnosed disabling spasticity in 4% of survivors by evaluating
performance in activities of daily living.[17]

Table 2. Selection of scales used to measure functioning

Scale	Measures	Description
Motricity Index[8]	Motor functioning	Range of movement in arms and legs tested and assigned scores. Scores are combined to give a total ranging from 0–100.
Modified Ashworth Scale (MAS)[9]	Spasticity	Six-point ordinal scale against which resistance to stretching of effecting muscle is measured.
Tone Assessment Scale (TAS)[10]	Spasticity	Contains 15 items split over three sections. Section A assesses posture at rest, Section B measures responses to passive movement using scoring system based on the Modified Ashworth Scale and Section C measures reactions to active movement.
Fatigue Assessment Scale[11]	Fatigue	Ten-item scale in which the patient is asked to rate how often they experience the feelings described in a statement (e.g. 'I feel tired all the time') through a five-point Likert scale scored from 1 (never) to 5 (always). Scores are summed to give an overall score.
Abbreviated Mental test[6]	Cognitive state	Ten-item scale with one point awarded to each item correctly answered.
Mini Mental State Exam[7]	Cognitive state	Contains 30 items assessing orientation, registration, attention and calculation, recall and language with each correctly completed item awarded one point.
Test of Everyday Attention[12]	Attention	Contains eight subtests which measure selective attention, sustained attention and attentional switching.
Hospital Anxiety and Depression Scale[13]	Anxiety and depression	Contains 14 items, half measuring depressive symptoms and half anxiety. Items scored from 0–3 and summed within each domain to give a depression and anxiety score each ranging from 0 (no symptoms) to 21.
Becks Depression Inventory[14]	Depression	Contains 21 items looking at symptoms associated with depression. Items scored from 0–3 according to severity and summed to give a total score 0–63. Symptoms include sense of failure, lack of satisfaction, guilt, loss of appetite and crying spells.

Incontinence has been shown to have an impact on quality of life and is associated with poorer psychological well-being.[18] Using data from the population based South London Stroke Register (SLSR), Patel *et al.* defined incontinence as 'losing bladder control at least once a week or having an indwelling catheter', and found approximately 15% of survivors at one year and 10% at two years after stroke were affected.[19] In the Erlangen Stroke Project, full urinary incontinence, defined as 'daily leakage of urine and/or leakage caused by triggers most of the time' was observed in 16% of one year survivors while a further 16% had partial incontinence, defined as 'weekly or monthly leakage of urine and/or leakage caused by triggers some of the time'.[20] In a study of faecal incontinence in 688 survivors from the SLSR, Harari *et al.* estimated that 'any degree of bowel leakage' affected 11% of survivors one year after stroke and 15% at three years. Further, they reported that late onset faecal incontinence was common, of those who were incontinent at one year, 63% had been continent at three months post-stroke.[21]

Appleros *et al.* estimated that the prevalence of pain considered by the survivor to be stroke related in a population-based study one year post-stroke to be 11%.[22] Post-stroke pain can be of several different types. Nociceptive pain can occur as a result of weakness or paralysis and there is a large range in the estimates of prevalence, with studies reporting between 5% and 84%.[23] Estimates of the prevalence of neuropathic pain range from 8% to 46% and, while it may be present immediately after stroke, Kumar *et al.* found that onset is typically between three and 12 months post-stroke.[24]

Fatigue is also commonly reported after stroke: a 2006 review by Colle *et al.* found reports of post-stroke fatigue affecting 39–72% of all stroke survivors.[25] A study by Smith *et al.*, which included a group of 80 Dutch stroke survivors on average seven months post-stroke, found levels of fatigue, measured using the Fatigue Assessment Scale, to be comparable to that in people with end-stage chronic heart failure and significantly higher than the general Dutch population.[26]

Stroke often results in a disruption of cognitive function, with memory, attention, language and orientation reported as the areas most commonly affected.[27] Patel *et al.* estimated the prevalence in South London using the Mini-Mental State Exam (MMSE) and found that approximately one-third of stroke survivors were cognitively impaired at three months, one, two and three years after stroke.[28] In Singapore, Tham *et al.* used the 'Vascular Dementia Battery' to give a more detailed representation of cognitive state, allowing for more subtle changes to be detected from baseline scores, within six months of stroke and follow-up one year later. They found that while the cognitive state of 77% of the 252 stroke survivors did not alter, a substantial proportion of survivors showed some improvement while others declined.[29] A similar approach was taken by Del *et al.* in a Spanish study of 193 stroke survivors, and similar trends were observed when follow-up was two years after stroke.[30]

Memory and attention are important in the rehabilitation process, which is often focused on the relearning of skills previously used in everyday life. To estimate the prevalence of attention deficits among community stroke survivors, Hyndmann *et al.* administered four sub-tests of the larger Test of Everyday Attention to 48 stroke survivors, who were on average four years post-stroke. They found deficits of sustained attention in 31%, auditory selective attention in 19%, visual selective attention in 35% and divided attention in 44%.[31] Teasdale *et al.* used a simpler approach, asking 450 stroke survivors at five, ten or 15 years after stroke to state whether or not they had difficulties in the areas of attention, memory or emotional control. The proportion reporting problems did not vary significantly across time points with attention problems experienced by 54–60%, memory by 59–62% and emotional control by 44–56%.[32] Language impairments are also common following a stroke and studies have highlighted that as many as 43% of individuals who experience language impairments in the acute phase have not recovered at 18 months post-stroke.[33]

Following the acute stroke event, about one-third of stroke survivors experience symptoms of depression.[34] However, defining depression without a clinical diagnosis can be difficult and prevalence studies report varying rates depending on the assessment tool used.[34] A systematic review of observational studies reporting post-stroke depression by Hackett *et al.* found 10 different mood scales and 4 psychiatric interview schedules in the 51 included studies. Further, where mood scales were used, the cut off points to detect depression varied across studies.[34]

Table 3. Summary of studies estimating prevalence of body impairments

Impairment	Prevalence	Time Point	Measurement Tool	Study Type	Sample Size
Spasticity	27–36%[16]	1 year	Modified Ashworth Scale and Tone Assessment Scale	Hospital based	106
Spasticity	17% + 4% (disabling spasticity)[17]	1 year	Modified Ashworth Scale	Cross sectional	140
Urinary incontinence	19%, 15%, 10%[19]	3 months, 1 and 2 years, respectively	Losing bladder control at least once a week	Population based	235
Urinary incontinence	16% (full), 16% (partial)[20]	1 year	Loss of control most of the time (full) or some of the time (partial)	Population based	752
Faecal incontinence	11%, 11%, 15%[21]	3 months, 1 and 3 years, respectively	Any degree of bowel leakage	Population based	1563
Pain	11%[22]	1 year	Participants asked if they had any pain considered to be stroke related	Population based	377
Fatigue	39–72%[25]	Non-specific	Mixed	Review	
Cognitive impairment	39%, 35%, 30% and 32%[28]	3 month, 1, 2 and 3 years, respectively	Mini-mental state exam	Population based	163
Attention deficit	19–44%[31]	4 years (mean)	Test of everyday attention	Cross sectional	48
Attention	59%, 54%, 60%[32]	5, 10 and 15 years, respectively	Yes/no response to 'Do you have problems with attention?'	Population based	450
Memory	62%, 59%, 59%[32]	5, 10 and 15 years, respectively	Yes/no response to 'Do you have problems with attention?'	Population based	450
Emotional control	56%, 58%, 44%[32]	5, 10 and 15 years, respectively	Yes/no response to 'Do you have problems with emotional control?'	Population based	450
Depression	30%[34]	Non-specific	Mixed	Review	

Activity (Table 4)

Activities are the execution of tasks or actions while activity limitations are difficulties an individual encounters while performing tasks or actions.[4]

Table 4. Scales used to measure activity

Scale	Measures	Description
Barthel Index[35]	Activities of Daily living (ADL)	Ten items with each scored according to extent of assistance required to perform each activity. Items include feeding, bathing, grooming, dressing, bowel control, bladder control, toilet use, stairs climbing, chair transfer and mobility. Scores are summed giving a total between 0 and 100, with 100 indicating functional independence.
Frenchay Activity Index[36]	Instrumental Activities of Daily living (IADL)	A 15-item scale which can be separated into three subscales; domestic activities (e.g. housework), leisure and work activities (e.g. social outings or participating in a hobby) and outdoor activities (e.g. walking outdoors or gardening). The frequency of each activity over the past three or six months is considered and each given a score from 1 (lowest) to 4 (highest), which are summed to give an overall and sub-scale scores.
Functional Independence Measure[37]	Functional independence	Contains 18 items assessing motor and cognitive functioning. A seven-point Likert scale (from 1 = complete dependence to 7 = total independence) is used to score each item. Within the motor domain, the items assess self-care, sphincter control, transfer and locomotion. In the cognition domain, communication and social cognition are assessed.
Modified Rankin Scale[38]	Functional independence	Single item scale. Guided interviews are used to assess patients' participation in activities in daily living as well as cognitive and speech deficits. Responses are combined and graded from 0, no symptoms, to 5, severe disability.

The ability to execute activities of daily living (ADL) is often used to assess an individual's capacity to independently carry out tasks necessary for their well-being. One of the most widely used measures to assess the ability to perform activities of daily living is the Barthel Index.[35] Hankey et al., using data from the Perth Community Stroke Study in Australia, estimated that 36% of five-year stroke survivors, who had been independent prior to stroke, were unable to independently perform all activities defined in the Barthel Index.[2] In an analysis of the South London Stroke Register in the UK, Patel et al., also using the Barthel Index, found that over 25% of stroke survivors were not independent in ADL at one and three years after stroke. With the use of the Frenchay Activity Index to assess functional activities, they also found that 50% of participants were classified as 'inactive' (i.e. a score of <16) at both time points.[39]

Secondary problems resulting from the original stroke impairment have been reported to affect the ability to function after stroke. Studies have shown that spasticity, pain and loss of bowel and bladder continence are associated with decreased activity and poor performance in activities of daily living.[16,40–43]

Participation (Table 5)

> Participation is the involvement in life situations whilst participation restrictions refer to problems individuals face when participating in life situations.[4]

Involvement in social activities and return to pre-stroke or modified activities are of importance to stroke survivors.[49–53] D'Alisa et al. assessed the extent of participation restrictions in 73 stroke survivors, who were on average five years post-stroke and ranged in age from 24 to 83 years, using the London Handicap Scale. They found the most severely affected domains were: occupation (45%), physical independence (40%), mobility (22%), and economic self-sufficiency (15%). Functional disability was independently associated with restrictions in the areas of mobility, physical independence and occupation. Meanwhile, depression was associated with restrictions in orientation and social integration.[54] Desrosiers et al.

Table 5. Scales used to assess participation and quality of life

Scale	Measures	Description
London Handicap Scale[44]	Participation	Contains six items each measuring disadvantage due to impairment in the following areas: mobility, physical independence, occupation, social integration, and economic self-sufficiency. Each item is measured on a six-point scale where disadvantage is rated from 'none' to 'extreme'. Weights are applied to give a final score ranging from 0 (maximum handicap) to 1 (no handicap).
36-item Short Form Health Survey (SF-36)[45]	Health related quality of life	Contains 36 items which assess quality of life in previous four weeks. Scores calculated for eight domains: physical functioning, role limitations due to physical problems, general health perceptions, vitality, social functioning, role limitations due to emotional problems, general mental health and health transition. Scores are then combined to give overall mental and physical summary scores. Summary scores range from 0–100 (mean = 50, s.d. = 10) with higher scored indicative of poorer outcome.
12-item Short Form Health Survey (SF-12)[46]	Health related quality of life	Abbreviated version of the SF-36 with 12 times taken from the original SF-36 items from which the physical and mental summary scores of the SF-36 have been shown to be reproducible using the SF-12.[47]
EuroQoL[48]	Health related quality of life	Contains 5 domains each scored by selecting one of three responses. Domains measure mobility, pain, anxiety/depression, self-care and usual activities. Weights are assigned to domains to give score from 0 (poorest state) to 1. Visual analogue scale also used to assess health status with a scale of 0 (worst status) to 100.

also investigated predictors of participation after stroke. They found that in addition to functional abilities related to motor coordination and upper extremity ability, increasing age and the presence of co-morbidities were predictors of lower levels of participation.[55]

The ability to participate in leisure activities can be important in maintaining quality of life after stroke. Niemi *et al.*, in a study of stroke survivors under 65 years, measured the quality of life of 46 individuals four years after stroke, across four domains of life. They found that the largest deterioration following stroke was in the participation in leisure time activities, such as social events, religious activities or other hobbies, while activities at home, including housework and participation in family life were least affected.[56]

Drummond surveyed stroke survivors 40 to 78 weeks post-stroke and found that leisure activities had decreased with regard to the number of activities and frequency of participation.[57] A cross-sectional study of Danish stroke survivors found 39% of five-year survivors reported leisure activities were 'very restricted'. However, this reduced to under a quarter in the ten- and 15-year survivors.[32]

A review by Bhogal *et al.* (2003) on social and leisure activities after stroke found that deterioration is most common in younger, better educated individuals.[58] The inability to return to paid employment following stroke is an important issue for many younger stroke patients. Using data from the South London Stroke Register, Busch *et al.* found that at one year after stroke, only 35% working before the stroke event had returned to paid employment.[59] In a cross-sectional Danish study of 450 stroke survivors, Teasdale *et al.* estimated that 55% of survivors at five years post-stroke, 39% at ten years and 32% at 15 years were not able to return to work.[32] Kersten *et al.* conducted a national survey to compare the needs of 18 to 45-year-olds with those aged 46 to 65 years in the UK. They found that the younger group reported significantly more unmet needs than the older group. These included holidays, intellectual fulfilment and family support. In the same study it was found that those who did not return to work had more unmet needs than those who reduced hours or changed jobs.[60] Furthermore, a systematic review by Daniel *et al.* found a wide range of estimates on the effect of stroke on sexual activity, with 5–76% of working age stroke survivors reporting a deterioration.[61]

There are currently no studies looking at participation restrictions specifically in older age survivors. However, it has been suggested that in older stroke survivors, reduction in participation is in part due to the process of normal ageing.[62]

Contextual factors

> Contextual factors include personal and environmental factors which may act as either barriers or facilitators to participation in daily life.[4]

Stroke survivors may face a variety of barriers to activity and participation. These can include personal factors such as age, socio-economic status, past illness experience, motivation and self-efficacy or environmental factors such as architectural barriers, organisational policies and practices, as well as social attitudes.[63,64] Other wider environmental barriers include living in an urban environment, crime, safety, weather, damaged pavements and lack of accessible transportation.[63]

Niemi *et al.* observed that individuals aged 51–64 years old experienced more severe deterioration in quality of life after stroke in comparison to younger patients aged 17–50 years.[56] Labi *et al.* observed that individuals with higher education and income levels had a lower quality of life after stroke, possibly due to the greater impact of decreased participation in social activities.[65]

A US study looked at barriers to participation in physical activity in 83 stroke survivors aged 30–70 years, who were at least six months poststroke. All participants could walk at least 50 feet without assistance and common barriers identified included the cost of programme, lack of awareness of location of a fitness centre, no means of transportation and lack of knowledge on how to exercise.[63]

Lack of information is one of the most widely reported problems faced by stroke survivors. A review of qualitative literature by Murray *et al.* concluded that service provision is one of the largest areas in need of development and found the availability of information after stroke to be of importance to survivors.[66] In an English community survey of 76 stroke survivors, O'Mahony *et al.* questioned respondents on whether they were satisfied with information provision in 18 different areas. Satisfaction was high in areas relating to general health and well-being.[67] However, 34% of respondents felt they had not received adequate information on health and social services, including those provided by the voluntary sector, available to them. There was also high dissatisfaction relating to provision of information on the emotional effects of a stroke, only 28% felt they had received enough information.[67]

In the UK, Hanger and Mulley carried out a study to identify the type and frequency of questions asked by stroke survivors, relatives and caregivers to Stroke Association centres during a four-month period. Nearly 2000 questions were asked, with almost a quarter relating to the nature of stroke. The second most common query, which was a theme in almost 10% of questions related to the availability of support for home care, while a similar number inquired about stroke support clubs. Speech help, recovery, personality changes and depression were themes in over 5% of all questions recorded.[68] In a longitudinal study in New Zealand, Hanger *et al.* asked 114 stroke survivors if they had any questions about their stroke. They found that the nature of the questions asked changed with time from stroke. For example, at two weeks post-stroke, 32% of the questions asked were about the nature of the stroke, falling to 14% and 8% at six months and two years, respectively. Questions on memory, psychological and cognitive problems became more prevalent at two years, making up one-third of the questions.[69]

It is indicated that during times of stress, individuals need to perceive that others are supportive or will be there if necessary to help cope with demands posed by the environment.[70] Social support has shown a significant, positive association with participation and quality of life.[71] A study of 86 stroke survivors by King *et al.* found similar associations between perceived social support and quality of life at one and three years after stroke.[72] In addition to formal social support, informal networks such as the family and other social networks, have been linked to better outcomes.[73] However, caregiving often results in mental and physical strain, and support for caregivers is an area which needs to be developed.[74,75] The needs of caregivers are further explored in Chapter 10.

Effective Interventions in the Longer Term to Improve Outcome

Interventions to improve recovery and rehabilitation have tended to concentrate on functional activities within the first few months after stroke, and there is little evidence in the long-term on which services can be based.[76] Wilkinson *et al.* observed that of stroke survivors whose Barthel Index scores were assessed at three months, 54% remained in the same category five years later and only 7% had improved.[1] However, it is widely acknowledged that the goals of rehabilitation cannot lie in recovery of function alone.[77] In the longer term, stroke survivors have reported involvement in social roles and return to pre-stroke or modified activities as being more important than the ability to carry out specific physical task.[78] Rehabilitation interventions can be classified in terms of the area which is being targeted within the ICF domains of body, activities and participation.

Body

Interventions aimed at improving impairments tend to concentrate on the early period following stroke; few studies look at increasing functions in the long-term. However, acupuncture and botulinum toxin-A have both been suggested as methods to improve spasticity after stroke. A systematic review of the use of acupuncture, which included patients 1 to 8.5 years post-stroke, found some evidence of improvement in neurological deficits. However, the overall number of patients included was low, totalling 368 and one trial showed no improvement.[79] The use of botulinum toxin-A has also been found to improve both upper and lower limb muscle tone and in a small sample of 20 patients, while muscle tone was improved, there was no associated improvement on functional outcomes.[80,81]

Activity

Mobility is important in an individual's ability to carry out activities independently. A review of the use of electromechanical and robotic-assisted gait training devices in survivors ranging from three weeks to three years post-stroke, suggests that training in combination with physiotherapy can increase the likelihood of walking independently and the distance covered.[82] In a review of repetitive task training of specific motor activities, similar improvements in walking abilities, and in the overall execution of activities of daily living, were found.[83] Ngan-Hing and Stretton, in a review of the home-based and outpatient physiotherapy for stroke survivors living in the community, found improvements in walking speed. However, these benefits were not maintained beyond three months following the completion of the treatment.[84] Two randomised controlled trials of survivors, with reduced mobility due to stroke, found physiotherapy initiated at least one year after stroke resulted in a small short-term improvement in mobility. However, the results were not maintained in the longer term.[85,86] A Cochrane review was conducted using 14 trials of stroke survivors living in the community, receiving therapy based interventions such as physiotherapy, occupational therapy, or multidisciplinary staff working with the patients on task orientated behaviour. It was found that some interventions resulted in an overall improvement in independence in personal ADL.[83]

A review by Legg *et al.* explored the benefits of occupational therapy on ADL and found an increase in ability to perform personal ADL. All studies included took place in the first year after stroke and recruited stroke survivors living at home.[87] However, another review of benefits of physiotherapy and/or occupational therapy by Aziz *et al.* found no evidence of a benefit when therapy was initiated more than a year after stroke.[88]

A study of stroke survivors attending two-hour sessions of aphasia therapy, followed by group activities including communication skills, use of different art forms and self-advocacy over a seven-week period, found improvements in quality of life and communication.[89] Similarly, a review of the intensity of aphasia therapy and recovery found a significant treatment benefit occurred for those who were provided with an intensive amount of therapy over a shorter time compared to those who were provided shorter sessions of therapy over a longer period of time.[90]

Participation

There is increased recognition of the importance of enabling participation. The majority of studies which aim to increase participation use interventions based on leisure and occupational therapy. Whilst several other studies have been conducted which consider the benefits of physiotherapy, multidisciplinary, educational and family functioning interventions.

A review of home-based and outpatient physiotherapy for stroke survivors living in the community consisting of nine-individual studies reported inconsistent improvements in social participation.[84] However, community-based occupational therapy intervention programmes offered at least six months post-stroke have shown significant improvements in levels of participation.[91] Some studies have looked at the use of leisure therapy, although these are much fewer in number compared to studies on occupational therapies. These studies have reported mixed results, with some showing an increase in participation in leisure activities as well as improvements in mood and overall satisfaction, whilst others showed no benefits. In the Nottingham Leisure Study, participants were randomised to leisure rehabilitation, conventional occupational therapy or a control group receiving existing hospital or social services.[57] It was found that those receiving leisure rehabilitation performed better in both mobility and psychological well-being than the other two groups. However, this study included stroke survivors who were between three and six months post-stroke. Parker *et al.*, however, found no long or short term benefits in their multicentre randomised control trial using the same interventions as the Nottingham Leisure Study in stroke survivors six to 12 months post-stroke.[92] Desrosiers *et al.*, using a leisure education intervention, observed increased participation in active leisure activities, such as social activities outside the house, and a reduction in passive activities such as watching TV. The sample consisted of stroke survivors who had been admitted to a rehabilitation or acute care facility at any point in the previous five years.[93] It is possible that differences in findings from various studies using occupational and leisure therapies may be due to the differences in provision of the actual interventions by individual therapists.

Harman-Maier *et al.* found that the use of a multidisciplinary intervention which included clients attending a wide range of group treatments provided by rehabilitation professionals (physical, occupational and speech therapists, art therapists, social workers and nurses) and volunteers two to four days a week resulted in increased participation in leisure activities. Life satisfaction rates amongst the participants

were significantly higher than the non-participants.[94] Following a study
of the role of social support, Beckley *et al.* determined that the quantity
of social support in comparison to the quality of social support had
a greater impact on social participation of stroke survivors three to
six months post-stroke.[95]

Stroke not only results in changing circumstance for the individual
but places much burden on the family.[96] Clark *et al.* carried out a randomised controlled trial in which education and counselling were used
for stroke patients and their families to determine whether this would fos-
ter a favourable environment in which functional recovery could occur.
The intervention consisted of a stroke information package containing
information about stroke and its consequences; practical coping suggestions; information about community services and other support
structures; and three one-hour visits from a social worker trained in family counselling. The intervention resulted in better social recovery for the
stroke survivors who returned to almost their pre-stroke level of participation.[97] Kendall *et al.* carried out a study in which a 'chronic disease
management' educational course was adapted with a stroke specific
information session to assist individuals in actively managing their emotional, physical and social well-being following a stroke. The
intervention group maintained a relatively stable level of adjustment over
time in comparison to the control group who showed early decline.
However, the difference between the groups, which was particularly evident at nine months, had reached similar levels by twelve months due to
improvements in the control group.[77]

Contextual Factors

The home and community environments have the potential to pose a
challenge to stroke survivors and their carers. Contextual factors can
assist in offsetting the impact of impairments and in facilitating activity
and participation. For example, the use of assistive technology devices,
such as canes, walkers, wheel chairs and bath benches may be used and
environmental interventions may include the addition of ramps, lowering
of cabinets and removal of rugs can offer some benefit.[98] However, there
is a lack of published evidence in this area.

Current Service Provision for Stroke Survivors and Their Families in the Longer Term

The recommendations for, and provision of services aimed at long-term stroke survivors can vary between countries. For example, in the UK, the Department of Health Stroke Strategy focuses on the need for support services to be tailored towards the individual.[99] The National Service Framework for Older People calls for the provision of services which provide individuals with appropriate social and emotional support. These services should aim to help survivors deal with the consequences of stroke, loss of independence, and offer support and follow-up to reduce the risk of further strokes.[100] Both documents also call for coordination between the various providers of long-term care (e.g. health and social care, housing and employment). In the Australian Clinical Guidelines for Stroke Rehabilitation and Recovery, focus is given to self-management. It recommends that any survivor without cognitive impairment should receive information on peer-support groups and self-management programmes prior to discharge. It is also suggested that they be given adequate support once they have returned to the community to enable access to such programmes.[101] The American Heart Association statement on physical activity and exercise in 2004 recommended that stroke survivors should be prescribed a training programme with exercise sessions three to seven days a week and lasting 20 to 60 minutes, depending on fitness levels.[102]

Much of the support available to stroke survivors is through support groups often provided by the voluntary sector. In England and Wales, the Stroke Association currently deliver over 220 rehabilitation and support services, including family and carer support, support for people of working age and a long-term support service. The long-term support service aims to reduce isolation, build confidence and emotional well-being as well as encourage people to take responsibility for their own health. It offers help and support to enable stroke survivors and their carers to set up local support and activity groups.[103] In Scotland, Chest Heart and Stroke Scotland (CHSS) have established a network of stroke groups run largely by volunteers. There are groups offering support and activities which are open to all stroke survivors, as well as smaller groups offering support on, for example communication, to which people are referred by healthcare professionals.[104] The US National Stroke Association also facilitates access to support groups and provide information resources for stroke survivors and their carers or families. This includes a series of fact sheets aimed at recovery and a more detailed brochure titled *Hope: The Stroke Recovery Guide*, which contains examples of two detailed exercise routines aimed at those with varying levels of fitness.[103]

Patients' Perceptions

The needs of stroke survivors and their carers differ with age, severity of disability and time from the event, as do the services and support available. Understanding the challenges and factors which have helped in coping is essential in developing interventions to address their needs and supporting individuals in the long-term.[105] While quantitative studies can give estimates of the overall prevalence of clinical outcomes such as cognitive impairment, depression or deficits in motor functioning, the use of qualitative studies allow exploration of the context and an understanding of the complexities experienced by an individual following a stroke.[106] Subjective experiences and needs of individuals and their families can differ from those thought to be necessary by service providers and medical professionals. Furthermore, even the needs defined by stroke survivors and carers can differ.[107]

Some survivors see their stroke as a part of their ongoing life experience with studies showing that factors such as age, co-morbidities and past life experience influence individuals' expectations and response in the long-term.[108,109] However, others see the stroke as a catastrophic, disrupting and life-changing event.[110,111] Some survivors view their bodies as unreliable and separated from the self. The loss in physical functioning and communication can result in restrictions in social abilities such as the involvement in family life, work, leisure, driving, as well as communication and independence.[105,112] Nearly half of stroke survivors experience isolation post-stroke[113] and specific difficulties have been noted in terms of maintaining perceived gender roles in both men and women.[105,114]

In a review of 23 studies with approximately 500 survivors up to six years after stroke, problem areas were identified in five domains: hospital experience, transfer of care, communication, services, and social and emotional consequences. The largest area of concern was the social and emotional consequences of stroke, accounting for 39% of the identified problems. These included problems relating to mood, social change, attitudes to recovery and changes in self-perception and relationships. Service deficiencies in health and social care were the second largest domain, accounting for 29% of the problems.[66]

Several studies of need have been conducted using focus group, questionnaires and in-depth interviews with stroke survivors ranging in age from 43 to 88 years. Only two studies attempted to define 'need' by identifying four types: felt/perceived, expressed, normative and comparative needs.[107,115] A study by Kersten *et al.* used the Southampton needs assessment questionnaire for people with stroke, containing questions on the impact of the stroke, information received and needed, personal and community mobility and access, social activities, family life, sex life, financial difficulties, service usage and unmet needs.[60] In all studies, participants felt a need for better accessibility to care (physiotherapy, occupational therapy, speech therapy) and three of the studies reported a need for more information regarding availability of services. Other needs which were considered of importance but not being fully met included psychosocial and emotional support; adapted transport and alteration of the home; sexuality or sexual relations; and financial concerns.[60,107,115]

A study of personal experiences of stroke rehabilitation from the views of members of a community-based stroke club in the US highlighted similar problems, such as feelings of abandonment from the rehabilitation system following their return home. Several of the participants expressed the need for follow-up treatment on returning home as well as a need to learn about resources available in the community. Stroke survivors often felt isolated due to lack of knowledge of how to access stroke groups.[116]

Studies of patients perceptions' of long-term interventions have been conducted.[117–120] A randomised controlled trial of the UK Stroke Association's family support organiser (FSO) was carried out.[121] The FSO aims to fulfil unmet needs of patients and carers by providing information, emotional support and liaising with other services such as social services and benefit agencies. This study showed no significant benefit for patients and only moderate benefit for carers, however, a qualitative study by the same group found that the FSO was able to meet some of the gaps in service provision.[117] Patients felt that the presence of an FSO helped maintain a more reliable and systematic continuity of care between different parts of the stroke services for aftercare in the community. Hartman-Maeir *et al.* found that participation in a community rehabilitation programme in which stroke patients attended a wide range of group treatments such a physical, occupational, speech, art therapies with social workers and nurses showed an advantage over non-participants, their leisure activity participation and satisfaction scores were significantly higher than non-participants.[118]

Conclusion

This chapter has reviewed the physical, social and emotional consequences of stroke in the long term. To address needs and concerns of stroke survivors, a combination of input from health and social care services is required. Current research mainly focuses on interventions aimed at increasing activity and participation after stroke. In the UK and worldwide, many support services for long-term stroke survivors are community based, locally organised and provided by voluntary sector organisations.

Discrepancies exist between stroke survivors perceptions of the markers of their recovery and needs after stroke, compared to those of their caregivers and healthcare professionals. It is important that these differences in perceived needs are addressed sensitively yet realistically, to ensure that the long-term goals of stroke survivors are achieved in an environment that is supportive of their individual needs.

References

1. Wilkinson PR, Wolfe CD, Warburton FG, Rudd AG, Howard RS, Ross-Russell RW, Beech R. Longer term quality of life and outcome in stroke patients: is the Barthel index alone an adequate measure of outcome? *Qual Health Care* 1997; 6(3): 125–130.

2. Hankey GJ, Jamrozik K, Broadhurst RJ, Forbes S, Anderson CS. Long-term disability after first-ever stroke and related prognostic factors in the Perth Community Stroke Study, 1989–1990. *Stroke* 2002; 33(4): 1034–1040.

3. Royal College of Physicians Intercollegiate Stroke Working Party. National Clinical Guidelines for Stroke. 3rd Edn. London: Royal College of Physicians; 2008.

4. World Health Organisation. International Classification of Functioning, Disability and Health (ICF). Geneva: WHO; 2001.

5. World Health Organisation. International Classification of Impairments, Disabilities, and Handicaps. Geneva: WHO; 1980.

6. Hodkinson HM. Evaluation of a mental test score for assessment of mental impairment in the elderly. *Age Ageing* 1972; 1(4): 233–238.

7. Folstein MF, Folstein SE, McHugh PR. "Mini-mental state". A practical method for grading the cognitive state of patients for the clinician. *J Psychiatr Res* 1975; 12(3): 189–198.

8. Demeurisse G, Demol O, Robaye E. Motor evaluation in vascular hemiplegia. *Eur Neurol*; 19(6): 382–389.

9. Bohannon RW, Smith MB. Interrater reliability of a modified Ashworth scale of muscle spasticity. *Phys Ther* 1987; 67(2): 206–207.

10. Gregson JM, Leathley M, Moore AP, Sharma AK, Smith TL, Watkins CL. Reliability of the Tone Assessment Scale and the modified Ashworth scale as clinical tools for assessing poststroke spasticity. *Arch Phys Med Rehabil* 1999; 80(9): 1013–1016.

11. Michielsen HJ, De Vries J, Van Heck GL. Psychometric qualities of a brief self-rated fatigue measure: the fatigue assessment scale. *J Psychosom Res* 2003; 54(4): 345–352.

12. Robertson IH, Ward T, Ridgeway V, Nimmo-Smith I. The structure of normal human attention: the test of everyday attention. *J Int Neuropsychol Soc* 1996; 2(6): 525–534.

13. Zigmond AS, Snaith RP. The hospital anxiety and depression scale. *Acta Psychiatr Scand* 1983; 67(6): 361–370.

14. Beck AT, Ward CH, Mendelson M, Mock J, Erbaugh J. An inventory for measuring depression. *Arch Gen Psychiatry* 1961; 4: 561–571.

15. Hendricks HT, van LJ, Geurts AC, Zwarts MJ. Motor recovery after stroke: a systematic review of the literature. *Arch Phys Med Rehabil* 2002; 83(11): 1629–1637.

16. Watkins CL, Leathley MJ, Gregson JM, Moore AP, Smith TL, Sharma AK. Prevalence of spasticity post stroke. *Clin Rehabil* 2002; 16(5): 515–522.

17. Lundstrom E, Terent A, Borg J. Prevalence of disabling spasticity 1 year after first-ever stroke. *Eur J Neurol* 2008; 15(6): 533–539.

18. Broome BA. The impact of urinary incontinence on self-efficacy and quality of life. *Health Qual Life Outcomes* 2003; 1: 35.

19. Patel M, Coshall C, Rudd AG, Wolfe CD. Natural history and effects on 2-year outcomes of urinary incontinence after stroke. *Stroke* 2001; 32(1): 122–127.

20. Wein AJ. Impact of urinary incontinence after stroke: results from a prospective population-based stroke register. *J Urol* 2005; 173(6): 2057.

21. Harari D, Coshall C, Rudd AG, Wolfe CD. New-onset fecal incontinence after stroke: prevalence, natural history, risk factors, and impact. *Stroke* 2003; 34(1): 144–150.

22. Appelros P. Prevalence and predictors of pain and fatigue after stroke: a population-based study. *Int J Rehabil Res* 2006; 29(4): 329–333.

23. Widar M, Samuelsson L, Karlsson-Tivenius S, Ahlstrom G. Long-term pain conditions after a stroke. *J Rehabil Med* 2002; 34(4): 165–170.

24. Kumar G, Soni CR. Central post-stroke pain: Current evidence. *J Neurol Sci* 2009 May 4.

25. Colle F, Bonan I, Gellez Leman MC, Bradai N, Yelnik A. Fatigue after stroke. *Ann Readapt Med Phys* 2006; 49(6): 272–274.

26. Smith OR, van den Broek KC, Renkens M, Denollet J. Comparison of fatigue levels in patients with stroke and patients with end-stage heart failure: application of the fatigue assessment scale. *J Am Geriatr Soc* 2008; 56(10): 1915–1919.

27. Tatemichi TK, Desmond DW, Paik M, Figueroa M, Gropen TI, Stern Y, Sano M, Remien R, Williams JB, Mohr JP. Clinical determinants of dementia related to stroke. *Ann Neurol* 1993; 33(6): 568–575.

28. Patel M, Coshall C, Rudd AG, Wolfe CD. Natural history of cognitive impairment after stroke and factors associated with its recovery. *Clin Rehabil* 2003; 17(2): 158–166.

29. Tham W, Auchus AP, Thong M, Goh ML, Chang HM, Wong MC, Chen CP. Progression of cognitive impairment after stroke: one year results from a longitudinal study of Singaporean stroke patients. *J Neurol Sci* 2002; 203–204: 49–52.

30. del ST, Barba R, Morin MM, Domingo J, Cemillan C, Pondal M, Vivancos J. Evolution of cognitive impairment after stroke and risk factors for delayed progression. *Stroke* 2005; 36(12): 2670–2675.

31. Hyndman D, Ashburn A. People with stroke living in the community: attention deficits, balance, ADL ability and falls. *Disabil Rehabil* 2003; 25(15): 817–822.

32. Teasdale TW, Engberg AW. Psychosocial consequences of stroke: a long-term population-based follow-up. *Brain Inj* 2005; 19(12): 1049–1058.

33. Laska AC, Hellblom A, Murray V, Kahan T, von AM. Aphasia in acute stroke and relation to outcome. *J Intern Med* 2001; 249(5): 413–422.

34. Hackett ML, Yapa C, Parag V, Anderson CS. Frequency of depression after stroke: a systematic review of observational studies. *Stroke* 2005; 36(6): 1330–1340.

35. Collin C, Wade DT, Davies S, Horne V. The Barthel ADL Index: a reliability study. *Int Disabil Stud* 1988; 10(2): 61–63.

36. Holbrook M, Skilbeck CE. An activities index for use with stroke patients. *Age Ageing* 1983; 12(2): 166–170.

37. Keith RA, Granger CV, Hamilton BB, Sherwin FS. The functional independence measure: a new tool for rehabilitation. *Adv Clin Rehabil* 1987; 1: 6–18.

38. van Swieten JC, Koudstaal PJ, Visser MC, Schouten HJ, van Gijn J. Interobserver agreement for the assessment of handicap in stroke patients. *Stroke* 1988; 19(5): 604–607.

39. Patel MD, Tilling K, Lawrence E, Rudd AG, Wolfe CD, McKevitt C. Relationships between long-term stroke disability, handicap and health-related quality of life. *Age Ageing* 2006; 35(3): 273–279.

40. Welmer AK, von AM, Widen HL, Sommerfeld DK. Spasticity and its association with functioning and health-related quality of life 18 months after stroke. *Cerebrovasc Dis* 2006; 21(4): 247–253.

41. Kikuchi A, Niu K, Ikeda Y, Hozawa A, Nakagawa H, Guo H, Ohmori-Matsuda K, Yang G, Farmawati A, Sami A, Arai Y, Tsuji I, Nagatomi R. Association between physical activity and urinary incontinence in a community-based elderly population aged 70 years and over. *Eur Urol* 2007; 52(3): 868–874.

42. Tibaek S, Gard G, Klarskov P, Iversen HK, Dehlendorff C, Jensen R. Are activity limitations associated with lower urinary tract symptoms in stroke

patients? A cross-sectional, clinical survey. *Scand J Urol Nephrol* 2009; 43(5): 1–7.

43. Widar M, Ahlstrom G. Disability after a stroke and the influence of long-term pain on everyday life. *Scand J Caring Sci* 2002; 16(3): 302–310.

44. Harwood RH, Rogers A, Dickinson E, Ebrahim S. Measuring handicap: the London Handicap Scale, a new outcome measure for chronic disease. *Qual Health Care* 1994; 3(1): 11–16.

45. Ware JE, Jr., Sherbourne CD. The MOS 36-item short-form health survey (SF-36). I. Conceptual framework and item selection. *Med Care* 1992; 30(6): 473–483.

46. Ware J, Jr., Kosinski M, Keller SD. A 12-Item Short-Form Health Survey: construction of scales and preliminary tests of reliability and validity. *Med Care* 1996; 34(3): 220–233.

47. Ware JE, Kosinski M, Keller SD. *SF-12: How to Score the SF-12 Physical and Mental Health Summary Scales.* 3rd Edn. Lincoln, RI: QualityMetric Incorporated; 1998.

48. EuroQol — a new facility for the measurement of health-related quality of life. The EuroQol Group. *Health Policy* 1990; 16(3): 199–208.

49. Burton CR. Living with stroke: a phenomenological study. *J Adv Nurs* 2000; 32(2): 301–309.

50. Hafsteinsdottir TB, Grypdonck M. Being a stroke patient: a review of the literature. *J Adv Nurs* 1997; 26(3): 580–588.

51. Pajalic Z, Karlsson S, Westergren A. Functioning and subjective health among stroke survivors after discharge from hospital. *J Adv Nurs* 2006; 54(4): 457–466.

52. Sabari JS, Meisler J, Silver E. Reflections upon rehabilitation by members of a community based stroke club. *Disability and Rehabilitation* 2000; 22(7): 330–336.

53. Wade DT, Legh-Smith J, Hewer RL. Effects of living with and looking after survivors of a stroke. *Br Med J (Clin Res Ed)* 1986; 293(6544): 418–420.

54. D'Alisa S, Baudo S, Mauro A, Miscio G. How does stroke restrict participation in long-term post-stroke survivors? *Acta Neurol Scand* 2005; 112(3): 157–162.

55. Desrosiers J, Noreau L, Rochette A, Bourbonnais D, Bravo G, Bourget A. Predictors of long-term participation after stroke. *Disabil Rehabil* 2006; 28(4): 221–230.

56. Niemi ML, Laaksonen R, Kotila M, Waltimo O. Quality of life 4 years after stroke. *Stroke* 1988; 19(9): 1101–1107.

57. Drummond A. Leisure activity after stroke. *Int Disabil Stud* 1990; 12(4): 157–160.

58. Bhogal SK, Teasell RW, Foley NC, Speechley MR. Community reintegration after stroke. *Top Stroke Rehabil* 2003; 10(2): 107–129.

59. Busch MA, Coshall C, Heuschmann PU, McKevitt C, Wolfe CD. Sociodemographic differences in return to work after stroke: the South London Stroke Register (SLSR). *J Neurol Neurosurg Psychiatry* 2009; 80(8): 888–893.

60. Kersten P, Low JT, Ashburn A, George SL, McLellan DL. The unmet needs of young people who have had a stroke: results of a national UK survey. *Disabil Rehabil* 2002; 24(16): 860–866.

61. Daniel K, Wolfe CD, Busch MA, McKevitt C. What are the social consequences of stroke for working-aged adults? A systematic review. *Stroke* 2009; 40(6): e431–e440.

62. Desrosiers J, Bourbonnais D, Noreau L, Rochette A, Bravo G, Bourget A. Participation after stroke compared to normal aging. *J Rehabil Med* 2005; 37(6): 353–357.

63. Rimmer JH, Wang E, Smith D. Barriers associated with exercise and community access for individuals with stroke. *J Rehabil Res Dev* 2008; 45(2): 315–322.

64. Shaughnessy M, Resnick BM, Macko RF. Testing a model of post-stroke exercise behavior. *Rehabil Nurs* 2006; 31(1): 15–21.

65. Labi ML, Phillips TF, Greshman GE. Psychosocial disability in physically restored long-term stroke survivors. *Arch Phys Med Rehabil* 1980; 61(12): 561–565.

66. Murray J, Ashworth R, Forster A, Young J. Developing a primary care-based stroke service: a review of the qualitative literature. *Br J Gen Pract* 2003; 53(487): 137–142.

67. O'Mahony PG, Rodgers H, Thomson RG, Dobson R, James OF. Satisfaction with information and advice received by stroke patients. *Clin Rehabil* 1997; 11(1): 68–72.

68. Hanger HC, Mulley GP. Questions people ask about stroke. *Stroke* 1993; 24(4): 536–538.

69. Hanger HC, Walker G, Paterson LA, McBride S, Sainsbury R. What do patients and their carers want to know about stroke? A two-year follow-up study. *Clin Rehabil* 1998; 12(1): 45–52.

70. Kim P, Warren S, Madill H, Hadley M. Quality of life of stroke survivors. *Qual Life Res* 1999; 8(4): 293–301.

71. Gottlieb A, Golander H, Bar-Tal Y, Gottlieb D. The influence of social support and perceived control on handicap and quality of life after stroke. *Aging (Milano)* 2001; 13(1): 11–15.

72. King RB. Quality of Life After Stroke. *Stroke* 1996; 27(9): 1467–1472.

73. Kotila M, Numminen H, Waltimo O, Kaste M. Depression after stroke: results of the Finnstroke Study. *Stroke* 1998; 29(2): 368–372.

74. Berg A, Palomaki H, Lonnqvist J, Lehtihalmes M, Kaste M. Depression among caregivers of stroke survivors. *Stroke* 2005; 36(3): 639–643.

75. Han B, Haley WE. Family caregiving for patients with stroke. Review and analysis. *Stroke* 1999; 30(7): 1478–1485.

76. Wilkinson PR, Wolfe CD, Warburton FG, Rudd AG, Howard RS, Ross-Russell RW, Beech RR. A long-term follow-up of stroke patients. *Stroke* 1997; 28(3): 507–512.

77. Kendall E, Catalano T, Kuipers P, Posner N, Buys N, Charker J. Recovery following stroke: the role of self-management education. *Soc Sci Med* 2007; 64(3): 735–746.

78. Clark MS, Smith DS. Factors contributing to patient satisfaction with rehabilitation following stroke. *Int J Rehabil Res* 1998; 21(2): 143–154.

79. Wu HM, Tang JL, Lin XP, Lau JLP, Leung PC, Woo J, Li Y. Acupuncture for stroke rehabilitation. *Cochrane Database of Systematic Reviews* 2006; (3): CD004131.

80. Rosales RL, Chua-Yap AS. Evidence-based systematic review on the efficacy and safety of botulinum toxin-A therapy in post-stroke spasticity. *J Neural Transm* 2008; 115(4): 617–623.

81. Caty GD, Detrembleur C, Bleyenheuft C, Deltombe T, Lejeune TM. Effect of upper limb botulinum toxin injections on impairment, activity, participation, and quality of life among stroke patients. *Stroke* 2009; 40(7): 2589–2591.

82. Mehrholz J, Werner C, Kugler J, Pohl M. Electromechanical-assisted training for walking after stroke. *Cochrane Database Syst Rev* 2007; (4): CD006185.

83. French B, Thomas LH, Leathley MJ, Sutton CJ, McAdam J, Forster A, Langhorne P, Price CI, Walker A, Watkins CL. Repetitive task training for improving functional ability after stroke. *Cochrane Database Syst Rev* 2007; (4): CD006073.

84. Ngan-Hing L, Stretton C. Does rehabilitaion improve gait and quality of life for chronic survivors? *New Zealand Journal of Physiother* 2006; 34(3): 147.

85. Wade DT, Collen FM, Robb GF, Warlow CP. Physiotherapy intervention late after stroke and mobility. *BMJ* 1992; 304(6827): 609–613.

86. Green J, Forster A, Bogle S, Young J. Physiotherapy for patients with mobility problems more than 1 year after stroke: a randomised controlled trial. *Lancet* 2002; 359(9302): 199–203.

87. Legg LA, Drummond AE, Langhorne P. Occupational therapy for patients with problems in activities of daily living after stroke. *Cochrane Database Syst Rev* 2006; (4): CD003585.

88. Aziz NA, Leonardi-Bee J, Phillips M, Gladman JR, Legg L, Walker MF. Therapy-based rehabilitation services for patients living at home more than one year after stroke. *Cochrane Database Syst Rev* 2008; (2): CD005952.

89. van der Gaag A, Smith L, Davis S, Moss B, Cornelius V, Laing S, Mowles C. Therapy and support services for people with long-term stroke and aphasia and their relatives: a six-month follow-up study. *Clin Rehabil* 2005; 19(4): 372–380.

90. Bhogal SK, Teasell RW, Foley NC, Speechley MR. Rehabilitation of aphasia: more is better. *Top Stroke Rehabil* 2003; 10(2): 66–76.

91. Egan M, Kessler D, Laporte L, Metcalfe V, Carter M. A pilot randomized controlled trial of community-based occupational therapy in late stroke rehabilitation. *Top Stroke Rehabil* 2007; 14(5): 37–45.

92. Parker CJ, Gladman JR, Drummond AE, Dewey ME, Lincoln NB, Barer D, Logan PA, Radford KA. A multicentre randomized controlled trial of leisure therapy and conventional occupational therapy after stroke. TOTAL Study Group. Trial of Occupational Therapy and Leisure. *Clin Rehabil* 2001; 15(1): 42–52.

93. Desrosiers J, Noreau L, Rochette A, Carbonneau H, Fontaine L, Viscogliosi C, Bravo G. Effect of a home leisure education program after stroke: a randomized controlled trial. *Arch Phys Med Rehabil* 2007; 88(9): 1095–1100.

94. Hartman-Maeir A, Eliad Y, Kizoni R, Nahaloni I, Kelberman H, Katz N. Evaluation of a long-term community based rehabilitation program for adult stroke survivors. *NeuroRehabilitation* 2007; 22(4): 295–301.

95. Beckley MN. The influence of the quality and quantity of social support in the promotion of community participation following stroke. *Aust Occup Ther J* 2007; 54(3): 215.

96. Greveson GC, Gray CS, French JM, James OF. Long-term outcome for patients and carers following hospital admission for stroke. *Age Ageing* 1991; 20(5): 337–344.

97. Clark MS, Rubenach S, Winsor A. A randomized controlled trial of an education and counselling intervention for families after stroke. *Clin Rehabil* 2003; 17(7): 703–712.

98. Mann WC, Ottenbacher KJ, Fraas L, Tomita M, Granger CV. Effectiveness of assistive technology and environmental interventions in maintaining independence and reducing home care costs for the frail elderly. A randomized controlled trial. *Arch Fam Med* 1999; 8(3): 210–217.

99. Department of Health. National Stroke Strategy. Department of Health; 2007.

100. Department of Health. National service framework for older people. 2001.

101. National Stroke Foundation. Clinical Guidelines for Stroke Rehabilitation and Recovery. Melbourne 2005.

102. Gordon NF, Gulanick M, Costa F, Fletcher G, Franklin BA, Roth EJ, Shephard T. Physical activity and exercise recommendations for stroke survivors: an American Heart Association scientific statement from the Council on Clinical Cardiology, Subcommittee on Exercise, Cardiac Rehabilitation, and Prevention; the Council on Cardiovascular Nursing; the Council on Nutrition, Physical Activity, and Metabolism; and the Stroke Council. *Stroke* 2004; 35(5): 1230–1240.

103. http://www.stroke.org.uk

104. http://www.chss.org.uk/community_support/stroke_servies/index.php

105. Ch'Ng AM, French D, Mclean N. Coping with the challenges of recovery from stroke long term perspectives of stroke support group members. *J Health Psychol* 2008; 13(8): 1136–1146.

106. Mayo NE, Wood-Dauphinee S, Ahmed S, Gordon C, Higgins J, McEwen S, Salbach N. Disablement following stroke. *Disability and Rehabilitation* 1999; 21(5–6): 258–268.

107. Talbot LR, Viscogliosi C, Desrosiers J, Vincent C, Rousseau J, Robichaud L. Identification of rehabilitation needs after a stroke: an exploratory study. *Health Qual Life Outcomes* 2004; 2: 53.

108. Faircloth CA, Boylstein C, Rittman M, Young ME, Gubrium J. Sudden illness and biographical flow in narratives of stroke recovery. *Sociol Health Illn* 2004; 26(2): 242–261.

109. Pound P, Gompertz P, Ebrahim S. A patient-centred study of the consequences of stroke. *Clin Rehabil* 1998; 12(4): 338–347.

110. Becker G. Continuity after a stroke — implications of life-course disruption in old-age. *Gerontologist* 1993; 33(2): 148–158.

111. Salter K, Hellings C, Foley N, Teasell R. The experience of living with stroke: a qualitative meta-synthesis. *J Rehabil Med* 2008; 40(8): 595–602.

112. Lynch EB, Butt Z, Heinemann A, Victorson D, Nowinski CJ, Perez L, Cella D. A qualitative study of quality of life after stroke: the importance of social relationships. *J Rehabil Med* 2008; 40(7): 518–523.

113. Haun J, Rittman M, Sberna M. The continuum of connectedness and social isolation during post stroke recovery. *J Aging Stud* 2008; 22(1): 54–64.

114. Kvigne K, Kirkevold M, Gjengedal E. Fighting back — struggling to continue life and preserve the self following a stroke. *Health Care Women Int* 2004; 25(4): 370–387.

115. Vincent C, Deaudelin I, Robichaud L, Rousseau J, Viscogliosi C, Talbot L, Desrosiers J, other members of the BRAD group. Rehabilitation needs for older adults with stroke living at home: perceptions of four populations. *BMC Geriatrics* 2007; 7(1): 20.

116. Sabari JS, Meisler J, Silver E. Reflections upon rehabilitation by members of a community based stroke club. *Disabil Rehabil* 2000; 22(7): 330–336.

117. Lilley SA, Lincoln NB, Francis VM. A qualitative study of stroke patients' and carers' perceptions of the stroke family support organizer service. *Clin Rehabil* 2003; 17(5): 540–547.

118. Hartman-Maeir A, Soroker N, Ring H, Avni N, Katz N. Activities, participation and satisfaction one-year post stroke. *Disabil Rehabil* 2007; 29(7): 559.

119. Ownsworth T, Turpin M, Brook A, Fleming J. Patient perspectives of an individualised self-awareness intervention following stroke: a qualitative case study. *Neuropscychol Rehab* 2008; 18(5/6): 692–712.

120. Carin-Levy G, Kendall M, Young A, Mead G. The psychosocial effects of exercise and relaxation classes for persons surviving a stroke. *Can J Occup Ther* 2009; 76(2): 73–80.

121. Lincoln NB, Francis VM, Lilley SA, Sharma JC, Summerfield M. Evalution of a stroke family support organiser, a randomized controller trial. *Stroke* 2003; 34: 116–121.

10 Caregiver Needs and Their Management in Stroke

Anne Forster*

Chapter Summary

Stroke is a family illness generating considerable personal, financial and societal burdens. After initial hospital treatment, many patients will be dependent on informal caregivers, usually family members, to provide assistance with activities of daily living, including bathing, dressing, and toileting. This burden of care has an important effect on caregivers' physical and psychosocial well-being, with nearly a half of caregivers reporting health problems, and many demonstrating anxiety and emotional distress.

The successful rehabilitation and adjustment of patients and their caregivers to the aftermath of stroke are clearly interlinked. However, caregivers' central role is often given low priority in the management of stroke, and they may feel excluded from the rehabilitation process. Caregivers require appropriate and timely information on stroke, the services and financial support available. Advice and guidance on the practical management of the patients' physical abilities would be appreciated. The burden of care may be unremitting even two or three years after the initial event. However, the complex interplay of the patient's disability, patient's

*Academic Unit of Elderly Care and Rehabilitation, University of Leeds and Bradford Institute for Health Research, Bradford, UK

and caregiver's mood, caregiver's own health and environmental factors including service and family support available, makes it difficult to predict which caregivers will be at risk of poor psychological outcomes.

The increasing evidence base reflects the growing recognition of the importance of caregivers. A range of interventions have been evaluated by randomised trial. There are suggestions of benefit from a structured competency-based training programme and some problem-solving approaches.

Introduction

Stroke is a family illness. Despite major steps forward in stroke treatment and care, the impact of stroke remains challenging for many. These challenges include coming to terms with a sudden major illness, understanding the treatment offered and the services and support that may be available, in addition to the practical and psychological difficulties created by physical and cognitive impairment. Few patients face these challenge alone and many are supported by partners and family, who in the health and social service systems, become re-categorised as caregivers. These caregivers frequently play a central role in the continued rehabilitation of the stroke survivor assisting in the 'restoration of the individual to his (or her) fullest physical, mental and social capability'.[1]

Stroke Event

> "It never occurred to either of us that it would ever happen to us. So that
> was our main feeling. Astonishment, almost — even incredulity."

The early emotions after stroke are ones of shock and confusion. Robust evidence supports the recommendation that patients with moderate or severe symptoms should be referred to hospital with the expectation of admission to a stroke unit.[2] Caregiver support has been identified as a key component of stroke unit care, yet, as currently provided, it is not compatible with their expressed needs. Caregivers feel excluded from the rehabilitation process,[3,4] are reluctant to ask busy staff for information and find visiting tiring and stressful.[5,6] The need for clear appropriate information is a common theme which is often not adequately addressed.[3–5]

Preparation for Home

"They brought K home for a weekend and they said, we're discharging him next week. I thought, oh my God, what do I do?"

Caregivers' pre-discharge information priorities may be different from those of rehabilitation staff, with caregivers identifying falls prevention, nutrition, staying active/mobility, managing stress and dealing with patient mood changes as particular priorities.[6,7] Caregivers do not feel adequately prepared for their caring role, with little information provided to help inform decisions.[3] Advice and guidance on the practical management of the patient's physical abilities would be appreciated[3] and there are missed opportunities for structured skills training.[5]

A recent systematic review of information provision which included 17 randomised trials involving 1773 patients and 1058 caregivers reported that provision of information in the ways evaluated (for example, leaflets, information packs, multidisciplinary team meetings) enhanced patient and caregiver knowledge but did not impact on caregiver stress. Interactive educational strategies in which there were opportunities to ask questions had a greater effect on patient but not caregiver mood.[8] One study evaluated provision of educational sessions (one inpatient and six post-discharge), content included the nature of stroke, role of therapy, psychological effects of stroke and risk reduction.[9] Although the course was well-received by those attending and was successful in improving stroke knowledge, compliance was low with only a small proportion of the caregivers (20 out of 107) attending three or more post-discharge sessions, citing poor health, work commitments or lack of interest as reasons for non-attendance. A more recent study reported similar problems with attendance.[10] A telephone support group for caregivers, which involved eight one-hour sessions supported by printed materials, is feasible but had limited impact.[11]

A different approach is to provide more structured training to caregivers whilst the patient is an inpatient. Kalra and colleagues[12] have reported the effectiveness of a systematic and structured training programme for caregivers, which included assessment of competencies in skills essential for the day-to-day management of disabled stroke survivors. The intervention was effective in decreasing caregiver burden and in decreasing their anxiety and depression, improving psychological outcomes for patients and reducing overall costs.[13] However, there are limitations to the generalisability of the trial findings as the intervention was tested in a single middle class suburban area, delivered by a separate specialist team that might be expected to have heightened motivation and expertise. Whilst promising, the intervention awaits wider testing.

Discharge Home

"As a carer, I feel on my own. You feel abandoned when the physio stops."

"Of course my life has changed dramatically. Its hard; it's not a piece of cake. But saying that, I don't do so bad. I can pat myself on the back a bit."

Once discharged home, the majority of patients will be dependent on informal caregivers, usually family members, to provide assistance with activities of daily living.[14–16] The early weeks at home are particularly challenging as caregivers face practical difficulties providing assistance in activities such as walking to the toilet that seemed much simpler in the hospital setting. In a community based sample ($n = 84$), 52% of patients received assistance for dressing, 48% for bathing and 36% for feeding one year after the stroke.[14] The majority of patients (over 80%) require help for more general domestic activities such as household maintenance and house work and community activities such as shopping, providing transport and arranging services.[15]

Caregiving tasks may change over time with a gradual shift from practical tasks, for example, helping with medicine and finances to assisting with travel and leisure activities by one year post-stroke, reflecting patient improvement or an adjustment in priorities.[16] Considerable time is spent in caregiving activities with estimates of six hours a day even six month after the event,[16,17] increasing to over ten hours if general supervision of the patient is included.[18]

It has been demonstrated that the presence of a caregiver who is initially informed about stroke and not depressed is a predictor of a satisfactory home situation.[19]

Need for information remains a consistent theme post-discharge[7,20,21] and for many years later as information is requested on stroke, the services available, aids and adaptations as well as financial benefits available.[22] Caregivers are often unaware of the services and support that may be available to them.[17] Services that were expected did not arrive[23] and services that might have been appropriate were not offered.[22] It is difficult to say whether this was because information was given but not absorbed, or not given.[7] This compounds feelings of 'abandoned'[4] and isolation. The opportunity to talk to other people in similar situations[4] is valued.

Longer Term Outcome

"As a carer I feel on my own...absolutely on my own"

"I can't go out by myself. I don't...well actually I could, but I don't like to leave him."

A review of over 70 studies has indicated the range of physical, practical and emotional problems facing patients after stroke.[24] Approximately one-third suffer depression in the first year after stroke, and this may be linked with fatigue, pain, falling, cognitive impairment, urinary incontinence and sexual dysfunction, all of which are challenges for families to address. Few patients return to work and financial problems are common.[24]

A review of 39 stroke studies has highlighted the complexity of factors effecting carer outcomes.[25] Caregivers' health-related quality of life may improve over the first six months post-discharge but deteriorate over time, being worse at 12 months.[26] Their psychological well-being may become less linked to the patient's physical ability and more influenced by the patient's cognitive behavioural and emotional changes over time.[27] Poor psychological caregiver outcomes may not necessarily be linked to duration of caring.[28,29]

Time for social events, levels of energy and emotional well-being are adversely effected. Many struggle with the altered role which may involve undertaking new physical activities and financial responsibilities, but also a more fundamental shift from husband and wife to patient and caregiver.[5,30] Disparity between health professionals' and families' perceptions of the recovery process with patients and caregivers measuring recovery in relation to their lives before and after stroke rather than from the stroke event, leads to disappointment when therapy intervention is stopped.[31]

Depression is common with prevalence of up to 52%, depending on the measures used and is consistently higher than comparison control groups.[32,33] Anxiety and emotional distress are also prevalent, effecting about one-half of caregivers at six months after the stroke.[34]

Caregivers' general health may also suffer, with symptoms of reduced physical strength, headache, poor appetite, musculoskeletal pain, breathlessness,[20] with nearly a half of caregivers reporting health complaints resulting from their caring role.[21] Increase strain may also lead to other adverse events. In one exploratory survey of 124 caregivers with a mean of two and a half years caring, 37 (30%) reported accidents in the previous six months. These included cuts and bruises, falls, car accidents and burns whilst cooking. Women were significantly more likely to report accident than men, those reporting accidents were more likely to receive help from others, caring for longer and expressed greater personal strain than those not reporting accidents.[35]

Adjustment

"There is life after stroke. It depends on what you want to do. You can get a different view of the world."

"You've got to learn to laugh — you've got to be strong. Carers have to be strong."

Adjustment varies according to the patient's and caregiver's individual circumstances. Whilst the burden of caring may ease over time for some, for others, concerns for example, about another stroke, falls or leaving the patient alone, means that their caring role is unremitting.[14] Almost half of all caregivers describe themselves as poorly adjusted after two to three years.[36] Not surprisingly, the quality of the relationship can be adversely affected[37] but this is not always the case as in one cohort almost a-third of respondents report improvements in relationships.[38]

The Burden of Caregiving

"I always run out of hours in the day you know, so I just keep very very busy."

Burden is defined as 'something that is exacting, oppressive or difficult to bear'.[39] Objective burden relates to the tasks undertaken, such as assisting with washing and dressing, whilst subjective burden refers to the psychosocial impact of caring. Subjective burden may be related to the objective burden of number of tasks performed rather than time spent caregiving.[17,18] Less strain is associated with spending more time with the patient, which may suggest that caregivers under greater strain are those who are not normally with the patient and have to fit in providing care around other tasks (for example, work and family commitments).[17] This applies to young female caregivers who report feeling overlooked by staff and may be in particular need of attention.[29] Poor psychological outcomes for caregivers is associated with caregiver mood in the early post-stroke phase[33,34,40,41] and the perceived[40] and actual[34] physical disability of the patient. High burden has been linked to lower quality of life.[18,27,29]

Risk Factors for Poor Outcomes in Caregivers

It is difficult to confidently predict which caregivers may be at risk of poor psychological outcomes. The interplay of the patient's disability, patient's and caregiver's mood, caregiver's own health and environmental factors including service and family support available is complex. Different factors can be associated with strain at different time points.[17,26] Different studies identifying different factors, and cause and effect of the range of factors is difficult to determine.[25] Regression models rarely predict more than 50% of caregiver's psychological outcomes. In addition, many reported studies include selected populations, for example, patients discharged from rehabilitation, recruits to randomised trials, volunteers from stroke clubs, therefore generalisability is limited.[37] It is likely, however, that caregivers with health problems of their own while caring for more disabled patients experience most strain in the first six months after the event.[18]

Measurement of Caregiving Outcomes

Outcome measures relevant to caregiving have been subject to reviews, both generic[42] and stroke specific.[43,44] Deeken and colleagues[42] identified 28 measures (17 burden instruments; eight needs instruments; three caregiver specific quality of life measures). Whilst summarising the requirements of an appropriate assessment tool: relevant, valid, reliable and sensitive to change, they make the important point that an assessment tool itself should not increase the burden of caregivers. Visser-Meily and colleagues[43] identified 97 stroke studies which used 45 different outcome measures to assess the impact of stroke on the caregiver, including 16 different burden scales. Eleven different measures have been used to measure caregiver depression. Most of the scales demonstrated moderate to good quality but for some there was no information available on reliability and for many of the scales there was little information about sensitivity to change.

Interventions

The growing recognition of the importance of caregivers in the recovery and rehabilitation of patients after stroke is reflected in the increasing evidence base. A number of overlapping systematic reviews have summarised the literature.[32,45–50]

Based on the theories of coping, attempts have been made to reduce stress and enhance the inner resources of the caregivers. One approach is to teach problem-solving skills, in which identified problems are refined and defined into more manageable (and solvable) components. A recent review of theoretically-based psychosocial interventions identified seven trials, based on four different psychological models (family systems theory, cognitive behaviour therapy, social problem-solving training and stress coping model). There were inconsistencies in the outcome measures used, length of follow-up and results, making it difficult to draw conclusions; however, there was a suggestion of benefit from problem-solving approaches.[48]

A review of evidence specifically focused on problem-solving identified 11 studies, six of which were randomised trials (four included in ref. 48). A wide range of different approaches were used with limited information on the theoretical approaches informing the interventions, and there was limited evidence of benefit.[49] Individual studies have reported benefits. For example, a randomised trial by Grant and colleagues,[51] in which problem-solving skills training was provided through one home visit and seven subsequent telephone contacts, reported positive benefits for caregivers, with reduction in depression, and improvements in mental health and social functioning. The intervention had no effect on burden and whether the effects were sustained was not assessed. Problem-solving and goal-setting is challenging in a situation where patients and caregivers (and professionals) may have very different perceptions of achievement, with patients focusing on what they could not yet do rather than goals achieved.[31]

The evidence for the effectiveness of stroke liaison workers has been evaluated in a systematic review. Liaison workers included in the review came from a range of backgrounds: nursing, social work, psychology and allied health professionals, and generally provided emotional and social support as well as information to stroke patients and their families, and liaised with services with the aim of improving aspects of participation and quality of life for patients and/or their caregivers. The review included 16 trials ($n = 4916$) which reported no significant difference in caregiver subjective health status, extended activities of daily living or mental health. Caregivers did, however, report satisfaction that they were not neglected, that they had received adequate information about the causes of stroke and recovery from stroke and that someone had really listened.[52]

The largest and most inclusive review is that by Visser-Meily and colleagues[46] which included 22 studies, four of which were randomised trials focused only on the caregivers. Of the 22 studies, ten reported positive benefits on one or more of the outcome measures, the conclusion were similar to other reviews reporting modest benefits for problem-solving approaches.

Respite care (adult day care, in-home respite, and institutional care) is positively received by caregivers but reported benefits on caregiver burden and mental and physical health are small.[53]

The reviews outlined above have informed the development of guidelines.[54,55] The UK guidelines recommend that the patients' views be sought on the involvement of their family members, that caregivers be involved in the management processes and be given emotional and practical support. Caregivers should be encouraged to participate in an educational programme, and be assessed for their own needs and provided with appropriate support.

Conclusions

The need to provide appropriate and timely information, services and support for caregivers after stroke is clear. With the current emphasis on shorter hospital stays, caregivers will play an increasingly important role in the care and continued rehabilitation of patients after stroke. The evidence base is developing rapidly and some suggestions for the way forward are emerging. Caregivers have expressed need for specific training in nursing and personal care techniques, and such a programme delivered in stroke units has demonstrated advantages in a single centre study. Some problem-solving approaches seem to suggest positive gains, but methods of delivery require refinement.

References

1. Mair A. Report of a sub-committee of the Standing medical Advisory Committee, Scottish health Service Council on Medical Rehabilitation. Edinburgh, HMSO; 1972.
2. Stroke Unit Trialists' Collaboration. Collaborative systematic review of the randomised trials of organised inpatient (stroke unit) care after stroke. *BMJ* 1997; 314: 1151–1159.
3. Brereton L, Nolan M. 'You do know he's had a stroke don't you?' Preparation for family caregiving — the neglected dimension *J Clin Nursing* 2000; 9(4): 498–506.

4. Kerr S, Smith L. Stroke: an exploration of the experience of informal caregiving. *Clin Rehabil* 2001; 15: 428–436.
5. Smith LN, Lawrence M, Kerr SM, Langhorne P, Lees KR. Informal carers experience of caring for stroke survivors. *J Adv Nursing* 2004; 46(3): 235–244.
6. Mackenzie A, Perry L, Lockhart E, Cottee M, Cloud G, Mann H. Family carers of stroke survivors: needs, knowledge, satisfaction and competence in caring. *Disabil Rehabil* 2007; 29(2): 111–121.
7. Pierce LL, Finn MG, Steiner V. Families dealing with stroke desire information about self-care needs. *Rehabil Nursing* 2004; 29(1): 14–17.
8. Smith J, Forster A, House A, Knapp P, Wright JJ, Young J. Information provision for stroke patients and their caregivers. *Cochrane Database of Systematic Reviews* 2008; Issue 2.
9. Rodgers H, Atkinson C, Bond S, Suddes M, Dobson R, Curless R. Randomized controlled trial of a comprehensive stroke education program for patients and caregivers. *Stroke* 1999; 30(12): 2585–2591.
10. Larson J, Franzen-Dahlin A, Billing E, von Arbin M, Murray V, Wredling R. The impact of a nurse-led support and education programme for spouses of stroke patients: a randomized controlled trial. *J Clin Nursing* 2005; 14(8): 995–1003.
11. Hartke RJ, King RB. Telephone group intervention for older stroke caregivers. *Top Stroke Rehabil* 2003; 9(4): 65–81.
12. Kalra L, Evans A, Perez I, Melbourn A, Patel A, Knapp M, Donaldson N. Training carers of stroke patients: randomised controlled trial. *BMJ* 2004; 328: 1099–1104.
13. Patel A, Knapp M, Evans A, Perez I, Kalra L. Training care givers of stroke patients: economic evaluation. *BMJ* 2004; 328: 1102–1104.
14. Anderson CS, Linto J, Stewart-Wynne EG. A population based assessment of the impact and burden of caregiving for long-term stroke survivors. *Stroke* 1995; 26: 843–849.
15. Dewey HM, Thrift AG, Mihalopoulos C, Carter R, Macdonell RA, McNeil JJ *et al.* Informal care for stroke survivors: results from the North East Melbourne stroke incidence study (NEMESIS). *Stroke* 2002; 33: 1028–1033.
16. Tooth L, McKenna K, Barnett A, Prescott C, Murphy S. Caregiver burden, time spent caring and health status in the first 12 months following stroke. *Brain Injury* 2005; 19(12): 963–974.

17. Bugge C, Alexander H, Hagen S. Stroke patients' informal caregivers. Patient, caregiver, and service factors that affect caregiver strain. *Stroke* 1999; 30(8): 1517–1523.

18. van Exel NJ, Koopmanschap MA, van den Berg B, Brouwer WB, van den Bos GA. Burden of informal caregiving for stroke patients: identification of caregivers at risk of adverse health effects. *Cerebrovasc Dis* 2005; 19: 11–17.

19. Evans RL, Bishop DS, Haselkorn JK. Factors predicting satisfactory home care after stroke. *Arch Phys Med Rehabil* 1991; 72: 144–147.

20. Sit JWH, Wong TKS, Clinton M, Li LSW, Fong Y. Stroke care in the home: the impact of social support on the general health of family caregivers. *J Clin Nursing*. 2004; 13(7): 816–824.

21. Murray J, Young J, Forster A, Ashworth R. Developing a primary care-based stroke model: the prevalence of longer-term problems experienced by stroke patients and their carers. *Br J Gen Pract* 2003; 53: 803–807.

22. Hare R, Rogers H, Lester H, McManus R, Mant J. What do stroke patients and their carers want from community services? *Family Pract* 2006; 23(1): 131–136.

23. Brotheridge S, Young J, Dowswell G, Lawler J, Forster A. A preliminary investigation of patient and carer expectations of their general practitioner in longer-term stroke care. *J Eval Clin Pract* 1998; 4(3), 136–141.

24. Murray J, Young J, Forster A. Review of longer-term problems after a disabling stroke. *Rev Clin Gerontol* 2007; 17: 277–292.

25. Greenwood N, Mackenzie A, Cloud GC, Wilson N. Informal carers of stroke survivors — Factors influencing carers: a systematic review of quantitative studies. *Disabil Rehabil* 2008; 30(18): 1329–1349.

26. Schlote A, Richter M, Frank B, Wallesch CW. A longitudinal study of health-related quality of life of first stroke survivors' close relatives. *Cerebrovasc Dis* 2006; 22: 137–142.

27. Forsberg-Warleby G, Moller A, Blomstrand C. Psychological well-being of spouses of stroke patients during the first year after stroke. *Clin Rehabil* 2004; 18: 430–437.

28. McCullagh E, Brigstocke G, Donaldson N, Kalra L. Determinants of caregiving burden and quality of life in caregivers of stroke patients. *Stroke* 2005; 36(10): 2181–2186.

29. van den Heuvel ETP, de Witte LP, Schure LM, Sanderman R, Meyboom-de Jong B. Risk factors for burn-out in caregivers of stroke patients, and possibilities for intervention. *Clin Rehabil* 2001; 15(6): 669–677.

30. Dowswell G, Lawler J, Dowswell T, Young J, Forster A, Hearn J. Investigating recovery from stroke: a qualitative study. *J Clin Nursing* 2000; 9: 507–515.

31. Lawler J, Dowswell G, Hearn J, Forster A, Young J. Recovering from stroke: a qualitative investigation of the role of goal setting in late stroke recovery. *J Adv Nursing* 1999; 30(2): 401–409.

32. Han B, Haley W. Family caregiving for patients with stroke, review and analysis. *Stroke* 1999; 30: 1478–1485.

33. Berg A, Palomaki H, Lonnqvist J, Lehtihalmes M. Kaste M. Depression among caregivers of stroke survivors. *Stroke* 2005; 36: 639–643.

34. Dennis M, O'Rourke S, Lewis S, Sharpe M, Warlow C. A quantitative study of the emotional outcome of people caring for stroke survivors. *Stroke* 1998; 29: 1867–1872.

35. Hartke RJ, Heinemann AW, King RB, Semik P. Accidents in older caregivers of persons surviving stroke and their relation to caregiver stress. *Rehabil Psychol* 2006; 51(2): 150–156.

36. Greveson G, James O. Improving long-term outcome after stroke — the views of patients and carers. *Health Trends* 1991; 23: 161–162.

37. Murray J, Ashworth R, Forster A, Young J. Developing a primary care-based stroke service: a review of the qualitative literature. *Br J Gen Pract* 2003; 53: 137–142.

38. Parag V, Hackett ML, Yapa CM, Kerse N, McNaughton H, Feigin VL, Anderson CS. The impact of stroke on unpaid caregivers: results from The Auckland Regional Community Stroke study, 2002–2003. *Cerebrovasc Dis* 2008; 25(6): 548–554.

39. Collins Concise English Dictionary, Collins Publishing, London.

40. Blake H, Lincoln NB, Clarke DD. Caregiver strain in spouses of stroke patients. *Clin Rehabil* 2003; 17: 312–317.

41. Wyller TB, Thommessen B, Sodring KM, Sveen U, Pettersen AM, Bautz-Holter E, Laake K. Emotional well-being of close relatives to stroke survivors. *Clin Rehabil* 2003; 17: 410–417.

42. Deeken JF, Taylor KL, Mangan P, Yabroff KR, Ingham JM. Care for the caregivers: a review of self-report instruments developed to measure the

burden, needs, and quality of life of informal caregivers. *J Pain Symptom Manage* 2003; 26(4): 922–953.

43. Visser-Meily JMA, Post MWM, Riphagen II, Lindeman E. Measures used to assess burden among caregivers of stroke patients: a review. *Clin Rehabil* 2004; 18: 601–623.

44. van Exel NJA, Scholte op Reimer WJM, Brouwer WBF, van den Berg B, Koopmanschap MA, van den Bos GAM. Instruments for assessing the burden of informal caregiving for stroke patients in clinical practice: a comparison of CSI, CRA, SCQ and self-rated burden. *Clin Rehabil* 2004; 18(2): 203–214.

45. Low JT, Payne S, Roderick P. The impact of stroke on informal carers: a literature review. *Soc Sci Med* 1999; 49: 711–725.

46. Visser-Meily A, van Heugten C, Post M, Schepers V, Lindeman E. Intervention studies for caregivers of stroke survivors: a critical review. *Patient Educ Counse* 2005; 56: 257–267.

47. Rombough RE, Howse EL, Bagg SD, Bartfay WJ. A comparison of studies on the quality of life of primary caregivers of stroke survivors: a systematic review of the literature. *Top Stroke Rehabil* 2007; 14(3): 69–79.

48. Eldred C, Sykes C. Psychosocial interventions for carers of survivors of stroke: a systematic review of interventions based on psychological principles and theoretical frameworks. *Br J Health Psychol* 2008; 13(3): 563–581.

49. Lui MHL, Ross FM, Thompson DR. Supporting family caregivers in stroke care: a review of the evidence for problem solving. *Stroke* 2005; 36(11): 2514–2522.

50. Brereton L, Carroll C, Barnston S. Interventions for adult family carers of people who have had a stroke: a systematic review. *Clin Rehabil* 2007; 21(10): 867–884.

51. Grant JS, Elliott TR, Weaver M, Bartolucci AA, Giger JN. Telephone intervention with family caregivers of stroke survivors after rehabilitation. *Stroke* 2002; 33(8): 2060–2065.

52. Ellis G, on behalf of the Stroke Liaison Workers Collaboration. Meta-analysis of stroke liaison workers for patients and carers: results by intervention characteristic. *Cerebrovasc Dise* 2006; 21(Suppl 4): 120.

53. Mason A, Weatherly H, Spilsbury K *et al*. The effectiveness and cost-effectiveness of respite for caregivers of frail older people. *J Am Geriatr Soc* 2007; 55(2): 290–299.

54. Intercollegiate Stroke Working Party. National Clinical Guidelines for Stroke. Royal College of Physicians; 2008.

55. van Heugten CM, Visser-Meily A, Post M, Lindeman E. Care for carers of stroke patients: evidence-based clinical practice guidelines. *J Rehabil Med* 2006; 38(3): 153–158.

11 Meeting the Palliative Care Needs of Stroke Patients

Irene J. Higginson*,†

Chapter Summary

Despite significant improvements in treatments, stroke remains the second or third most common cause of death in many countries. Palliative and end-of-life care are important for people affected by stroke. Three groups of patients can be identified and they and their families have slightly different needs. There are: (1) those who die within a relatively short time period (days or a few weeks following the stroke); (2) those who die within the first six months; (3) those who survive the first six months but have profound impairments and are at a high risk of subsequent death, with around 50% dying in subsequent years. In palliative care, the emphasis of care is on improving quality of life and helping patients to live as well as possible for their remaining life, as well as helping to relieve suffering and supporting those approaching the end of life and their families. Palliative care support is often given using the 'rectangle' model, where palliative care can be an increasing part of care.

*Professor of Palliative Care and Policy, King's College London, Scientific Director, Cicely Saunders International, Director, WHO Collaborating Centre for Palliative Care in Older People
†Department of Palliative Care, Policy and Rehabilitation, Cicely Saunders Institute, Bessemer Road, Denmark Hill, London SE5 9PJ, UK

Commonly symptoms and problems are multiple and include: difficulties in assessment because of changes in consciousness and communication problems, pain, breathlessness, fatigue, incontinence, constipation, confusion, and psychological problems, including depression and anxiety. There is a need for support of the family and patient. Simple tools for palliative care assessment, for example the Palliative Outcome Scale (POS), can be used to aid assessment. It is important to diagnose when a patient may be dying and also to change the focus of treatment at this point. Guidelines are available to help this shift.

Introduction

Unfortunately, despite improved prevention and treatment, stroke remains a leading cause of death and disability. In the United States of America, stroke is listed as the third major cause of death. By itself stroke is the second single most common cause of death in Europe, accounting for 1.24 million deaths in Europe each year.[1] Over one in six women (17%) and one in ten men (11%) die from the disease.[2] Within the European Union countries, stroke remains the second most common cause of death.

Mortality and morbidity following a stroke remains high. A recent cohort study including 7,710 patients from the Oxfordshire Community Stroke Project, the Lothian Stroke Register and the International Stroke Trial found that six months after stroke onset, 1,749 (22%) patients had died. The study followed patients for up to 17 years following stroke and found that at the end of the follow-up period, 1,620 (47%) patients who were functionally dependent at six months after stroke onset had died, versus 711 (28%) of the independent patients.[3]

Therefore when considering the palliative care needs of stroke patients, there are at least three different groups:

1. Those who die within a relatively short time period (days or a few weeks following the stroke) — some may show 'a stroke in evolution' at assessment or on admission to hospital (perhaps around 10% of stroke patients);
2. Those who die within the first six months (around 12% of stroke patients);

3. Those who survive the first six months but have profound impairments and are at a high risk of subsequent death, with around 50% of dependent stroke survivors dying in subsequent years.

In Slot *et al.*'s (2009) study, those who initially survived and died subsequently, most commonly died following a further stroke, pneumonia, pulmonary embolism, or cardiac disease. A smaller number died from diseases unrelated to their stroke, including cancer. Of those who survive a stroke, some may develop post-stroke dementia. Because of the different trajectory, disability and symptoms, these patients and their families may have different palliative care needs.

How Commonly do Stroke Patients have Palliative Care Needs?

The palliative care needs of stroke patients and their families remains relatively unexplored. Most data from clinical practice comes from the US, where stroke patients are more commonly cared for by hospice and palliative care services than in other countries. A retrospective chart review of 177 patients with neurological conditions (most common was stroke) seen by a palliative care service in the US found that 75 patients (58%) had symptoms recorded. Reasons for palliative care referral included 'comfort measures' in 40 (39%) and 'hospice candidacy' in 38 (37%). The most common recommendation made by the palliative care service was morphine in 44 (42%). Sixty-three (49%) were deemed hospice appropriate.[4]

In a study in Switzerland, all charts of patients dying from stroke in a tertiary hospital, and referred consecutively to a palliative care consultant team from 2000 to 2005, were reviewed retrospectively. Forty-two patients who died from stroke were identified — their median NIH Stroke Scale on admission was 21. The most prevalent symptoms were breathlessness (81% — a symptom not commonly referred to in texts on the palliative management of stroke patients) and pain (69%). Difficulties or inability to communicate because of aphasia or altered level of consciousness were present in 93% of patients. Pharmacological respiratory treatments consisted of anti-muscarinic drugs (52%) and opioids (33%). Pain was mainly treated by opioids (69%). During the last 48 hours of life, the team documented that 81% of patients were free of pain and 48% free of respiratory distress. The main causes of death were neurological complications in 38% of patients, multiple medical complications in 36%, and specific medical causes in 26%.[5]

These more recent studies confirm an earlier retrospective survey of the families or friends of 237 persons who died from stroke in 1990 in the UK. Respondents reported that more than half of the patients had experienced pain (65%), mental confusion (51%), low mood (57%), and urinary incontinence (56%) in the last year of life. Pain control had been inadequate: 51% of those treated for pain by hospital doctors and 45% of those treated by general practitioners were reported to have received treatment that relieved pain partially if at all.[6] There had also been a greater need for community support and information.[7]

However, although patients with stroke will have specific needs that relate to their condition, research in palliative care suggests that patients with progressive chronic diseases often have quite similar symptom profiles and problems as death approaches. Analysing symptoms in a comparative table (a grid), Solano *et al.* found that the prevalence of the 11 symptoms was often widely but homogeneously spread across five common diseases — heart failure, renal failure, COPD, cancer and AIDS. Three symptoms — pain, breathlessness, and fatigue — were found among more than 50% of patients, for all five diseases.[8] This work suggests that there appears to be a common pathway toward death for both malignant and non-malignant diseases and that some approaches and management in palliative care adapted for patients with other diseases will be applicable to patients and families affected by stroke.

A further consideration is that those affected by stroke will often be in older age groups. This is especially so for those with the poorer prognosis, who may be older and have co-morbidities. Thus the principals of caring for older patients in palliative care[9] and those with other chronic and acute diseases, as well as potentially social and emotional problems associated with ageing, must be applied.

The Role of Palliative Care

Palliative care is a person centred approach to care, concentrating on the alleviation of symptoms and emotional, social and spiritual problems for patients and those close to them. It helps patients and their families to live as well as possible for their remaining life, as well as helping to relieve suffering and supporting those approaching death and at the end of life.[9] The principals of management in palliative care include:

- the patient and family considered as the unit of care
- rigorous assessment, review and anticipatory planning of care
- expert symptom management, recognising the interaction of symptoms, and of symptoms with emotional, social and spiritual concerns
- care of emotional, social and spiritual needs
- excellent listening, communication and giving of information
- attention to ethical considerations
- care for the family, including into bereavement. The term 'family' here is used in the broad sense and includes all those close to the patient.

The UK End of Life strategy, launched in 2008, specifically raises the profile of patients with conditions other than cancer.[10] It is to be expected that palliative care services in the UK will soon be required to extend their remit to patients with non-cancer conditions, providing this is funded.

When does Palliative or Terminal Care Start: Rectangles or Triangles?

Figure 1 illustrates two visions of palliative care. In the rectangle, as Fox calls it, palliative care begins only when attempts at cure have been abandoned.[11] But in the triangle, palliative care merges seamlessly with attempts at cure. The World Health Organization's definition of palliative care includes the statement: 'Many aspects of palliative care are also applicable earlier in the course of the illness, in conjunction with anti-disease curative treatment'.[9] The triangle model of palliative care is especially important for those stroke patients who initially survive and subsequently die over months or years.

However, not everyone could be cared for by a specialist palliative care service. Three levels of care are proposed:

- the palliative care approach employed ideally by every doctor and nurse

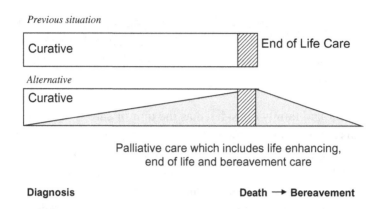

Figure 1. Alternative models of palliative and end of life care: rectangles or triangles?

- palliative care procedures and techniques (important adjuncts to care that are undertaken by relevant specialists)
- specialist palliative care, where doctors, nurses and other clinicians are specially trained.

The palliative care approach is something which many doctors and nurses can apply, and is often aided by education (which is increasingly being included in undergraduate programmes for student doctors and nurses, although it remains patchy) and by some of the recent checklists in management, although most of these are focussed on the end of life.

Specialist palliative care services, such as inpatient units, hospices and multiprofessional palliative care or hospice teams working in hospitals, at home and nursing homes, can work in collaboration with hospital clinicians and the primary care team to provide the extra support and expertise needed to care for patients with stroke. In some countries, for example the US, patients often need to choose whether to have hospice care or their existing community and hospital services. Note that US hospice care is primarily home based. However, in most European countries, and in Australia and New Zealand and Canada, patients can receive palliative care and hospice services alongside their usual hospital and community services.[12] Indeed, in the UK, palliative care teams in hospitals, and community teams and hospices in the community, offer care and support that is shared with existing doctors and nurses.[12]

Specialist palliative care services are usually multiprofessional, comprising doctors, nurses, and often social or psychosocial workers. Inpatient palliative care units offer care usually for short periods of time, with a median length of stay in the UK of less than two weeks. Around half of patients are discharged to supported care at home and the other half remain in the hospice to die. Palliative care home care and hospital teams care for patients at earlier stages of illness. They focus on dealing with patients with more complex needs, such as problematic symptoms, emotional, social or spiritual concerns.

Palliative Medicine became a specialty within medicine in the UK in 1987, and this has helped to drive forward the knowledge and skills base. Palliative clinicians experience seeing and caring for patients with complex symptoms and problems all the time and combined with their training, they are skilled and kept up-to-date especially in dealing with progressive or profound illness. A meta-analysis has shown benefits of multiprofessional specialist palliative care for patients in terms of pain and symptom control.[13,14] In this research, studies caring for non-cancer patients were included. Other research has suggested that although palliative care is rarely profitable by itself, palliative care in hospitals is associated with significant reductions in per diem costs and total costs, and can generate substantial savings to the health system by 'cost avoidance'.[15]

As Fig. 1 indicates, end-of-life or terminal care continues from and is part of good palliative care. The trajectory towards dying can vary: a patient may appear reasonably stable and then deteriorate, but then become stable again. Those stroke patients in group 1 (above) are likely to be on a trajectory where they will deteriorate and die in quite short a time; in contrast, those in the other two groups may need palliative care — to help improve symptoms, support the family and make plans — for a limited period and then will not need it again for a while.

Assessment and Measurement of Palliative Care Needs

Assessment is one of the cornerstones of palliative care. This involves listening to patients and families concerns. One of the particular challenges of assessing palliative care needs and problems among stroke patients is the high level of altered consciousness and communication difficulties.[16] This means that assessments which rely on patient reports cannot be completed in the most ill patients. Observation and proxy assessments (by the family and close staff) are required. Most severe strokes hamper communication, but this does not mean patients are not experiencing symptoms.

Initial assessment should consider the wakefulness of the patient, and his/her ability to communicate. Common symptoms include depression, anxiety, confusion and emotional lability, which can make assessment difficult.[17] Measurement of pulse, blood pressure, temperature and functional status are often inappropriate because they do not help to plan care. Appropriate assessment should emphasise pain and symptom control, the quality of life for the patient, fears and anxiety, psychological, social and spiritual concerns, any future wishes, and the circumstances and needs of the family members or carers. This breadth of assessment requires a multiprofessional approach to care. Excellent communication and listening is also needed.

It is important to determine the likely cause of the symptom or problem, and to assess its significance to the patient and family to plan treatment. Many patients, particularly older patients, have multiple health problems. So determining which problem is most important and should be dealt with first becomes a priority.

Not all symptoms may be due to the main disease. Symptoms may be caused because of secondary effects of the illness (for example, weakness or debility), because of side effects of treatment, or because of unrelated, concurrent illness. Good clinical assessment is necessary because in some instances it will affect the treatment used.

Clinical records are often helped by including a body chart on which pain and other symptoms are recorded at each visit. However, these are often charted only when patients are first seen, and re-assessment is missed. This can be improved by assessment and monitoring of key issues. Several such suitable assessment systems are available and several of these have been tested in primary care and or nursing homes as well as in hospices. Examples of assessment systems in common use are: the Support Team Assessment Schedule (STAS), Edmonton Symptom

Table 1. Example of one tool in palliative care: The Palliative Outcome Scale (POS)

Each item is graded 0 (no problem) to 4 (most severe / overwhelming problem), considering the last three days
* Open question, patients describe two most important concerns and grades the severity of these

A checklist then considers:

* Pain
* Other symptoms
* Patient anxiety
* Family anxiety
* Information
* Support
* Depression
* Self worth
* Wasted time
* Personal affairs

For further information on POS see:
http://www.kcl.ac.uk/schools/medicine/depts/palliative/qat/pos.html

For details of STAS see:
http://www.kcl.ac.uk/schools/medicine/depts/palliative/qat/stas.html

For ESAS see:
http://www.palliative.org/PC/ClinicalInfo/AssessmentTools/esas.pdf

Assessment System (ESAS), and the new Palliative Outcome Scale (POS) (Table 1).

The advantage of STAS is that it is completed by staff, based on their observations of patients and discussion with the family and patients, where possible. ESAS and POS have different formats that can be completed by patients, families, staff or observers. All of these assessment systems are short, and can be easily applied and integrated into the clinical interview, taking only around 5–8 minutes to complete. Yet, they give a picture of the nature and severity of palliative problems a patient and their family may have, covering physical, emotional, soul and spiritual/existential concerns. The Memorial Symptom Assessment

Schedule (MSAS) and the extended symptom schedule of POS (called POS-S) provide a more detailed assessment of symptoms which will be valuable among patients who appear to have palliative care needs.

Because psychological problems, especially depression and anxiety, are common following a stroke, a full psychological and social assessment is important. POS and ESAS can help with this, as can simple screening questions. The most recent National Institute for Clinical Excellence Guidance on managing depression in physical illness recommends that healthcare professionals should ask two questions to identify possible depression.[18] This should be at a person's first and subsequent contacts with services and after the completion of any rehabilitation programme. The questions are:

- During the last month, have you often been bothered by feeling down, depressed or hopeless?
- During the last month, have you often been bothered by having little interest or pleasure in doing things?

If a person answers 'yes' to either of the depression identification questions, healthcare professionals, when competent in basic mental health assessment, should:

- undertake a detailed clinical assessment including assessment of depressive symptoms, function and disability, and
- review and consider the role of both the current physical problem and any prescribed medication in the development or maintenance of the depression.

The POS and ESAS both include the first question about depression. In palliative and especially end-of-life care, when time is short, it may be appropriate to shorten the one-month period in the screening question to understand how the patient is feeling now. It is sometimes difficult to distinguish what is an understandably sad reaction to the losses of suffering a stroke from full depression. Work we have conducted to develop clinical guidelines on the management of depression as part of the European Palliative Care Research Collaborative has suggested that

(i) loss of enjoyment or pleasure is an important and consistent screening measure and (ii) treatment should consider whether there are depression symptoms that could be effectively treated (e.g. agitation, sleeplessness) using antidepressant drugs or other therapies, even at the end of life. A recent Cochrane Review has found that antidepressants are effective in patients with stroke and other physical illnesses (final review submitted, protocol).[19]

Management of Pain and Breathlessness

It is beyond the scope of this chapter to provide all the details of management of symptoms in the palliative care of stroke patients and so this section focusses on two common and very distressing symptoms, which are often not covered elsewhere. For a broader understanding of palliative care management, several good textbooks are available.[20]

Pain often develops following a stroke and can be central or focal. It is important to identify the cause of the pain and then plan the treatment. Pain in a hemiplegic arm is common and is associated with reduced quality of life. Physical therapy may be helpful and is essential in early stages of stroke. About 18–32% of patients have a post-stroke headache.[21] When patients have pain, appropriate analgesics should be given following the World Health Organization method. The key principals are that analgesics should be given:

- orally where possible, and subcutaneously (not by intramuscular injection, which is painful) when this is not possible
- regularly (lower doses are required when pain is prevented from becoming very severe leading to additional pain from psychological distress and muscle tension) with a provision for as required doses if the pain increases or breakthrough pain occurs
- by the ladder (see Table 2). This involves titrating the treatment against the pain until it is controlled to the patient's satisfaction. It increases from mild analgesics to opioids. In older people, opioid doses should start low and rise slowly. Note however that opioids have been shown to *not* have problems of addiction or tolerance when they are titrated against the pain.

Table 2. The World Health Organization approach to the management of chronic pain, the WHO Ladder

	Analgesics
Step 1: Pain	Non-opioid ± adjuvant (e.g. aspirin, paracetomol, acetaminophen, NSAID e.g. ibuprofen).
Step 2: Pain persists or increases	Weak opioid ± non-opioid ± adjuvant (e.g. dihydrocodeine, codeine, oxycodone (low dose), tramadol, dextropropoxyphene), NSAID may be used as well.
Step 3: Pain persists or increases	Strong opioids (e.g. morphine, hydromorphone, oxycodone) ± non-opioid ± adjuvant.

When pain is severe, it may be appropriate to move very quickly through the ladder directly to low dose opioids.[22] Then once on opioids, the dose can be increased against the pain. When adjusting or increasing the opioid dose, calculate the amount of opioid taken in the previous 24 hours (regular and additional as required doses) and adjust the new dose appropriately.

Now a wider range of opioid preparations are available. The mainstream opioids (such as morphine) should be used for first-line treatment, as doses can be increased, these opioids are widely available, are able to be given orally and subcutaneously and are well understood. Short acting opioids are helpful for breakthrough pain or pain on movement (when the opioid is given shortly before moving the patient) and increasingly are available using buccal or nasal routes which enter the bloodstream directly. However, they are not suitable for maintenance, except in the very rare situations that the patient *only* has incident pain. In patients with severe renal impairment, paracetamol, tramadol, and fentanyl or alfentanil (if subcutaneous) are the most appropriate medications for steps 1, 2 and 3 respectively. Switching between opioids can be considered if patients do not respond or develop toxicity, but this requires great care, as calculating the doses is complex and the evidence regarding appropriate dosage and time intervals is evolving. Therefore, clinicians not experienced in this should consult an expert (for example, a palliative care specialist) who is up to date in the latest information. In general, if patients are not responding to pain treatment following the WHO ladder, a full review should be undertaken and specialist help sought.

Not all pains respond equally well to opioids, so it is important to determine the cause of the pain. Pain caused by spasticity may be relieved by muscle relaxants (such as baclofen) of focal injections with botulinum toxin. Physical therapy may be needed to prevent contractures. Neuropathic pain is diagnosed by the presence of a burning or tingling type of pain, often with altered sensation and often in the area of a nerve. It is only partially responsive to opioids and is especially difficult to treat. Usually it requires additional treatment. Antidepressant and anticonvulsant drugs are usually the first-line treatment; other treatments include pregabalin, gabapentin lidoderm patches (not available in many countries) and tramadol, and specialist expertise is required. Note that when used in the treatment of neuropathic pain, antidepressant drugs are expected to start to have effects within 2–3 days — much more quickly than they do when treating depression. Central post-stroke pain is also best treated with antidepressants. Pressure sores can be very painful and may respond to topical treatments — there is some evidence to support the use of topic opioids[23] — and of course repositioning and prevention. However, oral or subcutaneous opioids may be needed.

As for all symptoms, the cornerstone to the management of breathlessness is accurate assessment as to the likely cause. In patients with stroke this may be infection, weakness, and other concurrent diseases, such as heart failure or chronic pulmonary disease. If treatment of the underlying cause improves the symptom, then it should be given. Optimum management in palliative care involves pharmacological treatment (principally opioids, occasionally oxygen and anxiolytics) and non-pharmacological interventions (including use of a fan, walking aids, a tailor-made exercise program, and psychoeducational support for patient and family)[24] with the use of parenteral opioids and sedation at the end of life when appropriate.[25] Effective care centres on the patient's needs and goals. As the patient becomes more breathless, eventually becoming breathless at rest, pharmacological treatments become more important. Opioids have the most extensive evidence base to guide their use, and are used in low doses, although most of the evidence relates to their use in cancer patients. Other pharmacological interventions may act partly by

helping breathlessness (by mechanisms still uncertain) or by treating concomitant precipitating and exacerbating conditions such as depression and
anxiety.

Nutrition and Hydration

Following a stroke, swallowing difficulties can affect 22–65% of patients.[26]
Dysphasia is a marker of poor prognosis.[27] Although in many patients, swallowing improves, in some it can persist for months. Poor nutrition in early
stroke may predispose to muscle weakness and fatigue, which will impair
rehabilitation and predispose the patient to pressure sores.[28] Artificial nutrition through a percutaneous gastrostomy may be short in patients with a
poor prognosis[28] and may have no benefit in these instances. For hydration
and nutrition in end-of-life care, see the later section in this chapter.
Involvement of the whole team and the family in decision-making is important, and specialist palliative care advice may be needed.[28]

Care of the Dying Stroke Patient

Diagnosing that a patient is dying?

Diagnosing dying is a neglected part of medical and nursing education. It
can be extremely difficult to identify when a patient is dying, but an
awareness that a patient might die and when that might be can be very
important for patients, families and healthcare professionals. It is also
valuable as it may reduce unnecessary tests.[29] Many patients and families
will ask about prognosis ('How long have I (or s/he) got?'), but it is usually better not to be too specific — all healthcare professionals are
notoriously inaccurate at predicting how long an individual has to live,
even close to death. It is helpful to consider the previous trajectory that a
patient has been on, for example, if a patient has been rapidly deteriorating, this is likely to continue. It is also helpful to think of days, or weeks,
rather than precise times, and also to help patients and families understand
what signs might signal approaching death.

Common signs of impending death include: profound weakness,
being confined to bed, drowsiness for extended periods, lack of interest in

food and fluids, disorientation with respect to time, limited attention span, and difficulty in swallowing medication. However, some patients do make a partial recovery following deterioration and a wide range of different trajectories can occur. It is sometimes helpful to discuss likely scenarios with the patient and the family, and to plan for both the best and the worst possible outcomes.

What is an 'appropriate' or 'good' death?

Experts in different countries have defined the principles of a 'good' death, and although the domains sometimes differ between and within countries and cultures, there are many similarities. Pain and symptom control and ensuring dignity are common priorities. There is no 'right' way to die and all studies identify the importance of an individual dying 'in character'. Thus, it is probably better to think of an 'appropriate', rather than a 'good', death. This needs to be reflected in individualised approaches to meeting need and care, taking account of culture, background, circumstances and preferences.

The family as the unit of care

Concern for the patient and family as the unit of care is an essential element in palliative and terminal care. The term 'family' is meant in its broad sense and encompasses those who are close to the patient, often a spouse, partner, child or sibling and close friend who are significant for the patient. The concerns of the family or friends need to be heard and discussed, wherever care is. Special efforts may need to be taken to meet with the family, as they may only be able to visit out of normal working hours (see below regarding care of the family).

Changing gear

Evidence-based guidelines have reviewed the need to 'change gear' when managing the care of patients who are dying.[30] During the terminal phase, the goals of care are redefined towards the alleviation of symptoms and distress as well as support for the patient and family at the time of death.

Existing symptoms may change or new symptoms arise, which require management. Patients often need more time to express what is important to them, and clinicians have to 'slow down' when dealing with the patient and family, and listening to their concerns.

Attention to detail, reassessment, and ensuring treatments and interventions are individualised are the cornerstones of successful management. Assessment can be aided by using standardised audit or assessment schedules (see earlier), especially if these are incorporated in a care pathway or protocol. Choose assessment schedules that are intended for the end of life and do not burden the patient.

In the dying patient, especially if s/he is unconscious, particular attention needs to be paid to mouth and pressure areas, comfort and dignity. The family or nearest carer's needs and their coping also need to be assessed, and often their perception of the symptoms and comfort is important.

A review of medication is needed. Some medications, such as those for pre-existing heart or respiratory disorders, or any other non-essential medication may become inappropriate, particularly if these are difficult for the patient to take.

Unnecessary or excessive tests, if uncomfortable, can increase rather than reduce suffering and should be avoided. Clinicians should always carefully assess patients to identify potentially reversible symptoms. Investigations should only be undertaken, however, where they are likely to inform management decisions and if further tests are in line with the patients' wishes.

At the very end of life, noisy breathing (death rattle) can become a problem. It is often more distressing for caregivers and relatives than it is for patients. Over-hydration can exacerbate the problem. Repositioning and explaining to the family is important. In clinical practice, hyoscine hydrobromide, hyoscine butylbromide and glycopyrrolate are commonly used (the latter two drugs often favoured as they are thought not to cross the blood brain barrier), but a recent systematic review showed lack of good randomised trials in this field.[31]

Care pathways including many of these steps have been developed to help clinicians plan end-of-life care. One such example, the Liverpool Care Pathway, is being increasingly used in hospitals across Europe.

Descriptive studies show that it improves documentation and may affect patient and caregiver outcomes.[32,33]

Planning of end-of-life care

Anticipatory planning of care, once it has been identified that a patient is likely to die, is crucial in order to facilitate patient and family choices. Factors that need to be considered are:

- Symptom control — anticipation of symptoms that might occur, particularly outside of normal working hours and the development of effective management plans to address these (including the prescribing of appropriate medication)
- Information and communication — it is vital that patients and families are given frequent opportunities to have questions answered and outstanding issues addressed
- End-of-life decisions — these can include treatment options or choices in place of care and of death as well as wishes regarding artificial feeding and hydration. Advance discussion and documentation of patients' wishes can reduce distress and facilitate appropriate care
- Equipment — as appropriate to facilitate safe care in all settings.

Oral and subcutaneous medication

A common difficulty is that dying patients become too weak to swallow oral medication. Ambulatory infusion devices, syringe drivers and other continuous delivery systems are useful in this situation. They allow either a continuous or regular infusion of opioid and other suitable medications, thus avoiding repeated injection. Patient controlled and spring operated delivery systems are also available and are particularly useful in countries where batteries to operate the delivery system cannot be obtained. The 24-hour dose for subcutaneous delivery should be calculated based on prior treatment. The most useful sites to insert the needle for subcutaneous infusions are the upper chest, outer aspect of the outer arm, abdomen and thighs. Patients should undergo frequent assessment of pain, cognition and other symptoms.

Pain control

While patients are dying, and even when they become unconscious, pain control using regular analgesics is still required if it was needed at an earlier stage of illness. For patients receiving strong opioids, the 24-hour morphine dose can then be recalculated to provide the equivalent dose subcutaneously. The dose of opioids and other adjuvants should be frequently titrated in order to prevent metabolite accumulation or drug interactions contributing to agitated delirium.

Feeding and hydration

In general, as death approaches, appetite reduces and many patients find it more comfortable to eat less, or little at all. This can cause great anxiety to families and, less commonly, patients. Explanation of the normality of reduced oral intake at the end of life, alongside a general 'shutting down' of the systems, is often required to support families.

Once the dying phase has been reached, there is no evidence that artificial feeding in patients with a progressive illness prolongs life, and insertion of intravenous, percutaneous and nasogastric feeding devices can cause iatrogenic disease. This does not mean, however, that good nursing care should not be continued, mouth care is especially important. Further good nursing care may encourage the patient to take pleasure from eating or drinking small amounts of things that they enjoy and contribute to improving quality of life.

The evidence regarding hydration is more complex. The sensation of thirst is probably not related to hydration or to sodium levels, and can be relieved by good mouth care, and sips of water or wetting the lips and mouth. Equally, intravenous hydration can be uncomfortable and restrictive in a dying patient, and can easily tip a patient into fluid overload. However, research has also shown that dehydration has been associated with increased confusion at the end of life, and giving relatively small amounts of fluid, (e.g. one litre per day) subcutaneously can reduce this. Thus, subcutaneous hydration may have a role for some patients.

Nursing care

Good nursing care of the dying patient is particularly important, especially in maintaining dignity. This includes care of pressure areas, mouth and skin care, bathing, as well as assessment and management of symptoms and support of the patient and family. Care should be orientated towards enabling the patient to 'live' with dignity until death. This can involve a wide and very individual range of aspects, in the last weeks or even days of life there may be new achievable activities, the creative activities of day care, attention to appearance (e.g. hair, teeth), the environment and surroundings, family gatherings or attending important functions, a reconciliation of existential and spiritual meanings.

Delirium

Delirium is a very distressing symptom for patients and family. Patients experiencing delirium may be aware of this, and they and their family may be very anxious. Sometimes referred to as acute confusional state, terminal restlessness or acute brain syndrome, it is characterised by acute onset cognitive impairment. Thresholds of detecting delirium vary, but some cognitive impairment, changing sleep-wake cycle, and fluctuating consciousness, are common in the terminal stages. Delirium is frequently undiagnosed and it is important to check the more distressing manifestations of delirium, such as misinterpretations, psychomotor agitation, hallucinations, delusions and other abnormalities of perception. Frequent causes include: urinary retention, infection, dehydration, constipation, metabolic abnormalities, toxicity of opioids, benzodiazepines and other drugs, and cytokine production. Where appropriate, underlying causes should be sought and actively treated.

Haloperidol is indicated in the symptomatic management of patients presenting with hyperactive forms of delirium, including psychomotor agitation, delusions, or hallucinations. It can be given orally or by subcutaneous infusion. Haloperidol should be considered a temporary measure while other strategies such as change in the type of opioid, hydration, or the management of metabolic or infectious complications are introduced.

If haloperidol fails to control symptoms, midazolam, which also can be included in a subcutaneous infusion, can be used.

Communication and information

Towards the end of life, patients, their families and those close to them may have specific concerns that they wish to discuss, or at least express. These may be related to the diagnosis, prognosis, or to particular things that s/he wishes to achieve or resolve before death. The skills needed for effective communication in palliative care include: listening, assessment, facilitation, techniques for handling difficult questions and self-awareness. Patients with a stroke and those who are dying need more time to express their concerns. Concerns can range widely, but some of the difficult issues may relate to fears about the process of death, how dying will happen, what will happen afterwards.[21] Some people may wish to plan their funerals in advance, but others may not wish to discuss death at all.

Psychological and emotional concerns

All of the emotional reactions found in palliative care (shock, anger, adjustment problems, depression, hopelessness) can be found in the patient who is dying. Fear of loss of control can be increased at this time. Fear of dying is a common and normal reaction. Nevertheless, a patient may be particularly upset or concerned by specific aspects of dying, the recognition of which allows the professional to intervene properly. Their fears may be about physical illness and suffering, treatments and their consequences, family, finances and social status, existential and religious concerns.

In order to understand the emotional process in response to dying, Buckman proposes a three-stage model:

1. The patient faces the threat of death and exhibits a combination of reactions, which depend on his/her previous personality and way of coping;
2. The second phase is characterised by resolution of the initial emotional response. The intensity of emotions may diminish, but depression and withdrawal can be common;

3. The final stage is defined by acceptance of death. Nevertheless, acceptance and full awareness of dying are not essential, especially if the patient is not distressed, has adequate relationships with family and friends and can make decisions as s/he wishes.

Care of the Family

The emotional concerns of family members or carers escalate as death approaches, and they are often more anxious than the patient. Those families most at risk of escalating anxiety are those who have been very anxious before. Other factors include: being a spouse of the patient, a patient diagnosis of breast cancer, young patient age, shorter time from diagnosis and low patient mobility.

The needs of the family are all too often overlooked; indeed family members and carers often feel ambiguous about asking for support. A recent study among the family members of patients who were close to death found that many report that they have put their own needs and life 'on hold', but at the same time they recognise that they long for support or a break.[34] As for the patient, communication and information about particular concerns or worries is important. It is likely that the family will need some time alone. In some instances, support groups or services have been found to help carers, and practical support and respite are important when patients are at home.

Care for family and friends does not stop with the death of the patient. The reaction of grief and bereavement is characterised by three aspects: the necessity to cry and search for the lost person; the necessity to repress crying or searching; and the necessity to review and modify internal models. A great variety of reactions during bereavement have been described. Grief is not a linear process with well-defined boundaries but an amalgamation of overlapping phases that vary between individuals. Modern interpretations of grief have identified components such as: numbness characterised by disbelief, panic, denial, anger (often early on, when death is anticipated even before the person dies); yearning characterised by search for the lost person, helplessness, despair, anxiety, restlessness, pangs of grief; despair characterised by the full awareness of the loss, reactive depression, apathy, social withdrawal and reorganisation and finally recovery. Contemporary theories of grief describe a Duel Process model, where adaptation during the grieving process allows the bereaved individual to face daily life whilst protecting against emotional anguish. Both confrontation (or 'loss') and avoidance (or 'restoration') of grief occur and are valid. Individuals may swing from one state to the other, sometimes within short spaces of time, possibly even in the same conversation. This process is individual both in people and in time.

Grief is a normal process and many individuals cope well within their own family support. However, bereavement is also responsible for high levels of morbidity and mortality.[35] Individuals particularly at risk of increased morbidity, mortality or complicated grief are those who are: male, older, have poorer physical functioning, expressed 'relief' at the death of the person they were caring for,[35] experienced an unexpected death, were highly stressed during care giving,[36] have low levels of social activities, small social networks, lower satisfaction with social support[37] or experienced multiple losses. In these instances referral to primary care or to other voluntary organisations offering bereavement support is helpful. Many hospices organise bereavement groups and visiting. In the rare instances when grief is very complicated or atypical psychiatric referral is required, and DSMIV categories include atypical grief.

Conclusions and Future Directions

Palliative and end-of-life care for people affected by stroke is an important but relatively neglected field. Multiple symptoms and psychological, social and spiritual concerns exist and are beginning to be more clearly identified. There are different groups of stroke patients who need palliative and end-of-life care, depending on the different trajectory and prognosis following a stroke and their degree of dependency and co-morbidity. Methods of assessment originally developed in other conditions can be adapted to aid stroke care, although further work among stroke patients and their caregivers is needed. Some guidance for 'changing gear' and care of the dying patient and their family is available. Future work should concentrate on testing ways to integrate and develop palliative care for patients with stroke and their families as well as the relief of symptoms and problems during this phase of life.

References

1. World Health Organisation. Mortality in Europe. 2009. www.who.int/whosis/database/mort/table1.cfm

2. British Heart Foundation Statistics. Total CVD mortality in Europe. 2009. www.heartstats.org/datapage.asp?id=754

3. Slot KB, Berge E, Sandercock P, Lewis SC, Dorman P, Dennis M. Causes of death by level of dependency at 6 months after ischemic stroke in 3 large cohorts. *Stroke* 2009; 40(5): 1585–1589.

4. Chahine LM, Malik B, Davis M. Palliative care needs of patients with neurologic or neurosurgical conditions. *Eur J Neurol* 2008; 15(12): 1265–1272.

5. Mazzocato C, Michel-Nemitz J, Anwar D, Michel P. The last days of dying stroke patients referred to a palliative care consult team in an acute hospital. *Eur J Neurol* 2009; 17(1): 73–77.

6. Addington-Hall J, Lay M, Altmann D, McCarthy M. Symptom control, communication with health professionals, and hospital care of stroke patients in the last year of life as reported by surviving family, friends, and officials. *Stroke* 1995; 26(12): 2242–2248.

7. Addington-Hall J, Lay M, Altmann D, McCarthy M. Community care for stroke patients in the last year of life: results of a national retrospective survey of surviving family, friends and officials. *Health Soc Care Community* 1998; 6(2): 112–119.

8. Solano JP, Gomes B, Higginson IJ. A comparison of symptom prevalence in far advanced cancer, AIDS, heart disease, chronic obstructive pulmonary disease and renal disease. *J Pain Symptom Manage* 2006; 31(1): 58–69.

9. Davies E, Higginson IJ. Better palliative care for older people. Denmark: World Health Organization 2004.

10. Department of Health. End of Life Care Strategy — promoting high quality care for all adults at the end of life 2008.

11. Fox R. From rectangles to triangles. *J R Soc Med* 2001; 94(9): 427.

12. Higginson IJ. End of life care: lessons from other nations. *J. Palliative Med* 2005; 8(S): S161–S173.

13. Higginson IJ, Finlay I, Goodwin DM, Cook AM, Hood K, Edwards AGK *et al.* Do hospital-based palliative teams improve care for patients or families at the end of life? *J Pain Symptom Manage* 2002; 23: 96–106.

14. Higginson IJ, Finlay IG, Goodwin DM, Hood K, Edwards AGK, Cook A *et al.* Is there evidence that palliative care teams alter end-of-life experiences

of patients and their caregivers? *J Pain Symptom Manage* 2003; 25: 150–168.

15. Smith TJ, Cassel JB. Cost and non-clinical outcomes of palliative care. *J Pain Symptom Manage* 2009; 38(1): 32–44.

16. Borasio GD, Rogers A, Voltz R. Palliative medicine in non-malignant neurological disorders. In Doyle D, Hanks G, Cherny N, Calman K (Eds.) *Oxford Textbook of Palliative Medicine.* 3rd Edn. 2005, 926–932.

17. Creutzfeldt C. Palliative care and the acute stroke patient. *J Hospice Palliative Nursing* 2009; 11(3): 141–143.

18. National Institute for Clinical Excellence (NICE). Depression in adults with a chronic health problem: treatment and management. final draft (July 2009) *Clinical Guideline.* London: National Institute for Clinical Excellence (NICE); 2009.

19. Rayner L, Price A, Evans A, Valsraj K, Higginson IJ, Hotopf M. Antidepressants for depression in physically ill people. *Cochrane Database of Systematic Reviews* 2008; (4): CD007503. DOI: 10.1002/14651858.CD007503.

20. Bruera E, Higginson IJ, Ripamonti C, von Gunten CF. *Textbook of Palliative Medicine.* London: Hodder Arnold; 2006.

21. Hamann G, Rogers A, Addington-Hall J. Palliative care in stroke. In Voltz R, Bernat JL, Borasio GD, Maddocks I, Oliver D, Portenoy RK (Eds.) *Palliative Care in Neurology.* Oxford University Press; 2004, 13–26.

22. Mercadante S. Opioid titration in cancer pain: a critical review. *Eur J Pain* 2007; 11(8): 823–830.

23. LeBon B, Zeppetella G, Higginson IJ. Effectiveness of topical administration of opioids in palliative care: a systematic review. *J Pain Symptom Manage* 2009; 37(5): 913–917.

24. Bausewein C, Booth S, Gysels M, Higginson I. Non-pharmacological interventions for breathlessness in advanced stages of malignant and non-malignant diseases. *Cochrane Database Syst Rev* 2008; (2): CD005623.

25. Booth S, Moosavi SH, Higginson IJ. The etiology and management of intractable breathlessness in patients with advanced cancer: a systematic review of pharmacological therapy. *Nat Clin Pract Oncol* 2008; 5(2): 90–100.

26. Ramsey DJC, Smithard DG, Kalra L. Early assessments of dysphagia and aspiration risk in acute stroke patients. *Stroke* 2003; 34: 1252–1257.

27. Smithard DG, Smeeton NC, Wolfe CD. Long-term outcome after stroke: does dysphagia matter? *Age Ageing* 2007; 36(1): 90–94.

28. Burman R. Neurological diseases. In Bruera E, Higginson IJ, Ripamonti C, von Gunten CF (Eds.) *Textbook of Palliative Medicine*. London: Hodder Arnold; 2006, 911–917.

29. Veerbeek L, Van ZL, Swart SJ, Jongeneel G, Van Der Maas PJ, Van Der Heide A. Does recognition of the dying phase have an effect on the use of medical interventions? *J Palliat Care* 2008; 24(2): 94–99.

30. Higginson IJ, Sen-Gupta G, Dunlop R. Changing Gear — Guidelines for managing the last days of life in adults. The Research Evidence. London: The National Council for Hospice and Specialist Palliative Care Services; 1997.

31. Wee B, Hillier R. Interventions for noisy breathing in patients near to death. *Cochrane Database Syst Rev* 2008; (1): CD005177.

32. Veerbeek L, Van Der Heide A, de Vogel-Voogt E, de BR, van der Rijt CC, Swart SJ *et al.* Using the LCP: bereaved relatives' assessments of communication and bereavement. *Am J Hosp Palliat Care* 2008; 25(3): 207–214.

33. Veerbeek L, Van ZL, Swart SJ, Van Der Maas PJ, de Vogel-Voogt E, van der Rijt CC *et al.* The effect of the Liverpool Care Pathway for the dying: a multi-centre study. *Palliat Med* 2008; 22(2): 145–151.

34. Harding R, Higginson IJ. Working with ambivalence: informal caregivers of patients at the end of life. *Support Care Cancer* 2001; 9: 642–645.

35. Bowling A. Predictors of mortality among a national sample of elderly widowed people: analysis of 28-year mortality rates. *Age Ageing* 2009; 38(5): 527–530.

36. Burton AM, Haley WE, Small BJ. Bereavement after caregiving or unexpected death: effects on elderly spouses. *Aging Ment Health* 2006; 10(3): 319–326.

37. Burton AM, Haley WE, Small BJ, Finley MR, Dillinger-Vasille M, Schonwetter R. Predictors of well-being in bereaved former hospice caregivers: the role of caregiving stressors, appraisals, and social resources. *Palliat Support Care* 2008; 6(2): 149–158.

12 Benchmarking and Improving Stroke Services

Anthony G. Rudd* and Alex Hoffman†

Chapter Summary

Stroke management is a rapidly developing area of medicine. Much of the important research demonstrating improved clinical outcomes has either tested specific models of healthcare delivery, e.g. stroke units, early supported discharge, or has tested interventions that require major restructuring of care, e.g. thrombolysis. Therefore, it is vital that all clinicians involved in delivering stroke care are expert and up to date in their field. This is where guidelines can be of particular benefit and services are configured in a way that ensures the best quality of care for all patients. Guidelines must, however, be of sufficient quality to be of value but unfortunately, many of those currently available are in many respects inadequate. Having set the standards through guidelines, it is important to objectively assess how well a service is performing. The ideal is to measure the outcomes of treatment; however, for many reasons this is often impracticable and therefore in most instances a combination of structure and process is the only viable option. Combined with patient reported outcomes, a comprehensive picture can be obtained as to what improvements

*Stroke Programme Director, Clinical Standards Department, Royal College of Physicians London, Stroke Physician Guy's and St. Thomas' Hospital, London, UK
†Stroke Programme Manager, Clinical Standards Department, Royal College of Physicians London

are needed to achieve high quality standards. This chapter describes the different methods available for measuring quality and subsequently effecting change, and gives examples of national audits and registers from around the world.

Introduction

No stroke service is perfect and therefore quality improvement should be integral to all aspects of care. This is essential to ensure that all patients and carers receive the treatment most likely to result in them surviving without disability and to be in a position to adopt new evidence-based forms of treatment. This chapter outlines the key components of a quality improvement programme and provides a framework which people can use to set standards, measure performance and rectify the deficits.

As illustrated in Fig. 1 the process of quality improvement involves a number of stages including:

- Setting the objectives for the service, for example developing an acute stroke unit.
- Defining the standards, which may require reviewing the literature, identifying a good service elsewhere that could be replicated or using existing evidence-based guidelines.
- Then deciding how quickly the change is going to take and therefore setting an appropriate monitoring schedule and conducting the first survey of current care. This stage involves the development of a tool with which to measure quality. This sounds easier than it is and wherever possible it is best to use existing tested and validated measures.
- Reporting results to all those that need to know and developing an action plan to rectify problems.
- Starting the cycle all over again by reviewing where you are and what needs to be done.

1. Setting the Objectives

The most important factor in determining the quality of a stroke service is knowing what it is you want to achieve. Having the vision to be able to

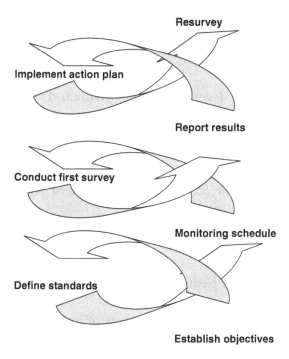

Figure 1. The quality spiral.

see what might be possible and the knowledge to know what, is desirable. There are a number of documents that can be used that clearly set out the key components of a stroke service, including the English National Stroke Strategy[1] and the Helsingborg Declaration.[2] However identifying good units and visiting them, talking to their staff and stealing their business plans, protocols and any other documentation they may have is an invaluable strategy. There is rarely a need to be completely original. Someone will have done it before, so learn from them.

2. Setting Standards: Guidelines

a. *Standards for development*

Translating evidence into routine practice remains a challenge for all health systems. One widely used method is the publication of guidelines;

however, it is important to be sure that the guidelines being used are of adequate quality. When assessing the quality of guidelines, it is important ask the following questions:

1. Was the guideline development group constituted appropriately? Did it include individuals who had the necessary expertise?
2. Was there a systematic review of the literature including all appropriate levels of evidence?
3. Is it clear what the purpose of the guideline is?
4. Is it up to date or has the evidence changed significantly since publication?
5. Was there a formal system of peer review that took account of contrary views?
6. Did the guideline have satisfactory input from those people who are going to be the recipients of the services, namely patients and their carers?
7. Is it clear that there were no conflicts of interest for the guideline developers that might have biased the recommendations and how was the guideline funded?

A systematic review of the quality of stroke guidelines makes depressing reading.[3] A hundred and seventeen documents were identified from the literature published between 1999 and 2005. Most guidelines received an overall score of 'would not recommend'. The lowest scoring domains were stakeholder involvement, rigor of development and applicability. Only five guidelines were highly recommended. In the UK, the NICE Guidelines on Acute Stroke and TIA[4] and the Intercollegiate National Clinical Guidelines for Stroke[4] are of high quality and can largely be relied upon.

b. *Why have guidelines?*

Not all stroke patients will be managed at all stages by experts and not all experts will know everything. There is robust evidence in many areas of stroke care to show that treatment works to both reduce mortality and morbidity. For other areas where evidence is less robust, appropriate management still requires the clinician do something. The British approach to evidence-based medicine has often in the past led to 'masterly' inactivity, not necessarily in the interests of the patient. For example, in the early hours after stroke, there is no randomised controlled trial evidence to show that maintaining normal levels of hydration, oxygenation, blood glucose and temperature is effective in improving outcomes. This is still being used as an argument to avoid the need to provide specialist acute stroke care. It sometimes seems that the price of adhering to evidence-based medicine is to sacrifice common sense. Thus national guidelines need not only to produce recommendations for areas where evidence exists but also for areas that are evidence free, developed from the consensus view of an expert committee.

Many guidelines on stroke have been produced around the world in recent years, with the majority concentrating on acute care and secondary prevention. The third edition of National Clinical Guidelines for Stroke was published in 2008[5] and attempted to cover the management of stroke from the acute event through to longer term problems and secondary prevention. Produced by the Intercollegiate Stroke Working Party, they are written to provide a resource for healthcare managers and purchasers, researchers as well as clinicians. One of their key functions is to identify the gaps in knowledge so as to encourage further research.

c. *Using guidelines*

Guidelines should not be used as a rulebook. The 80% rule is often cited, which means that guidelines should be applicable to 80% of patients, 80% of the time. In other words, there will often be instances when your patient will need to be treated in an unconventional way. In addition, there will be many instances when particular situations are not covered by guidelines at all or if they are, the level of evidence available to make a recommendation is weak. Under these circumstances there is no alternative but to rely on clinical experience and common sense. Research does not always address the most important issues in patient management. For example, there are plenty of papers that have studied the effects of botulinum toxin for spasticity after stroke but very few have looked at different physiotherapy techniques that might be used. The vast majority of patients will receive physiotherapy, very few will need botulinum toxin. The odd balance of research probably reflects the fact that pharmaceutical companies sponsor many studies of their products but there is no profit to be made from demonstrating that physical therapy is effective. Therefore guidelines can be of enormous help in defining standards but they need to be used with common sense and caution.

3. Measuring the Quality of Care

What should be measured?

The core principles for audit are to 'measure what counts: don't count what can be measured' and wherever possible, measure against predefined evidence-based standards.

Donabedian[6] defined three components of care that need to be evaluated to provide define quality.

- **Structure: How is care organised?** For example: Is there a stroke unit? How many staff are employed? Is there a weekend rehabilitation service, early supported discharge, systems in place to provide training for carers, etc?
- **Process: What happens to the patient?** For example: Was the patient admitted to a stroke unit and if so how long did it take? Did the patient have brain imaging and when, was thrombolysis given? Did the patient receive appropriate secondary prevention, etc?
- **Outcome: What was the end result?** For example: Did the patient die? What, if any, was the level of disability? Was the patient discharged home or did they need institutionalisation? Was the patient satisfied with the care provided, etc?

Measuring structure is relatively straightforward both for the auditor and those being audited. It requires a single piece of data collection at a particular point in time. Measuring process requires more time and effort and can be done prospectively or more easily, retrospectively, using the case notes to extract the data. Measuring outcome is fraught with difficulty. Stroke is a disease with such wide variability in pathology and severity and often affects people with a range of co-morbidites that each clinician or centre would need hundreds of cases to compare with others to be able to make meaningful assessments of quality of care based on outcome. In addition, the outcome, be it death or disability or recovery, will be the composite of large number of events and interventions delivered possibly over a long period of time by a wide range of different people. Interpreting what a high mortality rate means for a stroke population is very different from understanding why a large number of children having cardiac surgery are dying on the operating table. Research has shown a close link between the quality of care delivered and outcome for some interventions, such as stroke unit management and therefore wherever possible, these evidence-based process and structure issues should be used as proxies for outcome.

The outcome of stroke is not like a football match where the outcome is very clear at the end. Success in the treatment of a stroke needs to be measured in the context not just of the illness itself but also the patient's social and physical background. A patient previously disabled cannot expect to have as good an outcome as a patient previously fit and independent. Regaining independence is easier if the patient has a well-adapted, supportive environment to return to, as opposed to a seedy bedsit upstairs without a lift or heating. What may be perceived as a good outcome for one patient may not be accepted as such by another. Patient's perceptions and expectations must also be taken into consideration. Outcome measurement therefore needs to look at hospital care, the community health and social services, the physical environment, and social support. The effect of the illness on the physical, psychological and financial health of the carers also needs to be measured. Outcomes need to consider both short and more importantly, longer term effects of the illness.

Choosing outcome indicators for stroke is problematic. There are still many uncertainties about the epidemiology, the natural history and the most effective forms of therapy. Stroke is not a single disease; its natural history is enormously variable, and not always explicable. Sometimes, it is not clear why patients get better more quickly than others do. There are major difficulties in defining case-mix measures, which is a key area in interpreting any outcomes that are used. The patients who are having the strokes are often elderly and have a lot of co-morbidities, which complicate the whole picture.

There may be a conflict between the sensitivity and the feasibility of outcome indicators. It is important to define what the measure is intended to be used for. A measure that may have great use as a global outcome measure of use to clinicians and managers alike may not be useful as a tool for the routine monitoring of a patients progress with a physiotherapist or occupational therapist. For example, concern is often expressed about the widespread use of the Barthel Index, which is a crude but reliable 20- or 100-point measure of disability. What does it really tell you about the patient? It is not sensitive enough to be of obvious use to the physiotherapist treating the patient but nevertheless it does describe in broad terms some of the problems the person is going to have to deal with. It has been shown to be easily collected by a wide range of professionals, in a wide range of settings. More sensitive scores that therapists may prefer to collect are likely to be more time-consuming, less likely therefore to be completed consistently and are likely to have less inter-rater reliability. There is therefore a conflict between sensitivity and feasibility.

Meta-analysis has convincingly shown that patients managed on stroke units perform better in terms of disability and mortality than patients managed on general wards. To demonstrate within an individual trust that there were differences in these outcomes would take many years and could well be confounded by temporal changes in case mix. It therefore makes much more sense to opt for the measurement of the structure of the service and what interventions the patient has received. By using the process measure as a proxy of outcome, the issue about the case mix is avoided. Process measures such as these are also likely to be more acceptable to clinicians who might even welcome the opportunity to measure their service in order to provide ammunition to persuade managers in providing more resources.

Areas like patient satisfaction, carer burden, and patient knowledge of their disease, are areas where there needs to be a lot more work to develop reliable measures. Although they are important, there are few reliable scales that could be used.

Another crucial issue that needs to be addressed is how the results of outcome measurement should be interpreted. Two examples illustrate some of the difficulties involved. One study looked at the issue of patient satisfaction. A satisfaction survey was conducted in two services. One where there was a well coordinated stroke service where physicians, therapists and nursing staff felt that they were actually providing quite a good model of care, and one which was much less well coordinated in a community hospital.[7] The patient satisfaction survey did not show any significant difference between the two. The patients themselves were failing to identify what clinicians and the research literature thought was the good service. The other study looked at the influence of case-mix measurement on the interpretation of outcome.[8] In Scotland, stroke outcomes measurement has been undertaken for many years. A unit was studied before and after the introduction of a stroke unit comparing outcomes. Figure 2 shows the odds ratios (95% confidence intervals).

			Standard care	Stroke unit care	Odds ratio	p value
Outcome						
	★	Uncorrected	162/215	214/250	0.5 (0.3 to 0.8)	0.007
Alive at 30 days	✳	Age and sex			0.8 (0.6 to 1.0)	0.026
	✳	Case mix			0.9 (0.6 to 1.2)	0.454
	★	Uncorrected	131/215	181/249	0.6 (0.4 to 0.9)	0.01
Alive at 12 months	✳	Age and sex			0.8 (0.7 to 1.0)	0.046
	✳	Case mix			1.0 (0.7 to 1.2)	0.744
	★	Uncorrected	51/213	89/245	0.6 (0.4 to 0.9)	0.006
Independent at	✳	Age and sex			0.8 (0.6 to 0.9)	0.014
12 months	✳	Case mix			0.9 (0.7 to 1.3)	0.694
	★	Uncorrected	91/215		0.5 (0.3 to 0.7)	<0.001
Living at home	✳	Age and sex			0.7 (0.6 to 0.9)	0.001
at 12 months	✳	Case mix			0.9 (0.7 to 1.1)	0.252

Figure 2. Odds ratios (95% confidence intervals) comparing standard ward care with stroke service care; data for four outcomes before and after correction for age and sex only, and for 19 indicators of case mix.

Outcome data corrected for age and sex shows that the introduction of
the stroke unit produced a major benefit. Patients were surviving and
doing so in a fitter state than before the introduction of the stroke unit.
However, when multiple case-mix measures including conscious level at
admission, eye movements, urinary incontinence and other measures
known to be important in terms of defining how severe the stroke is, were
added into the model, there turned out to be no significant differences
before and after.

In summary therefore, when deciding how to measure the quality of a
service, the most straightforward option is to look at structure and process
and avoid venturing into the territory of outcome.

Examples of National Audit

Considerable resources have been devoted to local audit over the last three
decades without many concrete achievements. There are exceptions but in
general, local audit tools have not been subjected to rigorous development, samples are too small to answer the questions being asked and the
processes to effectively implement the findings have been missing.
National audit can overcome these problems and has the additional advantage of providing individual health providers with benchmarking data
enabling them to compare local performance with the rest of the country
(Figs. 3 and 4).

This combination of robust data tested for reliability[9] with large numbers (statistical power) and meaningful comparisons with one's peers, has
provoked genuine interest from clinicians of all disciplines, from managers and from patient groups. In England, Wales and Northern Ireland
national stroke audit has been performed on a two-yearly cycle since
1998. There is evidence to show that the audit has been a powerful driver
for change.[10–14]

The national audit of stroke is a snapshot of care across the country
(Fig. 5).[15] It collects data retrospectively from case notes about the care
provided from hospital admission to discharge, by all members of the
multidisciplinary team. Each participating trust provides information
about the organisation of services and the process of care of up to 60

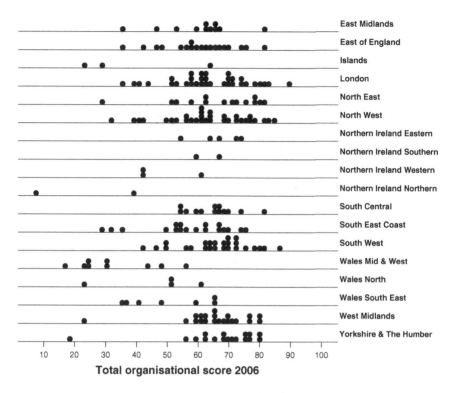

Figure 3. Individual hospital results organised by region of the audit of organisation of stroke care.

consecutive admissions with stroke. Until there is an electronic patient record, it will not be feasible to collect prospective data for a condition that often requires many weeks in hospital and involves so many different professionals in delivering treatment. Examples of data items collected are shown in the Appendix.

Results from the audit over the last ten years have shown a consistent improvement in the organisation and process of care. In 1998, only 18% of patients were managed for the majority of their stay on a stroke unit. By 2008, this has risen to over 60%. About 98% of hospitals in England now have a stroke unit, up from 40% ten years ago. Nearly all hospitals are now providing neurovascular clinics, although not all of

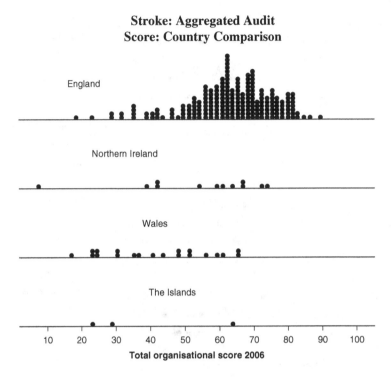

Figure 4. National sentinel audit results for organisational results 2006 displayed by country.

these are able to see and investigate patients within 14 days of presentation. Full details of the audit are available from www.rcplondon.ac.uk. There have been several drivers to the improved care, including the National Stroke Strategy,[1] the National Service Framework for Older People,[16] which included a chapter on stroke and the National Clinical Guidelines.[5]

There is a close correlation between the results of the audit of organisation of care the results a hospital gets when individual patient data are submitted for the process audit (Fig. 6). Given that the time and effort required preparing data for the clinical audit is so much higher than for the organisation of care, it does raise the possibility that the clinical audit may not be necessary to define the overall standards of a hospital. It does

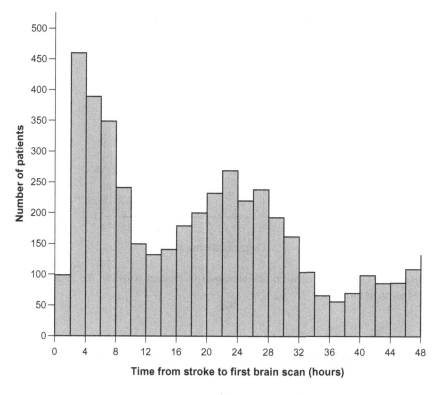

Figure 5. An example of national data from process of stroke care audit (National Sentinel Audit of Stroke 2008). Time from stroke to first brain scan for patients scanned within the first 48 hours.

however, provide a wealth of information about why a hospital is performing well or badly that is necessary to define what needs to be done to improve services.

National Stroke Registers: The RIKS Register (Sweden)

A few countries have national prospective registers for stroke rather than conducting episodic audit. Riks-Stroke[17] in Sweden is a tool for continuous quality improvement of stroke care (http:\\www.riks-stroke.org). The aim of the register is to support high and consistent

**"Structure" (Organisational) & "Process"
Indicator Totals by Trust**

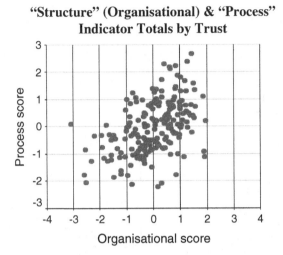

Figure 6. Correlation between organisational or process scores in the 2008 national sentinel audit for stroke.

quality of care for stroke patients throughout Sweden, ultimately to ensure patient benefit in the form of the best possible care. A second aim of Riks-Stroke is to provide a database for research on stroke. All hospitals contribute data and as of 2007, over 270,000 patients had been included on the register, with an estimated coverage of 82% of hospital admissions with stroke and about 77% of all strokes nationally. The data included is summarised in Table 1.

Results published in 2007 showed that there are wide variations between hospitals in the proportion of patients admitted to a stroke unit (Fig. 7), in secondary prevention and in the proportion of patients in institutional care at three months. Even after adjustment for available prognostic indicators, case fatality was lower and functional outcome was better in patients treated in stroke units than in patients treated in general wards.

While continuous registration of data clearly offers great advantages in being able to continuously monitor quality, there are disadvantages compared to intermittent retrospective data collection. It is more expensive to run, requires more time for data collection and it

Table 1. Data collected by the RIKS register.

Background Data	Process Indicators	Outcome Indicators
Living conditions (at home, in institution)	Admission to stroke unit*	Medical complications during hospital stay
Marital/cohabitant status	Diagnostic procedures	Discharge status
Primary ADL functions before stroke	Thrombolysis	Survival at three months
Previous stroke	Oral anticoagulants after cerebral embolism	Living conditions at three months
Co-morbidity	Other antithrombotic therapy	ADL dependency at three months
Smoking	Antihypertensive therapy	Support by next-of-kin
Level of consciousness on admission	Statins	Patient satisfaction with hospital stay and rehabilitation after discharge
Time to arrival in hospital	Access to rehabilitation after discharge	Low mood at three months
	Length of hospital stay	Perceived general health at three months

is difficult to maintain high levels of data entry and quality. A paper from one centre in Sweden that has contributed data to the RIKS register over the last 12 years raises important issues about interpretation of such long-term disease registers, particularly where the data are collected separately from routine clinical data.[18] There is variation in the completeness of case ascertainment and data completeness, particularly for follow-up data. Data are more likely to be submitted for patients admitted to a stroke unit bed than elsewhere. It is a major problem that the register does not record data on non-admitted patients as the number of these may be increasing as community services improve. It also highlights the difficulty of adjusting for variations over time in case severity.

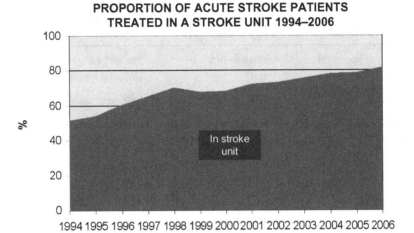

PROPORTION OF ACUTE STROKE PATIENTS
TREATED IN A STROKE UNIT 1994–2006

Figure 7.   An example of data produced by the RIKS stroke register. Proportion of
patients treated in a stroke unit 1994–2006.

Using routine data to monitor quality

The ideal way of monitoring quality would be to use routinely collected
information from the health services or insurance companies if such data
could be relied upon and if the data needed was available. In the UK, the
main source for routine data are the Hospital Episode Statistics (HES).
Unfortunately, the data is sparse and even such data as exists has been
shown often to be of poor quality. It is possible to obtain data such as mortality, inpatient complications and length of stay but information about
speed of access to imaging or therapies are not recorded. Considerable
investment in the UK is being made to develop a national electronic
patient record. However, this still seems likely to be some years away
from implementation. The plans are for this data set to contain the key
items for monitoring quality of care and may remove the need for specific
systems for audit.

Other Examples of National Audit

National audit is becoming more widespread and several papers have
reported their data highlighting particular issues that need addressing.

Argentina have developed a prospective multicentre countrywide stroke registry comprising 74 academic and non-academic institutions with 1991 patients included over two years.[19] They report low levels of thrombolysis and stroke unit admission (5.7%) and high levels of pneumonia. Outcomes are better in academic units, indicating the urgent need to develop a national stroke programme. Audit in Canada[20] has shown that patients from low income groups are more likely to be admitted to low volume hospitals and this group of patients had higher risk adjusted mortality than higher income groups admitted to high volume hospitals.

Ireland has introduced a similar system of audit to England, Wales and Northern Ireland but has extended it to include primary care.[21] Germany collects data prospectively, but mainly on care while still in the acute hospital (German Stroke Registers Study Group ADSR). By 2008 they had over 270,000 patients registered with the majority of acute hospitals contributing.[22]

Audit of Primary Care

The majority of the medical care that a stroke survivor receives will be from the primary care team after discharge from hospital. In the UK, this is likely to include secondary prevention and organisation of any longer term rehabilitation. Previous data following a relatively small number of patients up to six months after hospital discharge suggested that delivery of secondary prevention was in many cases inadequate.[23] An audit, conducted by QResearch[24] based in the Department of General Practice in Nottingham using data from routinely collected practice data systems from 200 practices with nearly 11,000 patients with a history of stroke, showed that 47% were normotensive (less than or equal to 140/85 mmHg), nearly 60% had a recorded cholesterol measurement within the previous 15 months, of whom 35% had a level over 5 mmol/l. Only half of all patients after stroke were on any form of lipid lowering drug. The full report available from the QResearch website[24] contains a wealth of similar data highlighting the importance of finding more effective ways of delivering effective secondary prevention to stroke patients than we currently have.

Audit of Transient Ischaemic Attack and Carotid Endarterectomy

A number of countries conduct regular audit of surgical management of carotid stenosis, including the UK,[25] Scotland and Germany. What has not yet been achieved satisfactorily has been evaluation of the quality of care of transient ischaemic attack (TIA) because of the difficulties in establishing the proportion of patients presenting and the quality of diagnosis in primary care.

Quality of Stroke Thrombolysis Services

A precondition of the license being given for Alteplase in Europe was that all patients being treated should have their data entered into the SITS (Safe Implementation of Thrombolysis) database (www.acutestroke. org). This collected detailed information on management of thrombolysed patients, including door to scan and needle times, appropriateness of treatment compared to the recommended criteria and outcomes in terms of neurological status at three months, haemorrhage rates and mortality. The results were published in 2007,[26] which confirmed that the results in routine practice were in line with the trial data. Since then, a full license has been given and data submission is no longer mandatory. However, the audit is still available and should be used for individual centres to monitor their practice and compare with national and international data.

Audit of Patient Satisfaction

Few attempts have been made to survey at a national level, stroke patients' perceptions of the quality of care they received. A paper published in 2007 in the UK attempted to determine the extent of correlation between stroke patients' experiences of hospital care with the quality of services assessed in the national sentinel audit.[27] Patients' assessments of their care derived from survey data were linked to data obtained in the National Sentinel Stroke Audit 2004 for 670 patients in 51 English NHS trusts. Patient experience scores were positively correlated with clinicians' assessment of the organisational quality of stroke care, but were largely unrelated to clinical process standards. Responses to individual questions regarding communication about diagnosis revealed a discrepancy between clinicians' and patients' reports. It did show that better organised stroke care is associated with more positive patient experiences. However, it confirmed that many of the aspects of care that the professionals regard as important are not those that the patients are most concerned about. Evaluation of the quality of stroke services should include a validated patient experience survey in addition to audit of clinical records.

Using data: implementing change and dissemination

Measuring quality is of little value unless something is done to deal with the issues that are identified. Providing information about local care compared to neighbouring hospitals and nationally is a powerful driver to encourage improvement. No one wants to be seen to be performing badly. However, there are additional ways apart from simply providing the data that can encourage change.

Producing reports

Producing the data from audits in different formats for the differing audiences is worth the effort. In the UK, reports are produced for the local hospitals, the Strategic Health Authorities (regional administrative bodies), the national Department of Health and Parliamentarians.

Education/Workshops

Bringing clinicians and managers together in local or regional workshops to discuss guidelines and audit, sharing examples of good practice, supporting colleagues having difficulties implementing change and helping develop working relationships between clinicians that, even though they may work in neighbouring hospitals and may have little or no routine contact, is of value.

Publicity

Publicising the results of the audit in the local and national press is a powerful driver for change. Anecdotally, there are several examples where clinicians had been attempting to improve the quality of their services but had been frustrated by lack of resources or management resistance, exposure to public scrutiny by a television or radio interview produced rapid results. 'I've been trying to get the trust to offer scanning for stroke patients for five years; within a day of receiving the audit report, the chief executive had convened a meeting with stroke service and radiology,' a stroke physician said after publication of performance indicators 2004 audit. Publication of data in peer-reviewed scientific journals can also have a positive impact, particularly at a central government level.

Using quality markers to reward or penalise health services

Several countries including the UK and Germany use audit data to reward or penalise hospitals performing well or badly. In England, stroke data are included in the annual 'health check' of hospitals, on which Chief Executives' performance related pay is partly based. In Germany, stroke units need to be accredited for insurance companies to fund acute stroke care. Poor performance on the audit puts accreditation at risk and therefore motivates quality improvement. The Quality Outcomes Framework (QOF) in primary care in England sets standards against which General Practitioners' pay is determined. A number of QOF targets have been set which relate to stroke care, mainly in the area of secondary prevention including blood pressure and lipid management. Since their introduction a few years ago, there has been a dramatic improvement in performance in these areas.[28]

Peer review

Provision of a system where health services can request a visit from a multidisciplinary team to provide advice on service improvement and support with implementation has been available for a number of specialties, including stroke in the UK, for some years. Formal evaluation of such schemes is rare but they appear to provide a useful addition to the service improvement armamentarium.

Developing leadership skills

The most common reason why services continue to perform badly is that there is inadequate vision and leadership within the team. Some aspects of leadership can be taught, so sending the relevant people on a leadership course can sometimes produce the necessary impetus for improvement.

Conclusion

An integral part of every stroke service should be a system for continuous quality improvement. This requires development of standards against which to measure performance (guidelines), measurement of current performance (structure, process and outcome) and methods to react to results that are aimed at rectifying deficits. No hospital should be working in isolation in this process as there is always much to be learnt from colleagues. National audit provides a powerful tool for clinicians, managers and commissioners to evaluate performance.

Appendix. Examples of organisational audit standards of stroke

Question number	Standard	Rationale	Audit help notes
		Staff Knowledge/Skills	
1.8	**Expertise** Patients' management and care is planned and provided by professionals with expertise in the management of stroke	Research evidence demonstrates the importance of medicine and nursing with specialist interest and knowledge of stroke[a] (Stroke Unit Trialists Collaboration, 1997).	**Medicine** — A physician with special interest in stroke manages or provides advice on the management of stroke patients. **Nursing** — The system of nursing facilitates the involvement of qualified nurses (with post-graduate/registration education in stroke rehabilitation) in direct patient care (Redfern, 1995; Waters, 1997).
	a) Medical treatment b) Nursing care c) Occupational Therapy d) Physiotherapy e) Speech/Language Therapy	The professional colleges' recommendations (RCS&LT, 1996; Chartered Society of Physiotherapists ACPIN, 1995; National Association of Neurological Occupational Therapies, 1996).	**Occupational Therapy** — The occupational therapy stroke service is under the overall supervision of a senior occupational therapist with at least five years experience, of which at least three is in Neurology (NANOT, 1996). **Physiotherapy** — Senior physiotherapist experienced in stroke rehabilitation or with access to specialist supervision (ACPIN, 1995). **Speech & Language Therapy** — specialist in acquired neurological communication and swallowing difficulties or with access to specialist supervision (RCSL&T, 1996).

(Continued)

Appendix. (*Continued*)

Question number	Standard	Rationale	Audit help notes
		Communication with Patients and Carers	
1.17	The organisation of the ward/unit ensures that patients and carers have access to their management plan.	So the patient/carer can understand the rehabilitation/treatment plan and participate actively in its achievement. Research suggests that the involvement of carers in the rehabilitation process may be a significant factor in clinical outcomes from rehabilitation.[a] (Stroke Unit Trialists Collaboration, 1997)	The management plan is kept near the patient's bed (e.g. end of bed) where she/he and the carer can refer to it.

(*Continued*)

Appendix. (*Continued*)

Question number	Standard	Rationale	Where most likely documented	Audit help notes
2.1	**Initial Assessment**			
2.1.1b i)	**Full neurological assessment (cont).** Patients are routinely screened with a standardised screening procedure to check for dysphagia.	The ability to swallow should be assessed within 24 hours of admission. Difficulties may be temporary but carry increased risk of complications. (Smithard, 1996; 1998).[b]	Team, medical or nursing records	Refers to a formal swallow screen (performed by any member of the team). Presence or absence of the gag reflex is not sufficient as it is proven to be of little prognostic value for the ability to swallow (Horner, 1988). (Cf. 2.2.1 for speech therapy assessment).
2.1.3	A brain scan is carried out within 24 hours where cerebral or subarachnoid haemorrhage is suspected, or if a patient is on warfarin, or if anticoagulation or thrombolysis is considered.	Haemorrhage is visible on CT scan immediately. Patients with haemorrhage may need surgical intervention. Imaging is also used to exclude haemorrhage before starting thrombolysis, aspirin, or anticoagulation (Warlow *et al.*, 1996).[b]	Team or medical records.	Notes mention suspected haemorrhage; and CT or MRI scan. NB: This refers only to *emergency* scanning and is relevant only in the cases *where haemorrhage is suspected in the first 24 hours after stroke*. Where haemorrhage is not suspected' the answer will be "No but…"

(*Continued*)

Appendix. *(Continued)*

Question number	Standard	Rationale	Where most likely documented	Audit help notes
3	Management plan			
3.1	There is written evidence of rehabilitation goals agreed by the multidisciplinary team.	Team goals (both short and longer term) promote forward planning and provide the framework for coordinated multidisciplinary care. If realistic, they can also help to motivate the patient.[c]	Team, medical, nursing or therapy notes.	This refers to the team goals for each patient, i.e. not those of individual disciplines. Auditors should identify with their clinicians how these would be documented within their Trust. Where it is documented that the team plan is palliative care, answer will be "No but…"

[a] Requires at least one randomised controlled trial as part of the body of evidence.
[b] Requires availability of well-conducted clinical studies but no randomised controlled trials in the body of evidence.
[c] Requires evidence from expert committee reports or opinions and/or clinical experience of respected authorities. Indicates absence of directly applicable studies of good quality.

References

1. National Stroke Strategy. Department of Health 2007. http://www.dh.gov.uk/en/Publicationsandstatistics/Publications/PublicationsPolicyAndGuidance/DH_081062

2. Norrving B; International Society of Internal Medicine; European Stroke Council; International Stroke Society; WHO Regional Office for European. The 2006 Helsingborg Consensus Conference on European Stroke Strategies: summary of conference proceedings and background to the 2nd Helsingborg Declaration. *Int J Stroke* 2007; 2(2): 139–143.

3. Puerto AN, Ibarluzea IG, Ruiz OG, Alvarez FM, Herreros RG, Pintiado RE, Dominguez AR. Analysis of the quality of clinical practice guidelines on established ischaemic stroke. *Int J Tech Assess Health Care* 2008; 24: 333–341.

4. Diagnosis and initial management of acute stroke and transient ischaemic attack (TIA) 2008. http://www.nice.org.uk/CG68

5. Royal College of Physicians, Intercollegiate Stroke Working Party. National Clinical Guidelines for Stroke 3rd Edn. London 2008. www.rcplondon.ac.uk

6. Donabedian A. Evaluating the quality of medical care. 1966. Milbank Q. 2005; 83(4): 691–729.

7. Pound P, Rudd AG, Wolfe CDA. Does patient satisfaction reflect differences in care received after stroke. *Stroke* 1999; 30: 49–55.

8. Davenport RJ, Dennis MS, Warlow CP. Effect of correcting outcome data for case mix: an example from stroke medicine. *BMJ* 1996; 312: 503–505.

9. Gompertz PH, Irwin P, Morris R, Rudd AG, Pearson M. Validity and reliability of Intercollegiate Stroke Audit Package. *J Evaluation Clin Pract* 2001; 7: 1–11.

10. Intercollegiate Stroke Working Party. Organisational Audit of Stroke Care in England, Wales and Northern Ireland. Royal College of Physicians 2008. www.rcplondon.ac.uk/stroke

11. Rudd AG, Hoffman A, Irwin P, Lowe D, Pearson MG. Stroke unit care and outcome: results from the 2001 National Sentinel Audit of Stroke (England, Wales, and Northern Ireland). *Stroke* 2005; 36(1): 103–106.

12. Rudd AG, Hoffman A, Irwin P, Lowe D, Pearson M. Stroke units: research and reality. Results from the National Sentinel Audit of Stroke. *Quality and safety in healthcare* 2005; 14: 7–12.

13. Irwin P, Hoffman A, Lowe D, Pearson M, Rudd AG. Improving clinical practice in stroke through audit: results of three rounds of National Stroke Audit. *J Evalu Clin Pract* 2005; 11(4): 306–314.
14. Rudd AG, Hoffman A, Down C, Pearson M, Lowe D. Access to stroke care in England, Wales and Northern Ireland; effect of age gender and weekend admission. *Age Ageing* 2007; 36: 247–255.
15. Rudd AG, Irwin P, Lowe D, Rutledge Z, Pearson M. National Clinical Audit. A tool for change. *Quality in Healthcare* 2001; 10: 141 151.
16. National service framework for older people. Department of Health 2001. http://www.dh.gov.uk/en/Publicationsandstatistics/Publications/Publications PolicyAndGuidance/DH_4003066
17. Asplund K, Hulter Asberg K, Norrving B, Stegmayr B, Terént A, Wester PO; Riks-Stroke Collaboration. Riks-stroke — a Swedish national quality register for stroke care. *Cerebrovasc Dis* 2003; 15 (Suppl 1): 5–7.
18. Appelros P, Samuelsson M, Karlsson-Tivenius S, Lokander M, Terént A. A national stroke quality register: 12 years experience from a participating hospital. *Eur J Neurol* 2007; 14(8): 890–894.
19. Sposato LA, Esnaola MM, Zamora R, Zurrú MC, Fustinoni O, Saposnik G; on behalf of ReNACer Investigators and the Argentinian Neurological Society. Quality of Ischaemic stroke care in emerging countries. The Argentinean National Stroke Registry (ReNACer). *Stroke* 2008; 39: STROKEAHA.108.521062v1
20. Lindsay P, Bayley M, McDonald A, Graham ID, Warner G, Phillips S. Towards a more effective approach to stroke: Canadian best practice recommendations for stroke care. *CMAJ* 2008; 178(11). Doi:10.1503/cmaj. 071253
21. Irish Heart Foundation National Audit of Stroke Care. http://www.irishheart. ie/iopen24/pub/strokereports/stroke_report.pdf
22. Heuschmann PU, Biegler MK, Busse O, Elsner S, Grau A, Hasenbein U, Hermanek P, Janzen RW, Kolominsky-Rabas PL, Kraywinkel K, Lowitzsch K, Misselwitz B, Nabavi DG, Otten K, Pientka L, von Reutern GM, Ringelstein EB, Sander D, Wagner M, Berger K. Development and implementation of evidence-based indicators for measuring quality of acute stroke care: the Quality Indicator Board of the German Stroke Registers Study Group (ADSR). *Stroke* 2006; 37(10): 2573–2578.

23. Rudd AG, Lowe D, Hoffman A, Irwin P, Pearson M. Secondary prevention for stroke in the United Kingdom: results from the National Sentinel Audit of Stroke. *Age Ageing* 2004; 33: 280–286.
24. National Stroke Audit in Primary Care. www.qresearch.org/.../National_ Stroke_Audit_Final_Report_2004.pdf
25. Halliday AW, Lees T, Kamugasha D, Grant R, Hoffman A, Rothwell PM, Potter JF, Horrocks M, Naylor R, Rudd AG. Long waiting times for carotid endarterectomy in the UK. *BMJ* 2009; 338: 1423–1425.
26. Wahlgren N, Ahmed N, Dávalos A, Ford GA, Grond M, Hacke W, Hennerici MG, Kaste M, Kuelkens S, Larrue V, Lees KR, Roine RO, Soinne L, Toni D, Vanhooren G; SITS-MOST investigators. Thrombolysis with alteplase for acute ischaemic stroke in the Safe Implementation of Thrombolysis in Stroke-Monitoring Study (SITS-MOST): an observational study. *Lancet* 2007; 369(9558): 275–282.
27. Howell E, Graham C, Hoffman A, Lowe D, McKevitt, Reeves R, Rudd AG. A comparison of patients' assessments of the quality of stroke care with audit findings. *Qua Safe Healthcare* 2007; 16: 450–455.
28. Simpson CR, Hannaford PC, Lefevre K, Williams D. Effect of the UK incentive-based contract on the management of patients with stroke in primary care. *Stroke* 2006; 37: 2354–2360.

13 New Horizons in Stroke

Lalit Kalra*

Chapter Summary

The last decade has seen an exponential growth in stroke literature and dramatic improvements in stroke care. This chapter touches upon the improvements in stroke care that can be expected over the next few years, the direction that research will take and some of the challenges that practitioners in stroke will have to face to deliver the promise of future advances in stroke. Prevention studies have shown that people who adhere to lifestyle recommendations to prevent vascular disease have dramatically lower stroke risks as compared to those who do not. The challenge then is to develop strategies that encourage healthy behaviours. A particularly challenging group is that of patients over 80 years of age. Most prevention studies have excluded such patients and the risk to benefit ratio of aggressive management remains open to debate. Data extrapolated from younger people and some recent studies suggest that this age group may have more to benefit compared with younger patients. However, the risks may also be greater and need further investigation. Predicting patients who will have the most successful outcomes after thrombolysis remains an imprecise science. New imaging techniques based on assessments of collateral circulation and cerebral haemodynamics may help select patients who are most likely to gain from

*Professor of Stroke Medicine, Academic Neuroscience Centre, King's College London, UK

thrombolytic treatments, even beyond conventional time windows. The future holds promise of new thrombolytic agents that may be more effective, safer or have a longer time window for intervention, intra-arterial techniques that may deliver better results and mechanical devices that aid recanalisation. In rehabilitation, imaging studies have provided new and unique insights into reorganisation after injury that have resulted in a paradigm shift in understanding recovery from stroke. These insights are being used to develop new interventions, many for impairments previously considered refractory to treatment. Regeneration therapy after ischaemic injury to the brain is another exciting development close to human testing. Finally, new systems such as telemedicine are being developed and tested to extend specialist healthcare to remote population, so that the benefits of advance in stroke reach out to the vast majority rather than being limited to selected populations who have access to specialist centres.

Introduction

The last decade has seen an exponential growth in stroke literature and dramatic improvements in stroke care, underpinned by new insights into the mechanisms of injury and recovery from stroke. Stroke care and research have both been benefited by the rapid advances in neuroimaging and therapeutics. The culture of randomised clinical trials for evaluation of stroke therapies is solidly planted and thriving. Given the advances in stroke described in the preceding chapters, it is tempting to speculate the improvements in stroke care that can be expected over the next few years, the direction that research will take and some of the challenges that practitioners in stroke will have to face to deliver the promise of advances in stroke in future.

Prevention

Prevention remains the cornerstone of reducing the burden of stroke on populations throughout the world and much is to be gained through better adherence to proven stroke prevention measures.[1] Stroke prevention guidelines developed by professional bodies, governmental agencies and voluntary organisations provide a variety of lifestyle and behavioural recommendations aimed at reducing stroke risk (Chapter 2). Recent studies from Scotland and Rome have shown that implementation of public health policies such as a ban on tobacco smoking in public indoor spaces have significantly reduced hospital admissions due to coronary heart disease.[2] It is likely that such policies will result in a similar decrease in the risk of stroke but this needs to be confirmed and in different settings. Research shows that people who adhere to lifestyle recommendations to prevent vascular disease have dramatically lower stroke risks as compared to those who do not. Subjects with a low-risk profile had a 69–79% reduction in the risk of all strokes and an 80–81% reduction in the risk of ischaemic stroke with a graded reduction related to level of adherence in the recently reported Health Professionals Follow-up Study.[3] Although these data are highly convincing, implementation of healthy lifestyles in the population remains a problem. The challenge remains in translating the benefits of what is already known into population health benefit, especially in the face of the growing epidemic of the metabolic syndrome and obesity across developed and developing countries.

A particular challenge in stroke prevention is posed by the worldwide growth of the population of individuals over 80 years of age.[4] The incidence of stroke increases sharply with older age and there is a doubling of stroke incidence with each successive decade after the age of 55 years.[5] Despite this increase in numbers and in the risk of stroke, studies show that older people are less likely to receive effective stroke prevention compared with younger people.[6] Some of this discrepancy between increased risk but decreased prevention may be attributable to fear of adverse events and interactions with drugs or perceptions of lack of capacity to benefit because of higher prevalence of disability, cognitive impairment and loss of autonomy.[7] However, it is equally true that there is a paucity of evidence-based studies in this population, simply because patients over 80 years of age were excluded from most studies and there are doubts about the cost-effectiveness of such therapies in this population.[4] Clinical outcomes in older patients tend to be much worse than for their younger counterparts even after adjusting for co-morbidities, favouring aggressive risk management.[8] Despite this, age disparities in prevention and treatment exist because older people are less intensively investigated and less well treated.

Most physicians adopt a paternalistic approach towards what is good and not good for older patients, which perhaps is not justified. These aspects of stroke and other vascular disease in older people as well as attitudes towards old age need to change if age disparities in prevention and treatment are to be successfully bridged.

Treatment for hypertension in patients over 80 years of age is a good example of the challenges facing reduction of stroke risk in older people. There is ample evidence that treatment of hypertension in elderly people can reduce stroke, improve quality of life and slow cognitive decline through attenuation of ischaemic vascular dementia, especially in the presence of early Alzheimer's disease.[4] Despite this, there is no single well-established goal for blood pressure levels in the very elderly and values of less than 140/90 mmHg or even less than 130/80 mmHg in people have been considered applicable for this population.[4] The Hypertension in the Very Elderly Trial (HYVET) showed that antihypertensive therapy reduced stroke incidence by 30% and mortality by 21% in individuals over 80 years of age with minimal risk.[9] However, the target blood pressure level of 150/80 mmHg for the HYVET was less intensive than in clinical trials done among younger individuals and the recommended treatment goal of 140/80 mmHg. Whether a more intensive systolic target would be associated with further reductions in risk as seen in younger patients or result in greater adverse events with decreased tolerability is less clear. This is important as some studies have indicated that over-intensive lowering of blood pressure below a certain critical level in elderly patients with long-standing hypertension might increase the risk of cerebral hypoperfusion and possibly precipitate cognitive decline.[10] A recent study of hypertensive patients aged 80 years or older, most of whom received antihypertensive treatment, has also shown a shorter survival time for those with systolic blood pressure below 140 mmHg, even after adjustment for known predictors of death.[11] Hence, there is very little prospective evidence specific to those over 80 years of age or over to argue for or against intensive management of blood pressure to recommended standards. It is also not known whether aggressive targets can be safely implemented in older patients outside inclusion criteria for randomised controlled studies. However, this does not preclude aiming for slightly higher blood pressure levels similar to those for the HYVET studies (150/80), as these are known to reduce risk specifically in the older population.

Imaging in Stroke

CT and MR imaging have revolutionised stroke research and practice over the last two decades. Several new modalities such as diffusion-weighted imaging (DWI), perfusion imaging and magnetic resonance angiography (MRA) made it possible to visualise evolving infarction and the effects of various interventions, which have had a dramatic effect on the management of stroke patients. In addition to structural CT or MRI scans to image neurovascular injury, many centres perform non-invasive assessments of key elements of ischaemic pathophysiology such as CT or MR angiography for vascular occlusion and CT or MR perfusion maps to measure haemodynamic compromise on initial presentation. Vascular imaging of carotid and vertebral arteries, the aortic arch and the heart may also be undertaken to define stroke aetiology.

Imaging of the collateral circulation

The effects of vessel occlusion may be significantly modulated by collateral networks that provide numerous alternative routes for blood flow in the setting of obstruction.[12] Recent correlative imaging studies of collateral circulation in acute and chronic ischaemia have demonstrated that the occlusive lesion may be incompletely characterised without consideration of collaterals. Collateral flow visible at conventional angiography is a potent determinant of tissue fate, even beyond measures of perfusion.[13] This critical adaptive response to ischaemia has been shown to be a sensitive sensing mechanism for up-regulation of arteriogenesis, which is predictive of the extent of tissue injury, vascular remodelling following occlusion and finally repair in the hours, days and weeks following stroke.[12] Hence, imaging of the compensatory collateral flow during initial assessment of stroke patients may have significant applications in selecting patients for recanalisation treatments, which can improve the effectiveness and safety of such procedures by targeting them to those most likely to benefit. However, it has not been possible to image this compensatory mechanism without the use of conventional angiography because of the small size of collateral anastomoses. Conventional angiography is not feasible as a 'first line' investigation in most stroke patients presenting acutely and visualising early collateral circulation has evaded many imaging approaches. Refinements in CT angiography (CTA) and MRA techniques have made it possible to assess this compensatory collateral circulation non-invasively in acute stroke patients on presentation.[14] The clinical utility of this imaging approach in informing recanalisation decisions needs to be investigated in clinical studies.

Penumbra and treatment time windows

Imaging of collaterals and cerebral haemodynamics (e.g. perfusion) may have significant implications for the treatment time windows for recanalisation. The dictum that 'time is brain' is accepted throughout the stroke community, but this is not an entirely accurate reflection of ischaemic pathophysiology. The time course of ischaemic injury varies markedly across individuals and time from symptom onset does not reflect stroke evolution.[12] Symptoms become manifest only once collaterals fail to compensate for hypoperfusion and in most cases, the time of vascular occlusion is never known. When time from symptom onset is measured, we are essentially resetting relative times to collateral failure. Tissue injury is not a linear function of time and the evolution of ischaemic injury can vary dramatically from hour to hour between individuals. However, clinical studies suggest that the amount of brain lost can be averaged based on time from symptom onset across populations, and that up to 4.5 hours between symptom onset and intravenous thrombolysis are associated with favourable patient outcomes (Chapter 5).

The important question is: If symptom onset does not correlate with the time of occlusion, why is there still a treatment effect on time windows based on symptom onset? The answer may be that the effectiveness of thrombolysis is dependent upon changes in collateral circulation and haemodynamic compromise following vessel occlusion that continue to evolve during this critical period. Recanalisation may be most effective early on because collateral perfusion is adequate and can maintain a degree of perfusion despite vessel occlusion. Several hours later, venous collapse and haemodynamic failure may limit reperfusion even if clot disruption is achieved. This may explain why some cases may benefit from recanalisation many hours after vessel occlusion whereas others show significant damage even when treated very early after symptom onset.[15] This would also be one of the reasons why basilar occlusions can be treated up to 24 hours from symptom onset.[15] New data suggests that the time course of haemodynamic failure and window for reperfusion may also vary across vascular territories, hence treatment to recanalise may also need to take into account the site of occlusion.[16] Finally, patients with unknown time of onset or those outside traditional time windows who show mismatch pose a significant therapeutic dilemma. Is thrombolysis indicated and will it be of benefit because of the mismatch or are these patients not prone to haemodynamic failure (benign oligaemia), thereby altering the risk/benefit ratio? Many of these questions will be answered by the use of more refined techniques to image the penumbra and haemodynamic compromise in newer intervention studies being designed currently.[17] These will be helped by the development of new technology such as whole-brain CT perfusion that offers increased spatial coverage with higher resolution, reduced contrast requirements, and minimised radiation; perfusion atlases that show regional variation in blood flow abnormalities and topography and software that can identify blood–brain barrier disruptions and flow in the microcirculation, in addition to the modalities already available for clinical use.[18]

Thrombolysis and Recanalisation

Recent years have not only shown that intravenous thrombolysis up to three hours after symptom onset in stroke patients results in 14% more patients being alive and independent, but also that thrombolysis in clinical practice is as safe and effective as in randomised clinical trials (Chapter 5). More recently, the time window for intervention has been extended to 4.5 hours after the publication of the European Cooperative Acute Stroke Study (ECASS-3),[19] the safety and benefit of which in clinical practice has been confirmed by the Safe Implementation of Thrombolysis in Stroke database.[20] The challenge is now to see if this time window can be extended up to six or nine hours and whether thrombolysis for stroke will have similar benefits for patients over 80 years of age, who have hitherto been excluded from the randomised controlled trials. These questions are being addressed in several ongoing studies.[21]

There is strong evidence that thrombolysis for acute stroke patients is safe and highly effective treatment but a minority have allowed their uncertainty over safety and doubts raised by individually neutral trials to restrict implementation of this potent therapy in clinical practice.[21] One of the major limitations of existing research is the tight patient selection criteria and the dependence upon very basic imaging as assessment for eligibility for thrombolysis. An important priority for the future is to develop assessment and treatment strategies which will enable more stroke patients to receive these treatments and extend the time window in which they can be treated. One of the most promising approaches for achieving this is the use of more advanced imaging in treatment decisions as described in the above section. The EPITHET study suggests that this approach will be productive both in research and clinical practice[22] The study used perfusion imaging to identify patients eligible for thrombolytic treatment beyond three hours and showed that thrombolysis in patients with mismatch was associated with increased reperfusion and better functional outcomes compared with controls. Although the study lacked the power for definitive conclusions, it does suggest that patient selection based on a physiological time clock established by imaging has the potential of extending thrombolytic treatments to patient groups hitherto excluded from treatment because of fixed time windows. Observational data from large registries support this concept; outcomes and bleeding rates in patients thrombolysed between 3–6 hours after stroke on the basis of perfusion–diffusion mismatch were no different from those thrombolysed within 0–3 hours using similar criteria, suggesting that fixed time windows may be irrelevant if these imaging modalities were to be applied.[23] There are several ongoing studies using perfusion–diffusion mismatch concept or angiographic evidence of occlusion in stroke patients up to nine hours after symptom onset. It is likely that the results of these studies will have a significant impact on practice.

The only intervention currently available for acute thrombolysis is alteplase and other approaches are being investigated. An early study using another thrombolytic agent, tenectaplase, showed encouraging preliminary results with better rates of recanalisation and functional outcome at three months.[24] However, there was a trend toward increased haemorrhage rates, which need further investigation. Desmoteplase from vampire bat saliva has shown promise in two phase 2 ischaemic stroke trials enrolling patients 3–9 h after onset when an MRI diffusion–perfusion mismatch pattern is present.[25] However, DIAS II, a phase 3 trial showed that the proportion of patients who achieved good outcome at three months was comparable in patients who received 90 mg/kg and placebo (45%) and surprisingly lower in those treated with the highest dose. Ultrasound-assisted thrombolysis has been shown to increase recanalisation rates, but again at an increased risk of bleeding.[26] Further studies are being undertaken to evaluate the safety and efficacy of continuous insonation of the occluded middle cerebral artery in patients with ischaemic stroke given intravenous alteplase.

Evidence on intra-arterial thrombolysis is limited and the role of this approach remains open to question.[27] There is extensive observational data implying efficacy of intra-arterial thrombolysis,[21] but very little evidence from randomised controlled studies apart from the PROACT II studies nearly a decade ago (Chapter 5). Furthermore, there are no comparative studies against intravenous administration of thrombolytic agents. There is one ongoing study on the intra-arterial thrombolysis in acute stroke management (IMS 3) and others are being planned.[21] Clot retrieval devices physically grasp cerebral thrombi and pull them out of the cerebral circulation. These devices can be used on their own or combined with intra-venous or intra-arterial thrombolysis. The MERCI Retriever devices were tested in the Mechanical Embolus Removal in Cerebral Ischaemia trial,[28] in patients with occlusion of the carotid, middle cerebral, vertebral or basilar arteries within eight hours of onset. Partial or complete revascularisation was achieved in 54%; successful recanalisation was associated with markedly improved clinical outcomes in 53% compared with 6% of non-recanalisers. The feasibility, safety and effectiveness of mechanical devices, with or without other thrombolytic therapies, need to be confirmed in other studies and in clinical practice.

Rehabilitation

Stroke rehabilitation has been the cornerstone of recovery for the last two decades and significant strides have been made in the development of interventions to facilitate stroke recovery and the organisation of rehabilitation (Chapter 8). Major achievements in this area include a large body of research to show that early, intensive and task-specific therapy interventions after stroke improve and expedite recovery from stroke[29] and their successful implementation in clinical practice through professional guidelines and national benchmarking audits.[30] The role of stroke units in achieving good patient outcomes and improving the quality of care is also well established.[31] Functional magnetic imaging and transcranial magnetic stimulation studies have also shown that the opportunity for rehabilitation extends well beyond the traditional short time windows and many patients can benefit by intensive treatment inputs years after the initial event.[32]

The era of randomised clinical trial for evaluation of therapies aimed at improving recovery from the impairments caused by stroke is now firmly established in clinical practice. Many new and exciting interventions have been or are being investigated in large, well-designed multicentre studies. A notable success was the Effect of Constraint-Induced Movement Therapy on Upper Extremity (EXCITE) trial, a large multicentre trial that showed clinically relevant motor gains in the paretic arm in patients three to nine months post-stroke.[33] A recent survey (2009) of the clinical trials listed under the heading of stroke and rehabilitation [clinical trials.gov], shows that there are 176 stroke rehabilitation trials in various stages from active and recruiting to completed with the results still pending publication. These studies include the use of electrical stimulation, constraint-induced therapy, bilateral and unilateral tasks, new orthotics, strengthening exercises, robots, psychosocial interventions, family-mediated exercise, acupuncture, cycle training with progressive resistance training, aerobic cardiovascular fitness training, and pharmacologic therapies including levodopa, botulinum toxin type-A, and escitalopram.

'Neglected' impairments

The new frontiers that need to be addressed in the coming years are addressing rehabilitation of 'neglected' impairments. An example of this is hemianopia, which is common after stroke and adversely affects performance on many functional tasks. Despite its impact, nihilism pervades the management of hemianopia on the assumption that visual system damage is not amenable to external interventions. These assumptions have been challenged by emerging literature, which suggests that visual systems may be partially repairable and visual rehabilitative strategies may reduce visual field defects and improve function.[34] Strategies to improve hemianopia include optical interventions with prismatic lenses, eye movement therapy and visual field restitution.[35] Optical interventions and eye movement therapy compensate for the deficit by bringing stimuli from the damaged visual field into the intact visual field. In contrast, visual field restitution is designed to restore function within the damaged visual field. Visual search training can achieve modest improvements in hemianopia within a relatively short period and compares favourably with rehabilitation techniques routinely used for other cortical impairments such as aphasia or neglect. Although small studies claim success, there is considerable controversy on the mechanisms and the pathways involved as well as long-term effectiveness in improving vision.[35,36] Investigation of these pathways and the potential to modulate them using various rehabilitative techniques are prime areas for future research.[35,36]

Similarly, sensory impairments may affect up to 60% of stroke patients but their management has taken a back seat both in research and practice. As with other aspects of rehabilitation research, studies on sensory interventions are small, heterogeneous and limited because of methodological problems. A review of active and passive sensory rehabilitation reported this year showed evidence to support the effectiveness of passive sensory training methods but not for active sensory training protocols.[37] Furthermore, there was not enough evidence to suggest that improvements in sensory impairments translate into functional improvements. Again, the time is ripe for high-quality studies with meaningful clinical measures to assess the effectiveness of sensory retraining following stroke.

Advanced imaging studies have also provided new insights into the rehabilitation of neglect. A recent study has shown that breakdown of functional connectivity in ventral frontoparietal networks, known to be associated with non-spatial attention, underlies behavioural deficits in spatial neglect.[38] Furthermore, the study showed that non-spatial attention training that raised overall attentional abilities was associated with improvements in neglect. This improvement was underpinned by changes in cortical activation patterns in these and other areas known to be associated with attention, thus suggesting that new cortical–subcortical connections may be formed to overcome this impairment. It is well-known but less recognised that neglect may be associated with motor impairments. Many patients with neglect have directional hypokinesia and are slower to initiate a motor response to targets appearing in the left hemispace, even when using their unaffected arm. The precise anatomical location of this impairment is debated but a recent paper has localised these motor deficits associated with neglect to the basal ganglia, suggesting that a relative depletion of dopamine in the nigrostriatal pathway on the same side of the lesion may be an important pathophysiological mechanism and potentially amenable to intervention.[39] A meta-analysis of magnetic resonance perfusion imaging studies in neglect patients has shown that hypoperfusion of the right angular and/or the superior temporal gyrus may be an important cause of neglect.[40] Furthermore, fluctuations in neglect in the acute–subacute period after stroke are often due to changes in blood flow caused by changes in blood pressure, emphasising the importance of vascular assessments and appropriate management to ameliorate such impairments during rehabilitation.

Technology in rehabilitation

The last decade has seen a number of stimulation, robotic, virtual reality and feedback devices being developed to support stroke rehabilitation. Significant improvements in motor function and strength of the paretic arm have been shown with electromechanical and robot-assisted arm training but these do not necessarily translate into improvements in activities of daily living.[41] Furthermore, there is no robust evidence to suggest that the robotic properties of these interventions have inherent therapeutic value.[42] Although variations in the patient characteristics, duration and amount of training or other concomitant treatments may be important confounders of any gain with robotic assisted devices, further research is needed to establish their place in stroke rehabilitation. In addition, the mechanisms by which these devices enhance movement recovery are not fully understood.[42] The same is also true for virtual reality techniques, where existing data potentially support their application in the treatment of the paretic upper limb after stroke, but their superiority over existing and widely used conventional treatments remains unproven.[43]

Virtual reality or robotics may have important applications in the assessment of impairments but these have not been investigated to the same extent as their role in treatment. Current diagnostic methods for higher level impairments are relatively crude and do not assess patients in everyday tasks.[44] Virtual reality technologies hold promise for the development of effective assessment techniques by providing rich, multimodal, and highly controllable environments to assess such impairments. In addition, robotic devices and virtual reality environments can measure performance objectively and contribute to a detailed phenotype of stroke recovery.[45] These technologies have also provided a new insight into the mechanisms of stroke recovery. Robotic and virtual reality studies have shown that the performance plateau exhibited by patients at the end of the 'standard' rehabilitation phase may represent a period of consolidation rather than a performance optimum.[45] A recent study on mirror feedback techniques suggests a paradigm shift away from neurological deficits in stroke being entirely due to irreversible damage to specialised brain modules towards some impairments resulting from short-term functional shifts that are potentially reversible.[46] Further investigation of these paradigms will pave the way to new treatments for the future.

Neuroregeneration

Since the pivotal studies highlighting the treatment benefits of thrombolytic treatments, there have been no major therapeutic advances, despite a large number of studies. This failure to develop successful new therapies has highlighted the need for a completely different approach, such as promoting regeneration and repair. Replacing cells following stroke makes sense. As the common final pathway of electrical and chemical signalling in the brain, neurons should be replaced to optimally reduce disability and handicaps. The main approaches proposed for human application include promoting endogenous neuogenesis using pharmacological agents or implanting exogenous stem cells, each with its challenges and champions.[47,48] Critical and as yet unanswered questions are only beginning to be addressed: Which cells do we transplant? When do we transplant them? Where do we transplant them?[49] The most exciting development in stem cell research is the finding that fibroblasts can be reprogrammed to make embryonic stem cells.[50] These reprogrammed cells meet the most stringent definition of stem cells and theoretically a single cell could give rise to a whole organism. The findings are exciting for stem cell research in regeneration after stroke because they overcome the limitations posed by the dependence on foetal tissues for such cells and offer a strategy for developing embryonic stem cells that are genetically identical to their recipient.

The other area of development in neuroregeneration that is closer to human testing involves the use of growth factors or drugs to increase production of neural progenitors in the subventricular zone of the brain following stroke. A number of distinct growth factors can increase neurogenesis in central nervous system germinal zones following injury: erythropoietin, stromal cell-derived factor-1 (SDF-1), and GCSF.[51] Studies from a number of groups have identified small molecule activators of the Hypoxia Inducible Factor (HIF) pathway that are ripe for testing in this context.[52] Some of these drugs are already in Phase II human clinical trials for other diseases and could be tested in preclinical recovery studies within the next 2–3 years. A potentially groundbreaking study has shown that polymorphisims in the gene for the growth factor — brain derived neurotrophic factor (BDNF) — are associated with differences in plasticity and recovery after stroke.[53] This suggests that those with this mutation will respond more poorly to stroke rehabilitation. Affirmation that the 'val66met' mutation reduces efficacy of motor rehabilitation in humans would ignite a search for drugs that overcome the BDNF secretion defect associated with this mutation.

Common to both approaches is the challenge of translating preclinical testing in animals to human trials. Methods that can definitively demonstrate the therapeutic effect of newly introduced neural cells or pharmacological interventions in the living human brain are lacking and any future trials are likely to be confounded by the choice of appropriate outcome measures and controlling for the effects of other rehabilitation inputs. The prospect of surrogate outcomes using imaging techniques are attractive and will enhance understanding of mechanisms by which transplanted or endogenous stem cells lead to functional recovery and structural reorganisation. These issues have led to consensus on a coordinated approach to stem cell research and a common language for taking this exciting area of research forward.[54]

Delivery systems for enhancing neuroregeneration

Another important consideration in modulating endogenous Neural Stem Cells (NSC) is the development of vehicles to deliver specific molecules to specific sites in the brain so that the greatest effectiveness can be achieved with maximum safety. Preliminary work is underway in the development of nanosystems — subcellular sized biomaterial delivery systems that may be able to deliver specific molecules to specific sites in the brain, such as medication to the peri-infarct site to modify gene expression.[55] The concept is that small molecules and proteins can be packaged inside protein vaults and potentially delivered intracellularly in the brain. It may also be possible to use biomaterial implants, such as a gel matrix or silica microspheres, which may be used to fill the infarct core, imbedded with materials that may enhance neurovascular growth, providing a site-specific depot of therapeutic molecules.[56] Many of these techniques are in very early developmental stages in animal models but the collaboration of bioengineering and neuroscientists is paving the way to innovative and exciting new strategies to deliver new treatments closer to the site of injury in the brain and improving the extent and speed of recovery from stroke.

Other Horizons

An emerging trend in stroke care is the use of telemedicine; a system whereby the health status and needs of a patient can be reviewed remotely by experts using information technology systems.[57] Although stroke has become one of the most frequently used applications of telemedicine, its use is often restricted to specific purposes such as the initiation of thrombolysis or for the selection of patients eligible for surgical and neuroradiological interventions. In addition to this role, telemedicine has the potential to offer service providers the opportunity to access large numbers of stroke survivors for targeting secondary prevention interventions.[58] The ideal 'telestroke model' can provide service support, education for the patient and caregiver, as well as integration of specialist and primary care services. Despite these possible benefits, the use of telemedicine services is still limited to a few centres and remains fragmented. Many healthcare systems in the European Union and the United States have expressed their commitment to the wider deployment of telemedicine as a policy to improve healthcare. The reality remains that most telemedicine initiatives are no more than one-off, small-scale projects that are not integrated into existing healthcare systems.[57]

There are several reasons why telemedicine has not impacted on healthcare systems despite widespread political and policy support. Despite some successful studies in the assessment of patients suitable for thrombolysis,[59] the evidence base for telemedicine remains limited and the risks or benefits of telemedicine applications have not been sufficiently investigated in pre-hospital and post-acute stroke care. The economic impact of telestroke systems is also unknown.[57] Although many enthusiasts believe that these systems would be highly cost-effective, no systematic analysis has been published to date that takes into account the societal costs of telemedicine that include stroke care, running networks, staff training, data and hardware maintenance as well as telecommunication services. Similarly, the savings that may be achieved by successful implementation of telestroke network over and above well-organised stroke care in terms of reduced mortality or disability, reduced interhospital transfers and family travel times remain unknown. Little is also known about user acceptance and the quality of care aspects of such systems. The time is ripe for controlled studies to address these issues although it needs to be acknowledged that such trials would be logistically difficult because the introduction of telestroke systems even as an experimental intervention may result in permanent changes in healthcare delivery systems.

Implementation of telemedicine in routine clinical care is also not without problems. Telestroke should be systems and not technology-driven, a fact that sometimes gets ignored when such systems are introduced in clinical settings. Insufficient planning of IT infrastructure, lack of long-term vision for sustainability, a lack of contextual perspective, poor communication across domains, lack of acknowledgement of existing practices and lack of awareness of potential financial barriers can further limit implementation.[58] Even where telemedicine has been used successfully for early recognition of strokes, it cannot replace the time-critical initiation of therapy which may prove difficult on the distant, and possibly less well resourced site. A 'drip-and-ship' model has been advocated in several healthcare systems where therapy is started at the remote facility followed by immediate transfer to the stroke centre. There are currently no data from controlled studies on either the safety or efficacy of systemic thrombolysis in such systems, the impact of interhospital transfer in critically ill patients, or on the legal responsibilities if things were to go wrong.[57]

The future of telestroke models lies in providing effective action in an integrated model of care that is cost-effective, of high quality and involves all existing players and practices. This can only be made possible by well-designed randomised controlled trials and/or longitudinal observational studies of clinical outcomes to demonstrate the effective use of telemedicine in different settings, ranging from assessments for thrombolysis to managing vascular risk in stroke survivors discharged from hospital.[60]

References

1. Goldstein LB. How much can be gained by more systematic prevention of stroke? *Int J Stroke* 2008; 3: 266–271.
2. Goldstein LB, Rothwell PM. Advances in primary prevention and health services delivery. *Stroke* 2009; 40: 295–297.
3. Chiuve SE, Rexrode KM, Spiegelman D, Logroscino G, Manson JE, Rimm EB. Primary prevention of stroke by healthy lifestyle. *Circulation* 2008; 118: 947–954.
4. Sanossian N, Ovbiagele B. Prevention and management of stroke in very elderly patients. *Lancet Neurol* 2009; 8: 1031–1041.

5. Sacco RL, Adams R, Albers G *et al.* Guidelines for prevention of stroke in patients with ischemic stroke or transient ischemic attack: a statement for healthcare professionals from the American Heart Association/American Stroke Association Council on Stroke. *Stroke* 2006; 37: 577–617.

6. Lawlor DA, Whincup P, Emberson JR, Rees K, Walker M, Ebrahim S. The challenge of secondary prevention for coronary heart disease in older patients: findings from the British Women's Heart and Health Study and the British Regional Heart Study. *Fam Pract* 2004; 21: 582–586.

7. Schmader KE, Hanlon JT, Fillenbaum GG, Huber M, Pieper C, Horner R. Medication use patterns among demented, cognitively impaired and cognitively intact community-dwelling elderly people. *Age Ageing* 1998; 27: 493–501.

8. Saposnik G, Cote R, Phillips S *et al.* Stroke outcome in those over 80: a multicenter cohort study across Canada. *Stroke* 2008; 39: 2310–2317.

9. Beckett NS, Peters R, Fletcher AE, Staessen JA, Liu L, Dumitrascu D, Stoyanovsky V, Antikainen RL, Nikitin Y, Anderson C, Belhani A, Forette F, Rajkumar C, Thijs L, Banya W, Bulpitt CJ; HYVET Study Group. Treatment of hypertension in patients 80 years of age or older. *N Engl J Med* 2008; 358(18): 1887–1898. Epub 2008 Mar 31.

10. Birns J, Markus H, Kalra L. Blood pressure reduction for vascular risk: is there a price to be paid? *Stroke* 2005; 36(6): 1308–1313.

11. Oates DJ, Berlowitz DR, Glickman ME, Silliman RA, Borzecki AM. Blood pressure and survival in the oldest old. *J Am Geriatr Soc* 2007; 55: 383–388.

12. Liebeskind DS. Imaging the future of stroke: Ischemia. *Ann Neurol* 2009; 66: 574–590.

13. Bang OY, Saver JL, Buck BH *et al.* Impact of collateral flow on tissue fate in acute ischaemic stroke. *J Neurol Neurosurg Psychiatry* 2008; 79: 625–629.

14. Hendrikse J, Klijn CJ, van Huffelen AC *et al.* Diagnosing cerebral collateral flow patterns: accuracy of non-invasive testing. *Cerebrovasc Dis* 2008; 25: 430–437.

15. Wunderlich MT, Goertler M, Postert T *et al.* Recanalization after intravenous thrombolysis: does a recanalization time window exist? *Neurology* 2007; 68: 1364 –1368.

16. Liebeskind DS. Collateral therapeutics for cerebral ischemia. *Expert Rev Neurother* 2004; 4: 255–265.

17. Donnan GA, Baron JC, Ma H, Davis SM. Penumbral selection of patients for trials of acute stroke therapy. *Lancet Neurol* 2009; 8: 261–269.

18. Kamena A, Streitparth F, Grieser C *et al.* Dynamic perfusion CT: optimizing the temporal resolution for the calculation of perfusion CT parameters in stroke patients. *Eur J Radiol* 2007; 64: 111–118.

19. Hacke W, Kaste M, Bluhmki E, Brozman M, Da´valos A, Guidetti D, Larrue V, Lees KR, Medeghri Z, Machnig T, Schneider D, von Kummer R, Wahlgren N, Toni D, for the ECASS investigators. Thrombolysis with alteplase 3 to 4.5 hours after acute ischemic stroke. *N Engl J Med.* 2008; 359: 1317–1329.

20. Wahlgren N, Ahmed N, Davalos A, Hacke W, Millan M, Muir K, Risto Roine O, Toni D, Lees KR; for the SITS investigators. Thrombolysis with alteplase 5 h after acute ischaemic stroke (SITS-ISTR): an observational study. *Lancet* 2008; 372: 1303–1309.

21. Higgins P, Lees KR. Advances in emerging therapies. *Stroke* 2009; 40; 292–294.

22. Davis SM, Donnan GA, Parsons MW, Levi C, Butcher KS, Peeters A, Barber PA, Bladin C, De Silva DA, Byrnes G, Chalk JB, Fink JN, Kimber TE, Schultz D, Hand PJ, Frayne J, Hankey G, Muir K, Gerraty R, Tress BM, Desmond PM. EPITHET investigators. Effects of alteplase beyond 3 h after stroke in the Echoplanar Imaging Thrombolytic Evaluation Trial (EPITHET): a placebo-controlled randomised trial. *Lancet Neurol* 2008; 7: 299–309.

23. Schellinger PD, Thomalla G, Fiehler J, Köhrmann M, Molina CA, Neumann-Haefelin T, Ribo M, Singer OC, Zaro-Weber O, Sobesky J. MRI-based and CT-based thrombolytic therapy in acute stroke within and beyond established time windows: an analysis of 1210 patients. *Stroke* 2007; 38(10): 2640–2645. Epub 2007 Aug 16.

24. Molina CA, Alvarez-Sabin J. Recanalization and Reperfusion Therapies for Acute Ischemic Stroke. *Cerebrovasc Dis* 2009; 27(Suppl 1): 162–167.

25. Hacke W, Furlan AJ, Al-Rawi Y, Davalos A, Fiebach JB, Gruber F, Kaste M, Lipka LJ, Pedraza S, Ringleb PA, Rowley HA, Schneider D, Schwamm LH, Leal JS, Söhngen M, Teal PA, Wilhelm-Ogunbiyi K, Wintermark M, Warach S. Intravenous desmoteplase in patients with acute ischaemic stroke selected by MRI perfusion-diffusion weighted imaging or perfusion CT (DIAS-2): a prospective, randomised, double-blind, placebo-controlled study. *Lancet Neurol* 2009; 8(2): 141–150.

26. Eggers J, Konig IR, Koch B, Händler G, Seidel G. Sonothrombolysis with transcranial color-coded sonography and recombinant tissue-type plasminogen activator in acute middle cerebral artery main stem occlusion: results from a randomized study. *Stroke* 2008; 39: 1470–1475.

27. del Zoppo GJ, Higashida RT, Furlan AJ, Pessin MS, Rowley HA, Gent M. PROACT: a phase II randomized trial of recombinant pro-urokinase by direct arterial delivery in acute middle cerebral artery stroke. PROACT Investigators. Prolyse in acute cerebral thromboembolism. *Stroke* 1998; 29: 4–11.

28. Lin R, Vora N, Zaidi S, Aleu A, Jankowitz B, Thomas A, Gupta R, Horowitz M, Kim S, Reddy V, Hammer M, Uchino K, Wechsler LR, Jovin T. Mechanical approaches combined with intra-arterial pharmacological therapy are associated with higher recanalization rates than either intervention alone in revascularization of acute carotid terminus occlusion. *Stroke* 2009; 40(6): 2092–2097.

29. Richards L, Hanson C, Wellborn M, Sethi A. Driving motor recovery after stroke. *Top Stroke Rehabil* 2008; 15(5): 397–411.

30. Kalra L, Walker MF. Stroke rehabilitation in the United Kingdom. *Top Stroke Rehabil* 2009; 16(1): 27–33.

31. Kalra L, Langhorne P. Facilitating recovery: evidence for organised stroke care. *J Rehabil* 2007; 39: 97–102.

32. Stinear CM, Barber PA, Smale PR, Coxon JP, Fleming MK, Byblow WD. Functional potential in chronic stroke patients depends on corticospinal tract integrity. *Brain* 2007; 130(Pt 1): 170–180.

33. Wolf SL, Winstein CJ, Miller JP, Taub E, Uswatte G, Morris D, Giuliani C, Light KE, Nichols-Larsen D, for the EXCITE Investigators. Effect of constraint-induced movement therapy on upper extremity function 3 to 9 months after stroke: the excite randomized clinical trial: *JAMA* 2006; 296: 2095–2104.

34. Plow EB, Maguire S, Obretenova S, Pascual-Leone A, Merabet LB. Approaches to rehabilitation for visual field defects following brain lesions. *Expert Rev Med Devices* 2009; 6(3): 291–305.

35. Schofield TM, Leff AP. Rehabilitation of hemianopia. *Curr Opin Neurol* 2009; 22(1): 36–40.

36. Romano JG. Progress in rehabilitation of hemianopic visual field defects. *Cerebrovasc Dis* 2009; 27(Suppl 1): 187–190. Epub 2009 Apr 3.

37. Schabrun SM, Hillier S. Evidence for the retraining of sensation after stroke: a systematic review. *Clin Rehabil* 2009; 23(1): 27–39.
38. He BJ, Snyder AZ, Vincent JL, Epstein A, Shulman GL, Corbetta M. Breakdown of functional connectivity in frontoparietal networks underlies behavioral deficits in spatial neglect. *Neuron* 2007; 53: 905–918.
39. Sapir A, Kaplan JB, He BJ, Corbetta M. Anatomical correlates of directional hypokinesia in patients with hemispatial neglect. *J Neurosci* 2007; 27(15): 4045–4051.
40. Hillis AE. Rehabilitation of unilateral spatial neglect: new insights from magnetic resonance perfusion imaging. *Arch Phys Med Rehabil* 2006; 87(12 Suppl 2): S43–49.
41. Mehrholz J, Platz T, Kugler J, Pohl M. Electromechanical and robot-assisted arm training for improving arm function and activities of daily living after stroke. *Cochrane Database Syst Rev* 2008; 4: CD006876.
42. Reinkensmeyer DJ. Robotic assistance for upper extremity training after stroke. *Stud Health Technol Inform* 2009; 145: 25–39.
43. Lucca LF. Virtual reality and motor rehabilitation of the upper limb after stroke: a generation of progress? *J Rehabil Med* 2009; 41(12): 1003–1100.
44. Tsirlin I, Dupierrix E, Chokron S, Coquillart S, Ohlmann T. Uses of virtual reality for diagnosis, rehabilitation and study of unilateral spatial neglect: review and analysis. *Cyberpsychol Behav* 2009; 12(2): 175–181.
45. Volpe BT, Huerta PT, Zipse JL, Rykman A, Edwards D, Dipietro L, Hogan N, Krebs HI. Robotic devices as therapeutic and diagnostic tools for stroke recovery. *Arch Neurol* 2009; 66(9): 1086–1090.
46. Ramachandran VS, Altschuler EL. The use of visual feedback, in particular mirror visual feedback, in restoring brain function. *Brain* 2009; 132(Pt 7): 1693–1710.
47. Zhang ZG, Chopp M. Neurorestorative therapies for stroke: underlying mechanisms and translation to the clinic. *Lancet Neurol.* 2009; 8(5): 491–500.
48. Burns TC, Verfaillie CM, Low WC. Stem cells for ischemic brain injury: a critical review. *J Comp Neurol* 2009; 515(1): 125–144.
49. Kalra L, Ratan R. What's new and exciting in stroke regenerative medicine. *Stroke* 2008; 39(2): 273–275.
50. Tahashi K, Tanabe K, Ohruki M, Narita M, Ichisaka T, Tomoda K, Yamanaka S. Induction of pluripotent stem cells from adult human fibroblasts by defined factors. *Cell* 2007; 131(5): 861–872.

51. Zhang ZG, Chopp M. Neurorestorative therapies for stroke: underlying mechanisms and translation to the clinic. *Lancet Neurol:* 2009; 8(5): 491–500.
52. Ratan RR, Siddiq A, Smirnova N *et al.* Harnessing hypoxic adaptation to prevent, treat, and repair stroke. *J Mol Med* 2007; 85: 1331–1338.
53. Kleim J, Chan S, Pringle E, Schallert K, Procaccio V, Jimenez R, Cramer SC. BDNF val66met polymorphism is associated with modified experience-dependent plasticity in the human cortex. *Nature Neurosci* 2006; 9(6): 735–737.
54. Stem Cell Therapies as an Emerging Paradigm in Stroke (STEPS): bridging basic and clinical science for cellular and neurogenic factor therapy in treating stroke. *Stroke* 2009; 40(2): 510–515. Epub 2008 Dec 18.
55. Xia T, Rome L, Nel A. Nanobiology: particles slip cell security. 2008; 7: 519–520.
56. Bible E, Chau DY, Alexander MR, Price J, Shakesheff KM, Modo M. The support of neural stem cells transplanted into stroke-induced brain cavities by PLGA particles. *Biomaterials* 2009; 30(16): 2985–2994.
57. Medeiros de Bustos E, Moulin T, Audebert HJ. Barriers, legal issues, limitations and ongoing questions in telemedicine applied to stroke. *Cerebrovasc Dis* 2009; 27(Suppl 4): 36–39.
58. Joubert J, Joubert LB, Medeiros de Bustos E, Ware D, Jackson D, Harrison T, Cadilhac D. Telestroke in stroke survivors. *Cerebrovasc Dis* 2009; 27(Suppl 4): 28–35.
59. Levine SR, Gorman M. 'Telestroke': the application of telemedicine for stroke. *Stroke* 1999; 30: 464–469.
60. Lewis M, Trypuc J, Lindsay P, O'Callaghan C, Dishaw A. Has Ontario's stroke system really made a difference? *Healthc Q* 2006; 9: 50–59.

Index